D1029290

The Ethics of Consent

The Ethics of Consent

Theory and Practice

Edited by

Franklin G. Miller and Alan Wertheimer

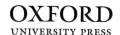

OXFORD
UNIVERSITY PRESS

2010

OXFORD
UNIVERSITY PRESS

Oxford University Press, Inc., publishes works that further
Oxford University's objective of excellence
in research, scholarship, and education.

Oxford   New York
Auckland   Cape Town   Dar es Salaam   Hong Kong   Karachi
Kuala Lumpur   Madrid   Melbourne   Mexico City   Nairobi
New Delhi   Shanghai   Taipei   Toronto

With offices in
Argentina   Austria   Brazil   Chile   Czech Republic   France   Greece
Guatemala   Hungary   Italy   Japan   Poland   Portugal   Singapore
South Korea   Switzerland   Thailand   Turkey   Ukraine   Vietnam

Published by Oxford University Press, Inc.
198 Madison Avenue, New York, New York 10016

www.oup.com

Oxford is a registered trademark of Oxford University Press

Library of Congress Cataloging-in-Publication Data
The ethics of consent : theory and practice / edited by Franklin G. Miller and
Alan Wertheimer.
p.   ;   cm.
Includes bibliographical references and index.
ISBN 978-0-19-533514-9 (hardback : alk. paper)
1. Consent (Law)   2. Informed consent (Medical law)   3. Ethics.   4. Medical ethics.
I. Miller, Franklin G.   II. Wertheimer, Alan.
[DNLM: 1. Informed Consent—ethics.   2. Interpersonal Relations.
W 20.55.H9 E8395 2009]
KZ1262.C65E84 2009
170'.42—dc22
2009009553

9 8 7 6 5 4 3 2

Printed in the United States of America
on acid-free paper

Contributors

Tom L. Beauchamp is Professor of Philosophy, Georgetown University.

Vera Bergelson is Professor of Law, Robert E. Knowlton Scholar, Rutgers University School of Law-Newark.

Brian H. Bix is Frederick W. Thomas Professor of Law and Philosophy, University of Minnesota.

Philip J. Candilis is Associate Professor of Psychiatry, University of Massachusetts Medical School.

Douglas Husak is Professor of Philosophy and Law, Rutgers University.

Steven Joffe is Assistant Professor of Pediatrics, Dana-Farber Cancer Institute, Children's Hospital, and Harvard Medical School.

David Johnston is Professor of Political Science, Columbia University.

John Kleinig is Professor of Philosophy, John Jay College of Criminal Justice, City University of New York, and Professorial Fellow, Centre for Applied Philosophy and Public Ethics, Charles Sturt University, Canberra, Australia.

Arthur Kuflik is Associate Professor of Philosophy, University of Vermont.

Charles W. Lidz is Research Professor of Psychiatry, University of Massachusetts Medical School.

Franklin G. Miller is on the Senior Faculty, Department of Bioethics, Clinical Center, National Institutes of Health.

Janet Radcliffe Richards is Professor of Practical Philosophy and Distinguished Research Fellow, Uehiro Centre for Practical Ethics, Faculty of Philosophy, University of Oxford.

A. John Simmons is Commonwealth Professor of Philosophy and Professor of Law, University of Virginia.

Robert D. Truog is Professor of Medical Ethics, Anaesthesia and Pediatrics, Harvard Medical School; and Senior Associate in Critical Care Medicine, Children's Hospital Boston.

Robin West is Professor of Law and Associate Dean of Research and Academic Programs, Georgetown University Law Center.

Alan Wertheimer is on the Senior Faculty, Department of Bioethics, Clinical Center, National Institutes of Health.

Contents

Preface

The Ethics of Consent: Theory and Practice

It is difficult to conceive of a moral code, especially within a civilized society, without some recognition to the requirement and moral force of consent. People simultaneously have an interest in control over their bodies and possessions and seek to engage in cooperative activities with others on terms that the cooperating parties can mutually accept. A requirement of consent, from a moral perspective, protects people from unauthorized invasions of their bodies and property. In addition to its protective function, consent is a facilitative moral power. Our consent makes interpersonal conduct permissible that would otherwise be prohibited as wrongful. And through our capacity to undertake obligations or bind oneself, consent makes possible cooperative activities in which one person must perform before another and also allows us to create expectations about one's future behavior. It is fair to say that modern liberal-democratic societies have been characterized by an ever-growing domain of personal sovereignty, making consent salient across a wide swath of human activities, including sexual relations, employment, medical care, buying and selling, medical research, professional relationships, and so forth.

The centrality of consent to our moral and legal lives is not matched by philosophical attention to the theory of consent. There is an extensive literature on the ethics of consent that is confined to one context or another, but few general treatments. For example, at least as far back as Plato and continuing through Locke (and beyond), it has been argued that citizens of (some) societies have an obligation to obey the law because they consent to do so. Other thinkers, starting at least with Hume, have contested that claim. Inspired in part by the feminist movement, there are now numerous treatments of consent to sexual relations. While not always couched in the language of consent, the entire corpus of contract law revolves around consent. And informed consent has played a central role in discussions of the ethics of medical treatment and participation in medical research.

Interestingly, despite a considerable literature on consent in different contexts, there is surprisingly little systematic analysis of the concept of consent and the moral and legal work that it performs. We know of no book-length monograph that ranges across contexts. Indeed, while Lawrence and Charlotte Becker's admirable *Encyclopedia of Ethics* contains a helpful discussion of consent by one of our contributors (John Kleinig), the equally admirable Internet-based Stanford *Encyclopedia of Philosophy* contains no entry at all (as of January 2009). And while the Nomos series published by the American Society for Political and Legal Philosophy contains volumes on some central concepts related to consent (coercion; political and legal obligation), there is no volume specifically devoted to consent. Perhaps more important, there has been a regrettable lack of cross-fertilization among the different contexts. Those who write about consent to medical treatment rarely ask what we might learn from the literature on consent to sexual relations (and vice versa). A major purpose of this volume is to stimulate such hybrid vigor.

This volume has its origins in what the editors regard as a most fortuitous academic relationship. Miller, a philosopher on the faculty of the Department of Bioethics at the National Institutes of Health, has focused on the ethics of research with human subjects. Among other things, he has been concerned with issues related to the character of "informed consent." Wertheimer, a political philosopher, was a visiting scholar in the Department of Bioethics in 2005–06 and has since joined its faculty. Although he had done little work in bioethics, he had previously worked on the concepts of coercion, exploitation, and consent (to sexual relations).

Wertheimer was intrigued by problems on which Miller had written extensively. Research ethicists have asked whether a subject can give informed consent if she is in the grips of a "therapeutic misconception," that is, a belief that she is receiving personalized medical care even when she has been informed that she will be participating in a randomized controlled trial. We were dissatisfied with the standard treatments. In response, we have developed what we call a theory of consent transactions (see Chapter 4). Along the way, we observed that bioethicists sometimes write as if the concept and principle of (informed) consent was first developed for their purposes and that there was no need to reflect on the way in which consent operates in other contexts in order to provide an adequate account of consent in medicine and clinical research. Accordingly, we thought there was much to be learned from a single volume that comprehensively discussed theoretical and practical issues relating to the ethics of consent. To that end, we engaged distinguished scholars in assembling an array of theoretical perspectives on the ethics of consent and more contextual analyses of consent within specific domains. We hope and expect that readers will share our delight with the breadth and depth of their contributions.

It is conventional for multiauthored volumes to begin with a summary of the included contributions. We confess to not finding these summaries generally useful and we have confidence that the contributions can speak for themselves. Still, tradition has its force, and so we will provide a brief sketch of what the reader will find here with the proviso that the reader is encouraged to proceed to the chapters themselves.

Part One includes seven chapters on the theory of consent. In Chapter 1, John Kleinig provides a general overview of the concept and the way in which it functions. Among other things, he considers the grammar of consent, the ontology of consent, means of signifying consent, and the limits to consent. In Chapter 2, David Johnston offers a brief history of the idea of consent in western political thought, going a long way toward filling a major gap in the literature. He traces the idea of consent from the Bible to the Greeks to Roman law and then to modern political philosophers such as Hobbes and Mill. In Chapter 3, Tom Beauchamp considers the relationship between consent and autonomy. In developing his "autonomous authorization" model of informed consent, he emphasizes voluntariness as well as information and then goes on to consider consent in the light of "split-level" theories of autonomy. In Chapter 4, Miller and Wertheimer argue that the fundamental question in many contexts is not whether a person gives valid consent, but whether the consent transaction is morally transformative—and that the answers to those questions are not always identical. In Chapter 5, Douglas Husak considers the relevance of consent to the justification of paternalism. As a general matter, A isn't acting paternalistically toward B if B consents to A's action. But what if B gives prior consent, as when a sober person tells a friend not to let him drive home if he is drunk? Contrary to the common view, Husak argues that B's prior consent has no bearing on whether A is justified in interfering. In Chapter 6, Arthur Kuflik considers the coherence and force of appeals to hypothetical consent—that to which a person would consent if she were in a position to do so. We might say it is permissible to perform surgery on an unconscious person because she would have consented had she been able to consent or arrange a person's posthumous affairs by reference to what she would have consented. Although the intuitive force of hypothetical consent is powerful, some philosophers have argued that such hypothetical consent not only is not real consent, but also that it can do no moral work. Arthur Kuflik argues that this view is too quick. In Chapter 7, Vera Bergelson asks whether we should accept the principle *volenti non fit injuria* (to one who consents no wrong is done). She considers the way in which the Model Penal Code treats the defense of consent and whether violations of dignity (as contrasted with physical harm) should be regarded as harms to which one cannot consent.

Part Two considers consent in a variety of specific contexts. In Chapter 8, Wertheimer focuses on the question as to when a person's consent to sexual relations is morally transformative. For example, if one consents while intoxicated or after one has been deceived, is it permissible for the other party to proceed? In Chapter 9, Robin West discusses the views of some radical feminists and queer theorists who have sought to undermine the distinction between consensual and nonconsensual sex. West argues that the distinction is important and can be sustained, but that consent does not immunize sexual relations from moral and political criticism. In Chapter 10, Brian Bix considers the role of consent in contract law. Although it is natural to think that contract law is based on consent, Bix observes that robust consent to the terms of a contract is more fiction than reality as revealed in the emphasis on "consideration" and in doctrines such as "implied terms." Bix also considers several principles for voiding contracts such as duress, undue influence, and unconscionability. In Chapter 11, Janet Radcliffe Richards examines the bearing of financial inducements on consent, focusing on the issue of selling kidneys for transplantation. How can it be considered unethical to sell kidneys if it is ethical to donate them? Radcliffe Richards contends that concerns about the validity of consent to sell kidneys cannot withstand critical scrutiny. In Chapter 12, A. John Simmons takes up the age-old question: Do we have an obligation to obey the law? It has long been argued that one has an obligation to obey the law if (Plato) and perhaps "only if" (Locke) one consents to do so. Simmons has no quarrel with the principle, but argues that citizens in a democratic polity do not consent to be governed and thus cannot acquire obligations in this way.

Chapters 13, 14, and 15 consider consent in the medical context. The doctrine of informed consent is well entrenched in medical care and medical research. But the requirements of consent arguably are different in these two medical contexts and may call for different moral and legal criteria. Chapter 13 begins with an empirical approach to consent. Conceptual clarity and analysis is important, but policies that regulate consent should be informed by empirical analysis. Philip Candilis and Charles Lidz review the most important findings from empirical studies of informed consent in medicine and research. For example, do people feel coerced to receive treatment? Do research participants understand that they are not receiving personalized medical care? In Chapter 14, Joffe and Truog analyze informed consent in medical treatment. Must patients consent to specific procedures? Does the physician's fiduciary obligation to her patient affect the importance of consent? Finally, in Chapter 15, Miller considers the scope and limits of consent to participate in research. Following discussion of a famous historical case of clinical research without informed consent, Miller examines the therapeutic misconception and the justifiability of research without consent.

We believe that both students and scholars from a variety of disciplines will find these discussions illuminating—philosophers, physicians, researchers, bioethicists, lawyers, and even the occasional layperson. Although it would be natural for readers to pick and choose, we hope that readers will share the conviction that motivated this volume. We hope that philosophers will read about consent in particular domains, that bioethicists will read about sexual consent and contracts, and that lawyers will read about informed consent in medicine and research. Finally, we anticipate that readers will find it interesting to compare thinking about the ethics of consent across the various domains and in light of the general theoretical approaches discussed in this volume.

A few words of thanks. First, we want to thank our contributors. We are thrilled that they shared our enthusiasm for the project and consented to write an original essay for the volume. Second, we want to thank Ezekiel Emanuel, who was Chair of the Department of Bioethics at the Clinical Center of the National Institutes of Health when this project was conceived and provided both personal and institutional support.

PART ONE

Theoretical Perspectives

1

The Nature of Consent[*]

John Kleinig

Introduction

Although consent has always had a role in moral and social discourse, that role has greatly expanded since the Renaissance and in particular with the development of liberal democratic societies.

In a post-Renaissance world, mature human relations (both individual and collective) are frequently assumed to be governed by a conception of personal flourishing whose realization is furthered through the recognition of various constraints on interpersonal behavior. Most critical have been those prohibiting people from acting toward each other in ways that are foreseeably detrimental to their interests—especially those that are central to the pursuit of what they conceive to be their good. Also, given the social nature of our development and the conditions for our continued flourishing, there are expectations that we contribute to the formation and maintenance of a social environment that will sustain our flourishing. Violations of such expectations are often characterized as violations of rights—a legally based discourse that identifies considerations worthy of coercive guarantees and whose breach is said to warrant a punitive response.

* I am grateful to Nick Evans and the editors for comments on an earlier draft of this chapter.

Against this background, consent plays an important moral role. In the contexts in which it is appropriately given, it may—and usually does—transform the normative expectations that hold between people and groups, whether directly or through various institutional arrangements. Where called for, consent can sometimes function like a proprietary gate that one opens to allow another's access, access that would be impermissible absent the act of voluntarily opening the gate. Thus, I may consent to another's sexual advance, use of my car, performance of an operative procedure, or dissemination of information concerning myself. Or, sometimes, consent can function like a normative rope whereby one binds oneself to another. Thus, I may consent to another's offer of marriage or request that I give a lecture or join a committee. In each case, whether the consent is viewed as opening a gate or as binding oneself, an act or outcome that would not be permissible absent the consent is given a normative sanction. Whether that sanction is sufficient to justify what is done is a further question, though there is usually a presumption that, in circumstances in which consent is normatively required and given, an important ground for complaint has been removed.

What is the nature of consent that enables it to work its "moral magic"?[1] And how much magic can it work? Although I will say something about both questions, my main purpose will be to engage with some of the complexities encountered by attempts to respond to the former. At first blush, that question might seem to divide into two: What is the nature of consent? and What gives consent its normative force? The two issues are, however, integrally related. Consent is not a neutral act that is then separately justified as having normative force, but is normative through and through even though it also has a descriptive content. To say that A consented to φ is not to report some evaluatively neutral doing, such as A's saying "yes," which is then to be followed by further discussion about the significance of saying "yes." Instead, it is intended to convey that whatever it was that A did to consent (including, perhaps, saying "yes"), it also possessed a certain normative force.

Some of the foregoing assertions are provocative and need to be addressed. At this point I offer a couple of preliminary explanations, though more substantial issues will be dealt with later. What I am concerned with articulating here is not everything that might be graced with the label of "consent" but with a core moral notion—that is, with genuine or, as it is sometimes referred to in more institutionalized circles, valid consent. Although consent figures quite importantly in certain formalized contexts—especially the law—it draws its strength in those contexts from the sense that I have characterized as morally transformative. Although I will refer to and draw upon such institutionalized renderings of consent, my concern here will be to illuminate its status as a transformative moral notion.[2] Moreover, as well as its more formalized renderings, the core notion of consent is surrounded by a penumbra of secondary meanings. For example, the suitor who seeks the "consent" of the woman's father is nowadays more likely to be seeking the father's approval (of the planned marriage) than his consent, because daughters are no longer (as they should never have been) considered as property.[3] And a consent decree is an arrangement whereby an organization that faces legal proceedings likely to lead to sanctions against it agrees to initiate certain reforms in exchange for their suspension. In addition to such secondary meanings, consent has also acquired various parasitical variants—such as imputed, tacit, future, implied, constructive, and hypothetical consent—some of which I discuss in the course of this chapter. The transformative power of consent is such that its moral authority is eagerly sought, sometimes in circumstances that do not warrant it.

The Grammar of Consent

So, then, what conditions need to be obtained if we are to be justified in saying "A consented to φ"? First, we should note that "A consented to φ" is incomplete as it stands. Consent is a three-place transaction in which consent to do something—φ—is always given to another party or agent, to whom we will refer as B. So, "A consented (to B) to φ." Although some accounts of consent countenance the idea that A might engage in an internal act of consenting, as though consent might simply express a certain kind of inner resolve or approval, I reject such an account. I argue for the view that consent is centrally and most appropriately a communicative act that serves to alter the moral relations in which A and B stand—and that for the moral relations to have been altered for B, a communicative act must have occurred.[4] But let us first give some brief consideration to each of the place holders in the transaction. What needs to be true of A, B, and φ, if it is to be justifiably said that "A consented (to B) to φ"? I will then discuss the substance of consent before turning to a number of remaining problems that need to be addressed.

(1) A

For A to consent, A must be an agent who has reached a certain level of maturity. (I explore that later in more detail.) Rocks and trees cannot consent; nor can infants. May dogs consent? I think not, even though they may willingly go along with some initiative of B ("Walk?") or show themselves to be enthusiastic participants in some activity (fetching balls). A dog's engagement in what is presented to it is not intended to alter the moral relations between the dog and *B*—in particular, to give *B* a permission he would not otherwise have or to obligate itself in some way. Those inclined to take issue with this almost certainly personalize dogs in ways that would tend to reinforce my initial claim about agency.

Nevertheless, consent is not limited to individual agents or persons, even if they constitute the paradigmatic subjects of consent. Consent may be given by "collective persons," whether as members of a particular class (such as the shareholders of a company) or as a collective unity (such as an orchestra). When a majority (or some relevant number) of shareholders signifies its agreement with the terms of a takeover offer, it consents to the takeover.[5] When an orchestra or band consents to perform in a certain location or to perform a particular piece of music, it does so as a collective unit, which may or may not reflect the preference of each individual member. In addition, we sometimes speak of corporations or organizations as quasi-persons capable of consenting to whatever options may be included in φ. Although some collective subjects of consent can be said to consent only by virtue of a set of preexisting institutional arrangements, they illustrate the general point that the subjects of consent need not be singular.

(2) B

As with *A*, the (implicit) *B* to whom *A* gives consent must also be a person, group of persons, or quasi-person—an agent of some kind who (most often) initiates the process of inquiry to which *A*'s consent is sought in response. *B* seeks from *A* either *A*'s permission to do something or *A*'s agreement to do something—something to which *B* had no moral right or entitlement.

Must consent always be in response to another's initiative? Suppose *A*, desirous of sexual intimacy with *B*, approaches *B*. *B* is agreeable and sexual intercourse takes place. Should a question later be raised whether *A* consented to the sexual contact, we would probably answer in the affirmative, though it would be more accurate—and we would be more likely—to respond by saying: "*B* did not merely consent; *B* initiated the contact." The sequence is more complex in cases in which a course of action has discrete parts. Suppose *A* makes an appointment with a physician with a view to getting cosmetic surgery. Even though *A* initiated the process, *A* will be asked to sign a consent form. This is because a decision to have the surgery is not presumed to be made until after a consultation in which the physician presents the terms under which he will perform the surgery, terms to which *A* consents, thus authorizing the physician to go forward.

Does anything hang on the initiation-response question? It may sometimes do so. A legal case will illustrate. If a 25-year-old man proposes sexual contact with a 13-year-old girl, and she consents to it, the fact that she has not reached the legal "age of consent" means that her consent will not do much to mitigate his offense.[6] If, however, she initiates the sexual contact and he consents to it, he is likely to fare better with the law (and probably morally) even though she has not reached the (legal) age of consent. In each case it is most likely that he will be found guilty of statutory rape (unless he had reason to believe she was considerably older). Nevertheless, her initiative offers a plausible ground for mitigating the penalty. He will be seen as opportunistic rather than predatory.

(3) φ

φ usually encompasses a course of action, one for whose pursuit A's authorization, permission, or agreement is required. The course of action may be one that B wishes to pursue—for example, performing a medical procedure on A or on someone for whom A has responsibility, entry to or use of A's property or property for which A has some responsibility, and so on. But the course of action may also be one that B wishes A to take, and which B has no right to expect of A absent A's consent. It may be for A to agree to give a lecture or attend a rally or visit someone. But if A is already under some obligation to do something, A's consent is not additionally required (though A's approval may be thought desirable). In cases in which B wishes A to take some course of action, A's consent obligates A to B.

Although consent alters the moral relations between A and B, the permissions granted or obligations created need not be of overriding or morally determinative importance. Indeed, A may consent to (do) things that it would be wrong for B or A to do. The prostitute who consents to paid intercourse will alter the moral relations between herself and B such that what B does will not constitute rape. It might, nevertheless, be argued that it is wrong for A to sell her body in this way (though whether, if that is the case, she should be prevented from doing so is another matter).

Consider, too, the case in which a woman consents to have intercourse with her therapist. He has not pressured her; indeed, she has become attracted to him and is welcoming of the proposition. Her consent has altered their relations to the extent that what they engage in does not constitute sexual assault. Yet we might still want to argue that the therapist has acted wrongly because he has corrupted the professional relationship he was obligated to maintain. True, there may be cases and cases. But the point is that the moral transformation brought about by consent may not be complete in the sense of making that which would have been a sexual assault into something morally acceptable. As a person, the patient had the moral authority to consent to sexual intercourse; as a professional in a professional relationship, the therapist had no moral authority to seek it.[7]

But what if B asks A to act as a hitman and A consents? Does this represent a case in which consent does not alter the moral relations between A and B, because B asks for something that he has no authority to give? Perhaps. It is not that A fails to consent, but that his consent mistakenly or illegitimately presumes that B is in a moral position to authorize what he requests. If the conversation has been monitored by police, A will not be able to claim that he failed to consent because B had no right to authorize what A was asked to do. If that appears to contradict the account of consent given so far, the point may be rephrased as follows. Given what A took to be the normative order governing gang behavior, B was authorized to arrange for a hit and, in terms of that normative order, A consented to do what B was authorized to request. He therefore transformed relations so far as that order was concerned. But within the larger frame of morally acceptable relations, the normative order represented by the gang had no traction.

Keeping in mind the complication just noted, to be the object of consent φ must identify some course of action to which the consented-to party would otherwise have no moral right. Or, more accurately, it must appear as though B has no right to φ without A's consent. If I consent to B's request that he borrow my car, it is implied that, without consent, B's using the car would constitute an unauthorized taking—indeed, a theft. Presuming that B is an eligible person, the consent constitutes a moral authorization to use the car.[8]

As we noted earlier, however, we sometimes perpetuate rituals of consent even though no authorization is necessary. Thus, a man who wishes to marry a particular woman may visit the woman's father to seek his "consent" to the arrangement, even though we no longer see daughters as the property of their fathers. What the man is really seeking in this ritualized act of consent getting is the approval of the father to the arrangement. Approval—or at least approval of—is not consent. Moreover, in cases in which consent is not morally required, A's disapproval of B's φ-ing will not constitute a refusal to consent. Furthermore, one may not approve of an arrangement to which one nevertheless consents. That no doubt occurs when fathers consent to their minor daughters getting tattoos, even though they consider their daughters beholden to the vagaries of fashion.

The action (φ) to which consent is given may be conclusive or continuous. If φ is a vote to be taken, then, once one's vote has been made, one cannot (usually) retract whatever it is that one has consented to. Even if voting is still in progress, one's pulling the lever or depositing a slip in the ballot box places one at a point of no return. One may regret the consent one has given, but that is another matter. That which signifies or expresses consent takes a form that does not allow for retraction. But in the case of a prolonged course of action, it may often be possible to withdraw one's consent. A person who consents to a medical procedure or therapeutic regimen may, after a time (though perhaps not any time), withdraw his or her consent. The person may have signed a consent form, but the form is likely to include a provision for withdrawal. A person who consents to sexual intimacy may withdraw that consent along the way, at least up to the point of intercourse, and maybe even beyond penetration. I may withdraw my consent to give a lecture at any point up to my giving it, though in this latter case, an obligation is created that, in the event of a withdrawal, requires at least an apology. In all cases, the initial act of consent will usually reflect an ongoing commitment.

Withdrawal is more problematic in some cases than in others. Though a withdrawal of consent may be technically possible, it may also have significant costs associated with it. Consent creates reliance and those who have obtained our consent may be seriously disadvantaged if consent is subsequently withdrawn. A late withdrawal of consent to giving a lecture may sometimes reasonably result in liability for the costs associated with setting it up. In the case of medical consent, however, patient autonomy is usually considered so important that withdrawal of consent during a procedure or a course of treatment is not only honored but also protected against reprisals.

The Ontology of Consent

Having said something about the parties to and object of consent, I turn now to the act of consenting. There is considerable disagreement about what constitutes the core of consent, and some of my earlier remarks will have been provocative precisely because they take a position on an issue that is hotly contested. It is time to make good on those claims. How, exactly, are we to conceive of consent? Does it consist primarily in a state of mind—in what Peter Westen speaks of as "a state of mind of acquiescence...a felt willingness to agree with—or to choose—what another person seeks or proposes"[9] or in what Hurd refers to as "an act of will—a subjective mental state akin to other morally and legally significant mens rea"?[10] Or is it constituted by a performative act or the conventional signification of agreement to some request or proposal? Or may it instead be some combination of these? Representatives of each of these possibilities may be found, though it is quite common in legal contexts to characterize the core of consent as a subjective mental state.

The position that I articulate and defend here is that there is always an expressive dimension to consent—that consent must be signified—and that only if consent takes the form of a communicative act can the moral relations between A and B be transformed. Absent such communication, B has no business doing that for which A's consent is needed even if A condones or would acquiesce to it. Consent is a social act in which A conveys something to B—something that, once communicated (and with my earlier caveats acknowledged), now gives B a moral right or entitlement that B previously lacked.

First, however, I offer some observations on subjective mental state accounts. These accounts range widely (and sometimes in a confused manner) from those in which consent is thought of as "being of a like mind with another" to those in which it involves merely a "willingness that others do as they request"—a tolerance of their wishes. Westen appears to run them together. To illustrate the core "factual attitudinal" meaning of consent, he appeals to the case of a child who, while pretending to be asleep, "secretly consents" when her grandmother leans over and kisses her.[11] But does what the child feels constitute consent, even of a secret kind? Are we merely denied knowledge of the child's consent or is her consent lacking? We need not deny that the child has "a welcoming state of mind." But many actions in which others engage us may create a welcoming state of mind without it being said that consent was involved. In the present case there is no way of distinguishing approval (of) from consent. But approving of and consenting are quite distinct, even if our consent to something is often contingent on our approval of it. The relevant kind of approval in the case of consent is not approving in the sense of approving of, as is the case when the little girl approves of what her grandmother is doing, but it is approval in the sense in which some authorization is given to the other to do as she seeks. In the case in question we need not deny that the child has consented or that this does not constitute an unconsented-to touching on the grandmother's part. But, if so, this is because we see past consent persisting into the present and not because it is now given.[12] As Westen construes it here, consent—a feeling of approval—is not morally transformative. It has been gutted of its moral significance. Were, for example, the child later to reveal that all the while she was secretly loathing her grandmother's kiss, what transpired would not ipso facto have constituted an unconsented-to touching. The grandmother was not to know that it would be unwelcome on this occasion, and might reasonably claim that an affectionate kiss of the kind she gave could have been expected to be welcome, given the relation that was presumed to exist between her and the child.

Let me be clear. I do not wish to argue that states of mind are irrelevant to consent, only that consent is not constituted primarily by a state of mind. There must surely be a certain willingness on A's part if A is to be said to have consented to B's φ-ing. What is critical is that A communicates with B such that B knows that A has authorized B to φ. Consent requires signification—not in the sense that a state of mind is reported but in the sense that a right or entitlement is created or permission given or obligation assumed. Consent is not about agreeing with but to, and the latter, as a morally transformative act, requires signification. Likewise, the withdrawal of consent is not simply a matter of changing one's mind but of communicating to another that a permission once given is now being withdrawn. Unless that communication occurs, the (presumption of) consent remains.[13]

Signification

Let me say more about signification. Because, as I have been arguing, consent is a communicative act requiring, for consent to occur, that A signifies it to B, a good deal of attention is often paid to the issue of its form or *morphe*. The form taken by the act of consent may vary considerably, though it will commonly be constituted by some gesture, word, or other recordable behavior that conventionally and contextually expresses it. Precisely because consent is a *communicative* act, there must be a convention whereby consent given is recognized as such. Moreover, because we have developed different conventions for different contexts, its conventional expression must be contextualized. Raising one's hand or shouting "yes" may express one's consent at a rally, but it will not do when election time comes round and a voting ballot paper must be filled out. Context will also allow for consent to be signified by a negative act—such as the act of remaining silent when called upon to indicate if one has any objections to a proposal. Presuming that one has heard the call and been able to make known any objection one has, one's silence may be a legitimate expression of consent.

Nevertheless, because ambiguity is often possible with more truncated forms of signification, it may be important that for some matters the conventions of signification (as well, of course, as the preparations for seeking consent) are more complex. Silence, for example, can sometimes indicate abstention, acquiescence,[14] and lack of interest as well as consent, and it may be risky to interpret it as consent. And words such as "yes" may fail to indicate the scope of one's consent.

I have already made it clear that in focusing on the critical importance of signification—an importance that arises from the fact that consent is a communicative act—I do not thereby want to argue the extreme position that consent is simply a matter of engaging in signifying behavior. For one might do what would ordinarily be taken to signify consent without actually consenting. This occurs when a person is coerced into agreeing to something. We may more appropriately speak of this person as assenting than as consenting. Because consent transforms the moral relations that exist between persons, the signification must be voluntary. Assent that is given under duress does not have the moral force of consent. When Joel Valdez broke into Elizabeth Wilson's apartment and sought to rape her at knife point, she agreed to submit if he wore a condom. He had sex with her for an hour until she was able to flee to a neighbor's apartment. But a Texas grand jury decided that her agreement to have sex if Valdez wore a condom constituted consent to intercourse and therefore that she was not sexually assaulted.[15] Given that Wilson negotiated her agreement under the threat of serious injury, her assent did not possess the moral force of consent. Coerced responses need not be strategically bereft, and evidence of physical resistance is no prerequisite of refusal to consent.

There may be cases in which, without a deeper understanding of the circumstances, one may be misled regarding consent. Suppose a CCTV camera picks up an encounter in which a man approaches a woman in a stairwell, grabs her, puts a knife to her neck, and then has sex with her. Our inclination would be to say that the sexual intercourse was nonconsensual and that she was raped. But we might well revise that judgment if we later learn that the "attack" was staged as part of a pornographic movie. There was only an appearance of duress; the sex was consensual.[16]

Sexual relations have proven particularly treacherous so far as signification is concerned. Not only are social conventions somewhat confused, confusing, and still often permeated by sexist prejudices, but the processual or continuing character of sexual relations allows for misunderstandings with regard to what is consented to as well as with regard to changes or withdrawals of permission.[17] The ambiguities and consequences of mistake have sometimes led to extreme requirements for consensual sex, even between those who may know each other quite well.[18]

Consent and Responsibility

In speaking of consent as a communicative act I have made it clear that I do not wish to deprive it of an inner dimension. All I have attempted to argue is that it is not exclusively or primarily a state of mind. As an act that morally transforms a situation, it must satisfy certain conditions—in particular, those for constituting it responsible behavior. If A cannot be held responsible for what gives the appearance of consent, then consent has not been given. So-called coerced consent is better characterized as assent: It does not authorize B to φ or alternatively obligate A to φ. Nor does it follow from what I am claiming that A may not irresponsibly consent, for one may be held responsible for one's irresponsible conduct.

If consent is to be a communicative act for which responsibility is presupposed, it must be the act of an agent who is competent to consent; it must be voluntary, in the sense of being free from coercion; it must be based on understanding, in the sense that it is appropriately informed; and it must be intentional.

The Competence Condition

As I pointed out earlier, young children lack the cognitive development to consent. They are not conceptually or emotionally equipped to provide the authorization or commitment for many of the situations that would ordinarily require their consent. As they develop, no doubt, they will acquire an increasing capacity for making determinations with regard to such matters. Until that time, though, we usually consider that parents or others who can be expected to have their best interests in view will provide the authorization—consent—that is needed. Nevertheless, we should not presume that the capacity to consent will occur all at once. The level of competence required to join a scout club is very different from that required to buy a house or accept an offer of marriage. As children become cognitively (and otherwise) capable of making certain kinds of decisions concerning interests over which they should have moral jurisdiction, the authority to consent should pass to them from their guardians. In cases in which there are serious learning disabilities, the capacity to give consent, at least with regard to those matters about which we are most inclined to demand consent, may never be reached.

But even if competence in the sense of a certain level of cognitive development has been reached, it may be subverted in other ways. Intoxication impairs one's ability to consent, though the impairment may be a matter of degree. Sometimes we hold people responsible for what they do under the influence of alcohol (or other drugs), and consider them to have acted irresponsibly rather than nonresponsibly, particularly if, prior to their impairment, they had reason to foresee what might occur.

Insanity and other forms of mental illness may also impair the capacity to consent to the point that what appears to be consent no longer transforms relations with others. Although there is no straight line from "mental illness" to "incapacity to consent," certain kinds and degrees of mental illness may undermine the various requisites of consent.

Cases of acute or chronic pain can also impair consent. We do not usually hold people responsible for what they agree to under torture because the pain of torture so consumes their consciousness that they can usually focus on little beyond what can be done to alleviate it. In certain circumstances the experience of intense pain may present others with something of a dilemma. If a person who is suffering unrelievable pain seeks to be put out of her misery, should we see that as a responsible request or as impelled by the pain?[19] There may not be any simple answer to such a question, and others might need to make a judgment about the likelihood of a change in the person's situation or whether, even if pain has overcome the person's capacity for rational thought, it would be in that person's interests to respond affirmatively to the request.

In other cases in which a person may have lost the capacity to consent to matters that would ordinarily require consent, decisions might be made not on the basis of what are deemed to be the person's best interests, but on the basis of what that person might have been expected to consent to, given what is known about her. This substituted judgment standard presumes that we know enough about the person to draw reasonable inferences about what that person would have consented to.

In cases in which the consent that A gives to φ concerns the affairs of another (call that other C) who would ordinarily be expected to give or withhold consent, we need to offer an argument for transferring the authority that would ordinarily belong to C to A. The expectation would be that the moral guardian would know enough about C either to make appropriate judgments about what C could have been expected to consent to (given her settled desires, values, and life plans) or, in the absence of that, what would be in C's best interests (something which, in the absence of better knowledge, C could be presumed to consent to having secured for her).

The Voluntariness Condition

If A is coerced into doing what ordinarily signifies consent—be it the raised hand or the uttered "yes"—he does not act voluntarily and what he does does not constitute consent. Some might argue that in such cases consent is given but, because it is coerced, it is not valid. But invalid consent no more counts as consent than an invalid vote counts as a vote. It has form but no substance. It is, I believe, more accurate to say that although *A* gave his assent, this did not amount to consent.

Lack of voluntariness may have a variety of sources—most dramatically from the knife to the throat but more subtly from the felt threat of social ostracism. Responsibility-defeating or responsibility-diminishing coercion takes many forms, and there is some dispute as to appropriate boundaries for its varied manifestations. It is generally agreed, for example, that assent given as a result of physical threats is coercive, but there is more debate about the coerciveness of moral and social pressures (say, social opprobrium and peer pressure); and even more contentious is the inclusion of certain "inner" forces (say, compulsions that affect what one agrees to). Furthermore, does coercion refer to threats that affect what one wills or may it include acts that make the will irrelevant? It is probably not necessary that we seek to resolve such questions here; what is important is the bearing that certain forces may have on the voluntariness of what we agree to and therefore on our responsibility for what would otherwise be taken to signify consent.[20]

Sometimes it may be very difficult to determine whether supposed acts of consent are voluntary and therefore genuine. Do prisoners who "volunteer" to participate in clinical trials give their consent, or do their circumstances subvert the voluntariness of their agreement or—not much less problematic for public policy purposes—mask it? It has often been argued that the inmates of total institutions, especially in cases in which improved conditions (material or social) may flow from participation and in which risks may be involved in participation, have their voluntariness for such decision making compromised or, if not compromised, that, given their situation, we are in no position to know whether their decision to participate would rise above an appropriate threshold of voluntariness. Plea bargains have also posed a problem for some writers. On the surface, the option of pleading guilty to a lesser charge in exchange for trial on other and more serious charges may not appear coercive. But if the penalties faced at trial are considerably greater than those offered through the plea agreement, even an innocent defendant may feel pressured to plead guilty.[21]

Although there is a tradition of thinking that coercion requires threats, there is some reason to think that, in appropriate circumstances, even offers may be coercive. They may be coercive either because a refusal of the offer is associated with some threat (what are sometimes referred to as "throffers"[22]) or, alternatively, because the baseline circumstances in which the offer is made are humanly unacceptable. If a factory owner takes advantage of economic conditions to advertise a subsistence wage for heavy work, we may see the offer as genuine but coercive.[23]

Ensuring the voluntariness of agreements is one of the conditions that enables acts of consent to constitute a responsible transformation of the moral landscape for those who are party to it.

The Knowledge Condition

The responsibility that undergirds the moral force of consent also requires that the act of signifying consent be a knowledgeable one. That is, for consent to have its force unqualified, it should be informed. "Unqualified" may mean a number of things. It may be uninformed and irresponsible (but valid) or it may be ill-informed or misinformed and by virtue of that either fail as consent or have its moral force qualified in some way.

Some people may choose to consent irresponsibly by refusing to inform themselves about the circumstances under which they are giving their consent. *A* may consent to enter into a business partnership with *B* without looking carefully at its financial prospects. Even though risk may be part of any such arrangement, the assumption of risk ought to be informed. One might be equally uninformed—and irresponsible—when voting for a political candidate. As long as one is eligible to vote and one's vote is voluntary, it may not matter (so far as the genuineness or the validity of the vote is concerned) if one's vote is ill-informed.[24] Those who vote irresponsibly may have themselves to blame for its outcome.

In medical contexts, however, there is usually some effort made to ensure that consent is not ill-informed. Institutionally, that now usually requires the signing of a consent form under certain conditions. Thus, for example, if consent to a medical procedure is to be regarded as valid, it needs to be described in adequate detail and in a language that is familiar to the patient; the costs and risks associated with the procedure need to be made clear and alternatives to the proposed procedure (where available) need to be noted, along with some indication of the prognosis. Although a morally adequate consent may require less or more than the formalities usually involved in medical consent, the point is that if an onus is to be shifted or obligation is to be assumed, the person whose consent is given ought to understand the nature and ramifications of what he is doing.

Deceptive knowledge failures may affect consent in more than one way. An old—albeit problematic—legal distinction between "fraud in the *factum*" and "fraud in the inducement" suggests how misinformation may sometimes negate consent but at other times not do so yet nevertheless provide the consenter with a significant cause for complaint.[25] An illustration often provided goes as follows: (1) A consents to a gynecological examination by B, who, she believes, inserts a vaginal speculum; in fact, he inserts his penis. (2) A consents to intercourse with her doctor B after he has deceptively induced her to believe that it will be therapeutically beneficial. On the traditional account, A's consent in (1) is negated by B's deception, and B is guilty of sexual assault. In (2), however, no sexual assault occurs, only a form of fraud. The reason usually given is that whereas the fraud in (1) goes to the very "fact" of what was done, in (2) it concerns only a "collateral matter." After all, in (2) A did consent to intercourse, albeit falsely believing it to be therapeutic, whereas in (1) A did not. But what might appear to be a clear-cut distinction between two types of fraud in (1) and (2) gets muddied once we introduce other cases. What if (3) A consents to intercourse with B, falsely believing that the man who (in the dark) has slipped into bed beside her is her husband? Has she been sexually assaulted or defrauded? Or, suppose (4) A consents to (her first) intercourse with B having been deceptively induced to believe that the papers she recently signed were marriage documents. Was A sexually assaulted or merely defrauded? What these and other cases tend to show is that underlying our judgments about the moral effect of misinformation are normative considerations concerning the seriousness of the deception. In cases (3) and (4), unlike case (2), there was consent to intercourse, although there was not—and it is assumed there would not have been—consent to extramarital intercourse. Even in cases similar to (2) distinctions might be drawn. Were it the case that (5) A, a prostitute, consented to intercourse with B after he deceptively led her to believe that he would pay, we might view it as simple economic fraud rather than as a sexual offense.

Leaving aside the varied ways in which the laws of different jurisdictions might view such cases, they indicate how normatively charged are our judgments concerning the impact of knowledge deficits. Moreover, given those varied ways, we should not assume that such normative undergirding will be uncontroversial. It may reflect cultural and other prejudices that stand in need of re-evaluation.

The Intention Condition

When A consents to φ, A consents to φ under a certain description. If A consents to B's using his car and (without A's knowing it) B uses the car to carry out a bank robbery, it would ordinarily be misleading to say that A consented to B's use of the getaway vehicle.[26] Consent is relatively determinate, and even though *A* did not explicitly exclude the possibility of its use as a getaway vehicle, some conventional expectations can usually be assumed to inform such acts of consent. In certain circumstances, it will be important to specify fairly precisely what is consented to. If *A* consents to engage in sexual intercourse with *B*, *A* does not thereby consent to (risk) contracting the STD with which *B* knows herself to be infected. *A* may be foolish not to inquire or take some prophylactic precaution, and *B* may be irresponsible in not informing *A*. But if *A* is aware that *B* is infected but nevertheless proceeds to have sex without a condom, we might want to argue that *A* voluntarily assumed the risk of contracting the STD. But this would still not amount to consenting to infection with the STD unless *A* stated that it was his intention to contract the STD. What we might say in such a case is that *A* consented to risk contracting an STD.

Though not incoherent, a so-called carte blanche consent would ordinarily be seen as either conventionally constrained or as irresponsible. "Whatever you wish," in response to a request that requires permission, is ordinarily bounded by the set of mutual understandings that is implicit in the relationship existing between *A* and *B*. Even so, a person who consents so generally may have to bear some moral responsibility for the risk that is implicit in giving such free rein to another.

Contact sports pose something of a challenge to what their participants consent to. It can be asserted with some confidence that those who play such sports professionally consent to certain risks inherent in the nature of the sport, and that injuries caused do not constitute either assaults or tortious harms. But what if the injury is caused as the result of deliberate breach of the rules of the game—such as the ice hockey player who slashes at an opponent's head with his stick? Here I would suggest that courts—in the United States, at least, though not so much in Canada—have compromised the moral force of consent for reasons that are not morally sustainable.[27] It does not seem reasonable to hold that those who have consented to participate in the game have consented to the risks associated with deliberate breaches of the rules—though here, as elsewhere, there will be cases and cases.

Political consent, insofar as it can be agreed to have been given, can be particularly treacherous. Except in referenda, which are often—though not necessarily—stated in fairly precise terms, the usual context for political consent—voting for a party or person—is necessarily open-ended, and we may find our consent abused. The party that we voted for because it promised not to raise taxes may decide, once in power, to raise taxes. Our consent is not easily withdrawn, given the institutional structures in place to give it effect, though we may wish to argue that the moral ramifications of our consent have been forfeited. Often, given the unsatisfactoriness of waiting for a next election, our best hope may be to protest the decision and seek to garner enough public support to lead to its revocation. In any case, our consent can be reconsidered and judged misguided or abused.

Political consent and voting are complex in other ways. When I vote for C in an election, it will not usually be said that I did not consent to D's election should C lose to D. Those who vote are ordinarily taken to have consented not simply to some particular person's election but to the outcome of the electoral process. That is what they intend. What we consent to is a particular decisional process (usually adopted in circumstances in which unanimity is unlikely) in which the outcome binds those who participate in it. There may be rare situations in which A takes the view that if C does not win he will not recognize D. But such a person will then have the burden of explaining why he participated in a particular process designed to resolve the issue of representation. Why not boycott the election altogether if only one candidate is deemed acceptable? The question is not rhetorical; nevertheless, the onus will be on A to make good his claim that participation did not amount to his consenting to the outcome (and hence to D's election in the event of D getting the most votes). In certain cases, that onus can surely be met. It will, nevertheless, be for A to meet it.[28]

This raises a further question with regard to those who do not participate in the electoral process. Presuming that participation is freely available to them, that they know of it and of what is at stake, can their failure to vote be taken as consenting to its outcome? I think not. At best it amounts to acquiescence, and with acquiescence, as with condonation, there may be some responsibility for the outcome. But this does not amount to consent, as is recognized by those who bemoan low participation rates and worry about the extent to which actual political outcomes can truly be said to manifest the "consent of the governed."

The issue of intention also comes into play in discussions about so-called tacit consent. Famously—or notoriously—Locke claimed:

> [E]very man, that hath any possessions, or enjoyment, of any part of the dominions of any government, doth thereby give his tacit consent, and is as far forth obliged to obedience to the laws of that government, during such enjoyment, as any one under it; whether this his possession be of land, to him and his heirs for ever, or a lodging only for a week; or whether it be barely travelling freely on the highway; and in effect, it reaches as far as the very being of any one within the territories of that government.[29]

If some overpsychologize consent, others fail to recognize the extent to which consent as a communicative act must be intended to convey to *B* a permission or entitlement. Tacit consent of the kind that Locke defends resolves consent into a signifying act that has been detached from that which it is intended to signify. There is no reason to think that the person who travels freely on the highway consents to the laws of the government within whose jurisdiction the highway is located. Perhaps such a person, in exchange for the ability to travel freely on the highway, ought to consent to such laws. But having good reason to consent is not to consent. And perhaps a person who enjoys the benefit of free passage has a duty to obey the laws of a jurisdiction that enables this to be so. But such a duty arises out of other considerations, not because consent to them has been given.

It is not that the idea of tacit consent is incoherent. It is coherent, but it is narrowly bounded by intention. When a person makes no response to the question "Any objections?" when it is asked in relation to a proposal that is to be voted on and we have every reason to think that she heard the question and was capable of responding to it, then her silence can be taken as tacit (as distinguished from express) consent to the proposal. But here the conventions regarding signification are clearly understood. Of course, to remove all possible ambiguity, the person conducting the vote may call for ayes and nays or hands. But often that will not be necessary.

What about deceptively intended consent? If *A* consents to *B*'s request for permission to enter premises and then calls the police to report an intruder, can he deny that he consented because he intended revenge? I think such cases reinforce the view that consent is a communicative act, not simply a state of mind. *B* did receive *A*'s consent. Had the proceedings been taped or had *A* given permission in his handwriting, then, barring some exotic set of circumstances, *A* consented to *B*'s entering the premises. A somewhat more complicated case would be one in which an undercover narcotics detective "consents" to be part of a drug trade, but then turns the other participants in. Does he simply pretend to consent or is the consent genuine? What we might say here is that in relation to the norms operative within the drug ring the detective consented to participate, but that in relation to the larger structure of societal expectations he did not consent and so cannot be held to be *particeps criminis*. Nevertheless, the fact that consent is genuine at some level in such cases can create a problem for police, for it can amount to breaking the law to enforce it.

Limits to Consent's Moral Magic

The moral magic of consent will not work if, as we earlier saw, the normative order against whose background it was given is morally bankrupt. The mafia hitman who consents to do a job has no moral authorization to go ahead with it, even though the rules of the organization now permit it. True, if the hitman eliminates someone without first receiving authorization to do so, he may have to contend with the normative order that operates within the criminal organization. But insofar as that organization has no moral standing, any moral magic will only be simulated.

More contentious are situations in which *A*'s consent is to what will be reasonably believed to harm *A* or otherwise be to *A*'s detriment. An ancient legal maxim, *volenti non fit injuria*, though sometimes given close to full rein in civil cases, has often been limited when it comes to criminal law. If *A* consents to *B*'s beating or killing him, the law has frequently refused to recognize its transformative power. Practical policy reasons might of course be advanced for this: There may be reason to doubt the genuineness of consent to self-harm, and it may be difficult to sort out those cases in which the consent is genuine from those in which it is not. But cases in which the consent is both genuine and known to be so no doubt exist, and yet criminal law and sometimes moral judgment resist the transformative power of that consent.

In the case of criminal law at least, it may sometimes be argued—albeit controversially—that people have social responsibilities that would be breached were they permitted to consent to self-harming behavior (some variant on the old idea that the king has a right to the aid and assistance of his subjects[30]), or that whatever right individuals may have to harm themselves, they have no overriding right to have others act as their agents in such matters, and that they and the other party have even less right to consent when the harmful course of action is at the initiative of someone other than the person who is harmed. In other words, whatever we say about *A* voluntarily and intentionally harming himself, it is more problematic if *B* agrees to *A*'s request that *B* harm him, and even more problematic for *B* if *A* consents to *B*'s request that *B* harm him.

This is not the place to explore these arguments in detail.[31] They indicate, however, that consent's moral magic may have some limitations—limitations that, even if particularly controversial when embedded in law, may sometimes function more plausibly in a purely moral setting. Whether or not the law should forbid consensual cannibalism or self-enslavement, there is something morally problematic both about seeking to have another consent to self-harming behavior and about using one's powers of consent to permit harm to be done to oneself. Our reservations may ultimately go back to the view that the value of consent is rooted in a conception of the social conditions under which humans may best flourish, conditions that will ordinarily support the magical power that consent is able to display. When consent functions otherwise, it seems to have uprooted itself from that which sustains it.

Notes

1. Heidi M. Hurd, "The Moral Magic of Consent," *Legal Theory* 2 (1996): 121–46. I do not, however, want to make Hurd's distinction between consent as "morally transformative" and as "giving stained permission." The focus of my account is what consent achieves by way of the relations between *A* and the person to whom *A* gives consent and not the moral quality of the acts to which permission is given. I say more about this later.

2. What we might argue, in view of the gap between legal and moral consent, is that legal consent is open to criticism to the extent that it fails to mirror moral consent. Such criticism need not be decisive, however, because law has social purposes that pure morality does not. In particular, law is designed to provide societal-wide guidance and closure, and to satisfy its public functions it must sometimes draw brighter lines than morally nuanced assessments would suggest.

3. That we are still inclined to speak of "consent" in such cases may have more to do with lingering conventions concerning the payment for wedding festivities and of course the fact that weddings usually remain extended-family occasions. Even if consent is not needed—either morally or legally—it may be good form to act as though it is. There may also be situations in which *B* may be legally entitled to φ, but not consider himself morally justified in φ-ing without *A*'s consent (as, for example, in the days when marriage was thought to constitute consent to sex whenever the husband desired it).

4. Does that mean that the communication has to have been with *B*? I think so— though there may be problematic cases in which, say, a letter of consent has been signed but not delivered. Even there, though, I would be inclined to argue that until notified, it would be presumptuous of *B* to φ.

5. Individually, the shareholders may consent to their votes being used in a count. Collectively, they consent to the terms of a takeover.

6. The "age of consent" represents a legal determination that prior to reaching a certain age a person cannot—for legal purposes—be said to have consented to some course of action (say, sexual intercourse, a medical procedure, or

contractual arrangement) even if the person has done what would ordinarily have been taken as giving consent. The theory behind such determinations—and what links them to consent as a natural moral notion—is that prior to the nominated age of consent the person could not be, or could not be taken to be, capable of grasping the nature of φ with the sophistication necessary to enable the act of consenting to be one for which A should be held responsible.

7. For a more extensive discussion of consent in such contexts, see Alan Wertheimer, "Sexual Exploitation in Psychotherapy," in *Exploitation* (Princeton, NJ: Princeton University Press, 1996), ch. 6.

8. However, it would be a moral authorization only in the sense that B could not claim that A had stolen the car or used it without permission. There may be other countervailing factors that make it improper for A to use it—A is too young, unlicensed, disqualified from driving, etc. Although these are essentially formal or legal disqualifiers, we generally presume that they track morally relevant considerations, such as the ability to drive a car safely.

9. Peter Westen, *The Logic of Consent: The Diversity and Deceptiveness of Consent as a Defense to Criminal Conduct* (Aldershot: Ashgate, 2003), 5.

10. Hurd, "The Moral Magic of Consent," 121.

11. Westen, *The Logic of Consent*, 4.

12. Grammatical confusion is easy: "A approves of B's doing φ" is to be distinguished from "A approves B's doing φ," as is "A agrees with B's doing φ" from "A agrees to B's doing φ."

13. The point may, however, be rendered moot, if B brings it about that A is no longer able to communicate any withdrawal.

14. Does acquiescence constitute a form of consent? I am inclined to say that it depends. Where consent is called for and refusal to consent is easily signified, then acquiescence might reasonably be taken to constitute consent. But in cases in which it may be costly to refuse consent, acquiescence may not always be taken to signify consent.

15. The case is discussed in Westen, *The Logic of Consent*, 1–2.

16. I assume of course that there were not other features of the situation (for example, participation in the making of the pornographic movie) that were coercive.

17. For two good discussions of the subtleties of consent in sexual contexts, see Stephen J. Schulhofer, *Unwanted Sex* (Cambridge, MA: Harvard University Press, 1998); and Alan Wertheimer, *Consent to Sexual Relations* (Cambridge, UK: Cambridge University Press, 2003).

18. A great deal of controversy surrounded a sexual consent policy developed in the 1990s at Antioch College, accessible at http://www.mit.edu/activities/safe/data/other/antioch-code.

19. Of course, this is also a case—the more usual one—in which *A* takes the initiative, though we could structure it so that *A* could consent to *B*'s request whether *A* would like to be put out of her misery.

20. For a valuable discussion of the subtleties of coercion, see Alan Wertheimer, *Coercion* (Princeton, NJ: Princeton University Press, 1987).

21. See Candace McCoy, "Plea Bargaining as Coercion: The Trial Penalty and Plea Bargaining Reform," *Criminal Law Quarterly* 50 (2005): 67–107.

22. See Hillel Steiner, "Individual Liberty," *Proceedings of the Aristotelian Society* 75 (1974–75): 39.

23. Some are unwilling to go as far as this, seeing such offers as unconscionable or exploitative and therefore grossly unfair rather than as coercive. For a longer discussion of the intricacies, see Wertheimer, *Consent to Sexual Relations*, 171–77.

24. Voting, indeed, is so often corrupted from without as well as within that political consent theorists have some difficulty in claiming that political legitimacy is a function of the "consent of the governed."

25. Rollin M. Perkins, *Criminal Law*, 2nd ed. (Mineola, NY: Foundation Press, 1969), 964–66.

26. This is not necessarily to relieve *A* of all culpability. If *A* consents to lend *B* his firearm, it might be reasonable to expect *A* to inquire what *B* wants it for.

27. The gladiatorial aspects of some contact sports are an important part of their popular appeal. But that makes them no more acceptable than were public executions. On Canadian developments, see Diane V. White, "Sports Violence as Criminal Assault: Development of the Doctrine by Canadian Courts," *Duke Law Journal* 6 (1986): 1030–54.

28. Consider the situation in which a person, though committed to the idea of a binding vote, believes that the actual electoral process has been so gerrymandered and corrupted by political tactics that the outcome of a voting process is at best a distorted representation of the considered judgment of those who have participated in it. The gap between the ideal and real may leave a person with reasonable doubts about whether an outcome represents the consent of the governed.

29. *Second Treatise Of Civil Government*, ch. 8, § 119.

30. This doctrine can be traced back to Aristotle, who argues that the person who harms himself commits an injustice, because he violates *public* law forbidding such action. See *Nicomachean Ethics*, V, ix. 6. The critical question of course is whether there should be such law.

31. For a valuable discussion, see Vera Bergelson, "The Right to Be Hurt: Testing the Boundaries of Consent," *George Washington Law Review* 75 (2007): 165–236.

2

A History of Consent in Western Thought[1]

David Johnston

In western thought, the concept of consent has been deployed in two major ways. In one of these, the notion of consent is applied to relations among individuals—or more precisely, among persons. In this context, it is widely accepted that acts of consent establish entitlements, create obligations, and shift risks and responsibilities from some persons to others. The principal issues that have arisen concerning this kind of consent have clustered around questions about the range of entitlements and obligations that can be created or transferred through acts of consent and about the kinds of persons who should be considered competent to give consent (as well as questions about the kinds of human individuals and groups who should be considered persons). These questions have long played central roles in legal and social thought.

The concept of consent has also been deployed in discussions of the relationship between governments and the collectivities over which they rule. When people have thought to ask whether their government is legitimate—a question of considerable antiquity—one of the most prominent claims that have been made in (partial) response is that governments are legitimated by the collective consent of the governed. Although this claim now occupies a virtually hegemonic position in western thought, it has gained that position only quite recently. For most of the history of western thought, the idea of government by consent contended with major rivals. That contention comprises much of the substance of the history of political theory.

These two ways of applying the concept of consent have been intertwined with one another at numerous junctures. In Roman thought, for example, the term *lex*, which appears to be based on the idea of an explicit contract between two person or two groups, later came to signify a kind of law, and the Latin word is accordingly translated into English by the latter term.[2] Similarly, in the seventeenth century Grotius constructed a justification of private property by hypothesizing that an original state of common human ownership of all the land on earth had been supplanted by the institution of private property through an act of collective consent to the latter.[3] The way in which acts of consent among private parties have been conceived has been linked in a variety of ways to the notion of consent to governments or to other public institutions.

Overall, however, each of these two principal ways of applying the concept of consent has blazed its own path through the history of western thought. As a major theme, the idea of government by consent assumed a prominent and positive place in that history earlier than did the notion of individual consent as a basis for important obligations and entitlements. I will accordingly discuss the history of the concept of consent in political theory separately before moving on to the history of that concept in legal and social theory.

Consent in Political Theory

It is widely believed that the view that government is legitimated by the consent of the governed gained very little traction before the early modern era. Samuel Beer's observation is representative:

> For more than 2000 years nearly all leading minds had rejected
> popular government. Classical philosophy had taught the rule of the
> wise, Christian theology the rule of the holy. Medieval thinkers had
> combined the two ideas.[4]

Although Beer may be speaking here about a particular *form* of government rather than about the way in which a government gains *legitimation*, his observation is misleading at best. The idea that government is legitimated by consent of the governed–or at least by those among them who were considered capable of giving consent, a group that often excluded women, always excluded slaves, and frequently excluded other classes of human beings as well–has occupied a prominent, though not always dominant, position in western political thought from its beginnings onward. This idea plays central roles in the literatures of the ancient Israelites, Greeks, and Romans.

After the Israelites had escaped enslavement in Egypt and encamped near the foot of Mount Sinai, God asks Moses to tell the people that

> If only you will now listen to me and keep my covenant, then out of all peoples you shall become my special possession; for the whole earth is mine. You shall be my kingdom of priests, my holy nation.[5]

When Moses presents the covenant to the elders, the "people all answered together, 'Whatever the Lord has said we will do.' "[6] This covenant is one of the central topics in Hebrew Scriptures. The Hebrew prophets and other later writers refer to it and frequently report promises to renew it. In *Isaiah* 55 (second or pseudo-Isaiah) God promises to "make a covenant with you, this time for ever, to love you faithfully as I loved David."[7] The writer compares this key covenant with a marital contract:

> For, as a young man weds a maiden,
> so you shall wed him who rebuilds you,
> and your God shall rejoice over you
> as a bridegroom rejoices over the bride.[8]

In the covenant that is central to the narrative of the Hebrew Scriptures, the form of government God proposes to the Israelites is a theocracy, not a "popular" government. But it is also a government by consent of the governed. It is true that God is the author of that government in the sense that he defines its major provisions and fundamental laws. The people's role is limited to the act of consent to those provisions. Yet without that consent, there would be no covenant, the Israelites would not enjoy the benefits God promises to them, and God would not receive their acceptance of his terms.

It is true that the kind of consent God elicits in his covenant with the Israelites is quite constrained. God dictates the terms of the covenant and offers the Israelites no opportunity to bargain over those terms, a fact that is especially striking because of their prowess at bargaining in other contexts. It is also noteworthy that the Israelites' consent is a collective act in which a group of elders represents and speaks for the people, not an act in which the opinion or will of each individual is registered and the results are aggregated in a democratic process. These features are typical of the conception of consent that plays a role in the legitimation of government in the literatures of the Israelites, Greeks, and Romans. From a modern, democratic and individualistic viewpoint, that conception is shockingly inadequate, perhaps even farcical. Yet the conception of consent to government that runs through much of these ancient literatures was not mere window dressing. For the act of consent, even when collective and constrained, was understood to shift some portion of responsibility to those who had given their consent. Through their consent, a government became, in a meaningful sense, *their* government, and its acts became *their* acts.

The idea that government is legitimated by consent also plays a central role in Greek political thought. Through a series of institutional reforms, the Athenians created a distinctive democratic form of government—actually a series of such governments—during the fifth century BCE. In the *Republic*, written early in the fourth century, Plato reports the following view through the mouthpiece of Glaucon, who in real life was Plato's brother and in the dialogue serves as principal interlocutor to Socrates, the main character in the text:

> They say that to do injustice is naturally good and to suffer injustice bad, but that the badness of suffering it so far exceeds the goodness of doing it that those who have done and suffered injustice and tasted both, but who lack the power to do it and avoid suffering it, decide that it is profitable to come to an agreement with each other neither to do injustice nor to suffer it. As a result, they begin to make laws and covenants, and what the law commands they call lawful and just. This, they say, is the origin and essence of justice.[9]

Here, Plato describes a view according to which government and indeed the whole of justice is legitimated by an act of collective consent. To be sure, the view he sketches is not his own. Although Plato developed a conception of political legitimacy rooted in consent in his earlier Socratic dialogue *Crito*, in the *Republic* he associates the notion of legitimation by consent with the sophists, a school of thinkers whom he often held up as his principal ideological antagonists. Even in this later work, however, the notion of government (and justice) by consent is the point of departure for the alternative conception he develops, and Plato clearly regarded this notion as a formidable competitor to his own theories. The idea that government is legitimated by the consent of the governed played a central role in the formation of Greek political philosophy, even if some of the most famous of those philosophers rejected that idea.

It is true that Plato was a vigorous opponent both of popular government and of the idea that government is legitimated by the consent of the governed. Plato, of course, has long been regarded as one of the greatest of all philosophers. Moreover, Plato's influence on subsequent political thinkers in antiquity was considerable. In this sense it might plausibly be claimed that nearly all "leading minds" in the ancient world rejected the ideas of popular government and government by consent of the governed. In reality, however, this claim is an artifact of an interpretation of the history of western thought that bestows an outsized part in that history to Greek philosophy, and especially to the philosophy of Plato.

Plato was in fact *the* principal critic of the idea that government is legitimated by the consent of the governed as well as the author of a major alternative to that idea. Most writers in the Greek traditions that preceded Plato assumed that the primary purpose of government is to enable all those involved in or affected by it—the governed as well as the governors—to pursue their worldly interests effectively. For Plato, by contrast, the purpose of government ideally is to cultivate an order in the city (which for him was the natural locus of the political association) and, even more important, in the soul, that accords with the divine, natural form of justice. In the *Republic*, speaking through the mouthpiece of his onetime mentor Socrates, Plato explains that his conception of justice can be attained only if rulers pursue a rigorous course of cultural purification or indoctrination and only if they are willing coercively to apply the prescriptions of justice to those who are ruled without the need to elicit the latter's consent. Plato's most stunning proposal for the coercive use of power is his suggestion that when a philosopher comes to power in a city, he or she should expel everyone over the age of 10 from the city.[10] This act of forcible relocation will leave the ruler free to impose upon the children who remain the culture, habits of thought, and practices that accord with Plato's idea of justice as reciprocal domination and submission among unequals and to form those few persons who are capable of being so formed into the internally harmonious, rigorously self-controlled individuals who embody justice, as he sees it, in its most perfect sense. For Plato, the political community is like a school for the tutelage of its members, not an association for the pursuit of their worldly interests.[11] Government is legitimated not by the consent of the governed–not even their constrained and collective consent–but by its adherence to standards that are distinct from and independent of their wills.

This conception of the purpose of government as tutelage remained vital in the history of western political thought from Plato's time onward, but neither this conception nor the sharp rejection of the idea of legitimation by consent it entailed dominated that history. While Aristotle followed Plato in emphasizing the educational purpose of political associations, he nonetheless breaks from Plato by according an important role in the legitimation of government to the collective consent of the major elements of society.[12] The principle that consent is the foundation of all governmental authority, again in the form of collective consent from the major elements of society, was fundamental to the constitution of the Roman Republic and this principle persisted in the theory of the Roman constitution for centuries after the

Republic had effectively been superseded by the Roman Empire. As in the case of the ancient Israelites, the consent in question was collective and was elicited from representatives who may often have had neither the interests nor the wills of the people in mind. Yet that ostensible consent was not meaningless. In Roman thought, the effect of a law–or at least of the kind of law that was based on *lex*, which was only one of several sources of law in ancient Rome–was that of a contract to which one has consented, and its violation was viewed as a breach of an obligation one has assumed by consent. The jurist Gaius, writing in the second century CE, defines a *lex* (again, *lex* was only one of several sources of law, alongside plebiscites, senatusconsults, constitutions of the emperor, edicts, and the opinions of jurists) as "a command and ordinance of the people."[13] Papinian, who is sometimes considered the greatest of Roman jurists, says that *lex* is a "communal covenant of the state" (*communis rei publicae sponsio*).[14] *Sponsio* was the essence of the formal, oral contract (*stipulatio*) at Rome. Hence to describe *lex* as a covenant was to call attention to the principle that the authority of at least that kind of law is derived from the consent of those to whom it applies. Imperial rule led to the gradual erosion of this principle, but centuries passed before it was discarded altogether. Not until the compilation of Justinian's *Institutes* some four centuries after Gaius do we find the principle of consent eclipsed by the idea that the emperor's will is the sole source of law.[15] In antiquity, the idea that government is legitimated by the consent of the governed, however constrained and collective, proved remarkably resilient.

With the effective demise of the Roman Republic, the principle of government by consent began to recede from its place at the center of western political thought. The fact that under imperial rule it became increasingly clear that this principle had become a mere fiction was one factor in its decline. However, another factor that proved even more significant in the long run was the spread of Christianity, especially in the centuries after it had been given a distinctive doctrinal form through the writings of St. Augustine. From the early years of its promulgation by the apostle Paul, Christianity had preached the devaluation of political affairs and indeed of all worldly things. Augustine incorporated this line of thinking into his exposition of Christian doctrine, but he combined it with a distinctive interpretation of the place of political affairs in human life. For Augustine, the principal purpose of a political association is to impose and maintain an external order upon unruly human beings. The maintenance of that order transmits to those subject to it an understanding of their equal status of radical domination by and subjection to God, a status on which the subjects' consent or lack thereof has no bearing whatsoever.[16] The differences between this conception of the political community and Plato's are sharp. Nevertheless, the consequences of Augustine's conception of the role of government in human life, which was disseminated widely throughout western Christendom in the centuries after his death, were as inimical to the principle of government by consent as Plato's political theory had been. In Augustine's view, governments are legitimated neither by the consent of the governed nor by their adherence to abstract standards that are prior to and higher than the wills of their members, but by the fact that their existence is willed by an omnipotent God. According to this view, the legitimacy of government is independent of the consent of the governed.

This view and variations thereupon dominated western political thought from roughly the middle of the first millennium CE to the early part of the second millennium. Although St. Thomas Aquinas, writing toward the end of this period, allocated a greater role to consent by the governed than had Augustine, for the most part he was a disciple of the Augustinian view who held that governments are legitimated by hierarchical relations that inhere in nature, not by the wills of human beings.[17] Yet Aquinas was only one of the great thinkers of the middle ages. Between roughly 1100 and 1350, a major shift occurred in the ideas of many medieval philosophers, theologians, and canon lawyers on the subject of government and its legitimation. For example, around 1300 Duns Scotus argued that political authority was justly derived from "the common consent and election of the community."[18] In a variation of early contract theories like the one Plato attributes to the sophists, Scotus imagines a group of strangers coming together to form a city. With no natural paternal authority to which to submit, he suggested that they might all submit themselves by consent to one ruler or each submit himself to the authority of the community as a whole. After several centuries of decline, the consent theory of political legitimacy was revived.

Scotus was hardly alone. Around 1315 Herveus Natalis, master-general of the Dominican Order, attempted to explain how it is possible that rulers are able to oblige their subjects. His argument is that ruling power can be held in only two ways, either by consent or by violence. Since violence cannot create right, he concludes that the right to impose obligations can originate only in the consent of the people. Like a number of later thinkers, Herveus envisages a two-stage process in which a people first consent to establish a government and then consent to install a particular person in the office they have created.[19] Marsilius of Padua, too, argued that government can be made legitimate only by consent of the governed. Marsilius specifically considers the Platonic claim that superior wisdom confers an entitlement to rule and specifically rejects that claim. For Marsilius, a ruler acquires legitimate power only by election, not by virtue of his personal qualities, however superior they might be.[20]

We find a similar viewpoint in the writings of many canon lawyers and legal commentators of the era, in part because of the resurgent influence of Roman legal writings. In the twelfth century Ranulph Glanvill, Henry II's chief justiciar, compiled his *Tractatus de Legibus et Consuetudinibus Regni Angliae* (*Treatise on the Laws and Customs of the Realm of England*), which he seems to have thought of as a kind of English equivalent of Justinian's *Institutes* of Roman law.[21] Glanvill understood the central principle of the Roman constitution to be the doctrine that the *populus* is the sole source of law, and he believed that this principle applied as fully to English institutions as to Roman ones. Some 60 years later Henry of Bracton, author of the most significant of all medieval books on English law, argued in his introduction to that work that

> these English laws . . . since they have been approved by the consent
> of those who use them and confirmed by the oath of kings, they
> cannot be changed without the common consent of all those by
> whose counsel and consent they were promulgated.[22]

From the twelfth century onward, a basic maxim derived from Roman private law, *quod omnes tangit ab omnibus approbetur* ("what touches all is to be approved by all") was invoked repeatedly by canonists and legists. While the point of this provision in its early form was to stipulate that persons affected by legal proceedings should be entitled to attend those proceedings, its sense was transformed over time, ultimately providing a basis for modern principles of representative government.[23]

As the process of state formation gathered force in the sixteenth, seventeenth, and eighteenth centuries, the principle of government by consent gradually gained ground by being invoked repeatedly by a series of groups who sought to obtain a share of emerging state power. In England, the beginnings of this process can be dated back at least as far as *Magna Carta* in 1215, but the most significant strides were made in the constitutional struggles of the sixteenth and seventeenth centuries. The English constitutional crisis of 1621 is an especially noteworthy episode. King James asserted that his subjects enjoyed their liberties, including the privilege of meeting as a parliamentary body, as a grant from the crown that could in principle be withdrawn. Leading members of the parliament of that year disputed this claim. Sir Thomas Wentworth, who was later to become Earl of Strafford and a principal target of the ire of the parliament of 1641, asserted that "We are they that represent the great bulk of the commonwealth," and the famous jurist Sir Edward Coke suggested that the authority of parliament rests on the fact that it "served for thousands and tens of thousands."[24] James claimed that his authority to govern was based on rights he had inherited from his predecessors that were not contingent on the consent of the governed. By contrast, the parliamentarians claimed the right to assemble and to deliberate on the ground that the people had consented for the parliament to represent them.

Western political thought had now started down a path that would lead to the doctrine of popular sovereignty and to the institutions of modern representative government. Old arguments about the basis of governmental authority that invoked inheritance, custom, or natural hierarchy gradually gave way to a line of reasoning that located the basis of that authority squarely and unambiguously in popular consent. By the mid-seventeenth century Thomas Hobbes, one of the most notorious defenders of political absolutism and ultimately the most influential political philosopher ever to have written in the English language, had seized firmly on the future direction of political thought. Despite his commitment to the idea that political authority must be "absolute and arbitrary"[25] and in no usual sense responsible to popular will, Hobbes declared that the only thing that can legitimate that authority is the consent of the governed. Moreover, and most important, Hobbes insisted that consent must be given by each member of the political association as an individual. On this point Hobbes's view marks a sharp break from Aristotle and from nearly all Roman and medieval political theory. In Roman political thought, the effect of a *lex* is that of a contract to which the citizen has agreed. But as we have seen, *lex* was only one of several sources of law in Rome. For Hobbes, in contrast, *every* law in a political association is binding on its individual members in the way in which a contract is binding because *every* law is the product of a contract to which *each* has agreed. Indeed this "is more than consent, or concord; it is a real unity of them all, in one and the same person, made by covenant of *every man with every man*..."[26]

Although Hobbes argued that only the consent of the governed can legitimate political (sovereign) authority, he did not endorse the doctrine of popular sovereignty, which holds that only the members of a political community as a collectivity can constitute a sovereign or ultimate ruler. That doctrine flowed several decades later from the pen of Hobbes's compatriot John Locke and received perhaps its most famous expression in the political theory of Jean-Jacques Rousseau.[27] Rousseau, like Hobbes, endorsed the idea that the extent of the authority that can be constituted through popular consent is virtually unlimited. Neither of these thinkers envisaged significant fetters on the scope of the authority that can be created through an act of popular will.

While Locke shares responsibility with Rousseau for the formation of the modern doctrine of popular sovereignty, he departed from both Hobbes and Rousseau by arguing that significant limits exist to the scope of legitimate political authority. This claim, which (again) can be dated back at least as far as *Magna carta*, has played a central role in modern western political thought. Most commonly, these limits are conceived as individual rights, often (but not always) as natural rights or universal human rights. Rights of these sorts have played a significant role in western political thought since the medieval period,[28] but that role has arguably become more important over the past few centuries as the power available to states has grown and (sometimes) received legitimation through the doctrine of popular sovereignty. In constitutional democracies, a form of government that originated in western political thought and practice and has now taken hold in a considerable portion of the world, it is generally assumed that some rights are inviolable, regardless of the content or the strength of popular will.

Constitutional democracy is now, barely two centuries after it was first conceived, the almost universally preferred form of government in western political thought. Indeed, this form now has no serious competitors within the western tradition.

The idea of constitutional democracy combines two major components. The first is the idea of legitimation by consent of the governed taken as individuals. In western thought, the alternatives to legitimation by popular consent with which this idea contended for centuries are now taken seriously by almost no one. Worldwide, numerous forms of government continue to exist, including hereditary monarchies, theocracies, and despotisms in various forms. To thinkers inculcated in western traditions, however, no form of government is considered fully legitimate unless it is based on popular consent, now conceived as something that must be renewed periodically through free and fair elections of political leaders.

The second major component of constitutional democracy is a set of limits on the scope of governmental authority. Sometimes, as in the written constitution of the United States, these limits are prescribed by a list of rights. At other times, they are evoked by provisions for an independent judiciary that it is assumed will enforce rights. Often both measures have been adopted. In any case, the essential principle is that there are some things no government can legitimately do. The notion that government can be made legitimate only through popular consent is central to modern western political thought,[29] but so is the notion that some acts and policies cannot be made legitimate by popular consent, no matter how powerful a consensus may exist in support of those policies or acts.

Consent and Relations among Persons

In the earliest writings in the western tradition, consent plays a limited role in shaping relations among individual persons, and when it does play a role, it is often cast in a negative light. When God bestows entitlements and obligations on the first man, according to the account in the Hebrew Scriptures, he bestows them by command. He does not ask Adam to consent to his terms. The first significant actions that result from individual consent are Eve's and Adam's eating of the fruit of the tree in the middle of the garden of Eden, actions that flow from deceptive promises made by the serpent and that constitute sinful disobedience to God's direct command.[30] When God makes a covenant with Abram, he simply explains the benefits that will accrue to Abram as well as the duties he expects Abram to perform, without asking for Abram's consent.[31] Only much later, when God proposes a covenant with the Israelites as a people at Mount Sinai, is consent to the arrangement asked for or given, and that act of consent, which is one of the most momentous events in all of Hebrew Scriptures, is collective, not individual.[32]

It is true that the narratives in *Genesis* and later books of Hebrew Scripture describe a number of instances in which entitlements and obligations are exchanged by acts of individual consent. But these exchanges, like the decisions of Adam and Eve to eat the forbidden fruit, are frequently marked by deception or other forms of unfair dealing. During a famine Abram journeys to Egypt with his wife Sarai. Fearing that Pharaoh might kill him, Abram tells Sarai to pretend that she is his sister, not his wife. Pharaoh takes Sarai into his own household to act as one of his wives, while Abram prospers during their time in Egypt. Only when Pharaoh and his household are struck down with diseases does Pharaoh discover the deception to which he has been exposed, at which point he expels Abram and Sarai from Egypt.[33] Later, Jacob agrees to work for his kinsman Laban for 7 years in return for the promise that he will be permitted to marry Laban's daughter Rachel at the end of that period. When Jacob completes his end of the bargain, Laban sends him his elder and less attractive daughter Leah in place of Rachel with the explanation that it is the custom in his country that an elder daughter must marry before a younger one. The transaction is consensual, but Laban obtains Jacob's consent through deception, and Jacob is forced to work for his father-in-law for an additional 7 years to earn Rachel's hand as well.[34] In the earlier Hebrew Scriptures, at least, the most important obligations and entitlements are allocated by command, not by individual consent. When consensual transactions are depicted, they are usually presented in a highly critical light, as if to suggest that entitlements and obligations that originate in consensual agreements among individuals are inherently suspect.

Individual consent fares no better in the other early literatures that have played a significant role in western thought. The transactions between individuals depicted in the *Iliad*, for example, are frequently tainted by deception and treachery.[35] The most significant bonds among people are those which flow from their membership in kinship groups. By comparison with these bonds, obligations that are assumed through voluntary acts are insignificant and unreliable. In both early Greek and early Hebrew literatures, the kinship group is the primary locus of ethical significance and the primary basis for allocating entitlements and obligations.

In both these literatures, responsibility for harmful actions is allocated on the basis of kinship groups as well. A harm or wrong perpetrated by one individual typically precipitated retaliation against that person's kin (usually male) and this liability to retaliation was transmitted to the wrongdoer's descendants. An early glimmering of a challenge to this basis for allocating responsibility occurs in *Genesis* 18, when Abraham bargains with God over the planned destruction of Sodom in collective punishment for its grievous sins. Abraham persuades God to spare the city if he can find just 50, then 45, then 40, and finally just 10 righteous men in Sodom. It is significant, though, that this story concludes with God's failure to find even 10 righteous men and that ultimately, only Abraham's brother Lot and his daughters are spared from destruction.[36]

The first clear assertion of a principle of individual rather than collective responsibility occurs in the writings of the prophet Ezekiel in the early sixth century BCE. Writing during a period of Babylonian rule over Israel, when the Israelites had begun to focus their energies more on commerce than on war, Ezekiel reports that God has told him that the old proverb

> The fathers have eaten sour grapes,
> and the children's teeth are set on edge

will never again be used in Israel. According to Ezekiel, God continues by explaining:

> You may ask, "Why is the son not punished for his father's iniquity?"
> Because he has always done what is just and right and has been
> careful to obey all my laws, therefore he shall live. It is the soul that
> sins, and no other, that shall die; a son shall not share a father's guilt,
> nor a father his son's. The righteous man shall reap the fruit of his
> own righteousness, and the wicked man the fruit of his own
> wickedness.[37]

This passage is among the most momentous in western literature. Acceptance of the principle of individual responsibility is an essential prerequisite to the formation of a society in which transactions between private persons can flourish and constitute a major basis for productive endeavors and other forms of social cooperation. Without the principle of individual responsibility, it is impossible for a system of legal and social relations in which entitlements and obligations are reliably created and transferred via individual consent to arise.

A related development can be discerned in Greek literature at a slightly later date. The value that is emphasized most strongly in early Greek thought is *areté* ("virtue" or "excellence"), which in the Homeric poems is associated closely with the qualities of a warrior. Although the concept of justice is present in this literature—it is invoked in a stage-setting scene depicted near the beginning of the *Iliad*—justice as a value is clearly subordinated to *areté*. The preeminence of *areté* in the Homeric scheme of values was rooted in the need for protection. In a society of scattered households without centralized political authority or the rule of law, the individual with outstanding warrior-like qualities of strength, cunning, and skill in the use of weapons would best be able to provide security to the (extended) household, and these qualities accordingly were the objects of greatest admiration. This association of *areté* with the qualities required for success in battle was loosened at a later stage of Greek culture. In the poet Hesiod's *Works and Days*, the principal subject of which is how to be a successful farmer, to avoid famine, and to be prosperous, the concept of *areté* takes on a decidedly less militaristic tone than it had assumed in the earlier heroic compositions. In neither case, however, is *areté* intrinsically connected to justice. And in neither case is justice ranked as highly in the scheme of values as *areté*.

We can see the beginning of a change in this order of valuation in a couplet attributed to the poet Theognis around the end of the sixth century BCE:

> The whole of *areté* (virtue or excellence) is summed up in *dikaiosuné* (justice); every man, Cyrnus, is *agathos* (virtuous) if he is *dikaios* (just).[38]

This statement, which Aristotle much later treats as a generally accepted and even anodyne proverb,[39] expresses a view that was probably held by a minority at the time of its composition. The writer appears to be claiming that justice—a quality that is associated with reciprocity and fair dealing and that is revealed in transactions between individuals rather than in unilateral actions—is not merely a necessary but also a sufficient condition for virtue, a claim that is incompatible with Homeric values. The growth of cities had changed the character of Greek society. Cities are best able to flourish when their residents are inclined to cooperate by making and keeping agreements and by restraining themselves from doing harm to one another, practices that cannot easily be reconciled with a scheme of values that exalts the virtues of outstanding warriors. This observation is especially applicable to Athens, which had begun to establish itself as a commercial power at the time this couplet was composed. The writer seems to have grasped this problem and accordingly suggests a striking revision of the values that dominated Greek culture at the time, one that places justice at the center of the Greek moral universe, sets the stage for a legal and social system in which responsibility is assessed to individuals rather than to kin groups, and makes it possible for decisions by and agreements among individuals to assume a major role in the organization of human affairs. A scheme of values that is compatible with a society in which individual consent plays a large role in the relations among persons had begun to emerge.[40]

Writing well over a century later, after Athens had achieved commercial preeminence and the new system of values had attained widespread acceptance, Plato became its most forceful and eminent critic, just as he was the principal critic of the idea that government is legitimated by the consent of the governed. In the *Republic*, he lampoons the democratic form of society in which individual choice, individual consent, and individual values play a dominant role in directing human actions. He essays the following description of the typical democratic man:

> ...so he lives on, yielding day by day to the desire at hand.
> Sometimes he drinks heavily while listening to the flute; at other
> times, he drinks only water and is on a diet...sometimes he even
> occupies himself with what he takes to be philosophy. He often
> engages in politics, leaping up from his seat and saying and doing
> whatever comes into his mind. If he happens to admire soldiers, he's
> carried in that direction, if money-makers, in that one. There's
> neither order nor necessity in his life, but he calls it pleasant, free, and
> blessedly happy...[41]

While Plato accepts that there is a place for market transactions and other consensual exchanges in a well-ordered polity, he devalues the element of consent that is central to those transactions and exchanges sharply. Earlier in the same work, he lays out a case for his alternative vision of society, which is based on the observation that different human beings are born with radically different aptitudes:

Socrates: . . . it occurred to me that, in the first place, we aren't all born alike, but each of us differs somewhat in nature from the others, one being suited to one task, another to another. Or don't you think so?

Glaucon: I do.

Socrates: Second, does one person do a better job if he practices many crafts or—since he's one person himself—if he practices one?

Glaucon: If he practices one . . .

Socrates: The result, then, is that more plentiful and better-quality goods are more easily produced if each person does one thing for which he is naturally suited, does it at the right time, and is released from having to do any of the others.[42]

"Doing it at the right time" is more replete with meaning than it first appears. Slightly later in the text, Socrates observes that

we prevented a cobbler from trying to be a farmer, weaver, or builder at the same time and said that he must remain a cobbler in order to produce fine work. And each of the others, too, was to work all his life at a single trade for which he had a natural aptitude and keep away from all the others, so as not to miss the right moment to practice his own work well.[43]

Despite superficial resemblances, Plato's conception of the allocation of functions in a city is fundamentally different from Adam Smith's notion of a division of labor. The assumption that a craftsman should work "all his life" at a single task and be prevented from attempting any other line of productive work is starkly incompatible with the "system of natural liberty" Smith championed and from the market principles most economists have favored from Smith's time onward.[44] Unlike Smith and many other modern thinkers, Plato appears to have believed that people are born with dramatically and unalterably diverse capabilities. For him it followed that a well-ordered society would compel its inhabitants to cultivate their distinctive capabilities and prevent them from wasting their efforts on pursuits to which they are not suited. This vision of society allows little room for individual choice or for social relations based on individual consent, and although it is clear that Plato recognizes a need for consensual market and social relations to have some place in such a society, it is equally clear that these relations are far from the center of his interest.[45] What matters is that individuals be directed to the tasks to which they are best suited, a direction that can best be accomplished by those few members of society who possess wisdom.

As events unfolded, however, it eventually came to seem that Plato was attempting to hold back an unstoppable tide. It is striking that Aristotle, lecturing soon after Plato's death and after having studied for a time at Plato's Academy, places enormous emphasis on social relations that are based on individual consent, relations that Plato had been inclined either to condemn or to ignore. Aristotle's account of justice is rooted in the idea of an association that is held together by repeated exchanges of goods and services among free and independent producers and consumers.[46] He takes it for granted that the innumerable transactions that take place in such an association will be consensual. Aristotle displays great interest in individual choice and responsibility as well as in the attributes that make an action voluntary or involuntary, reaching the conclusion (among others) that while ignorance about matters of fact may make an action involuntary, ignorance about what makes an action right or wrong makes an action simply wicked. Taking up the question whether it is possible for a person voluntarily to consent to unjust treatment, Aristotle concludes that no one can consent to be the recipient of injustice.[47] In short, the differences between Aristotle on the one hand and Plato and the earliest Greek writers on the other with regard to consent are dramatic. For Aristotle, the bonds that hold the political association together are forged through free economic exchanges and other consensual social relations. Aristotle certainly does not deny the importance of kinship groups, but in his ethical and political philosophy, he considers consensual transactions to be at least as important as a source of entitlements and obligations as kinship ties.

Emphasis on consensual transactions was similarly prominent in Roman thought. Although the modern, popular image of Rome highlights the militaristic characteristics of Roman society, ancient Rome was also a flourishing commercial center and the seat of developments in the law of contract that were of great significance both to Roman society and to many later societies in which Roman private law was revived. Contracts in Roman law can be divided into two main categories, formal and informal. The formal contract of *stipulatio* was made orally, not in writing, and was concluded by question and answer in which the formal terms had to correspond with one another precisely. As long as precise correspondence was achieved between the statements of the promisee and the promisor, a contract was created by those statements and a binding and enforceable obligation on the promisor came into being. If the correspondence between statements was not precise, then the putative contact was null and void. No legal restriction limited the possible content of this kind of contract, except that an illegal or immoral promise would be unenforceable. *Stipulatio* was therefore an extremely flexible form of contract that could give legal force to an agreement of any kind.

The principal exemplars of the other, informal type of contract are consensual contracts of sale, hire, partnership and the like. The essentials of these contracts were governed by preexisting law, which defined the range of matters that were subject to this type of contract. In an informal consensual contract of sale (*emptio venditio*), for example, the parties had only to identify the object to be sold and its price; the other terms of the contract were provided for by law.[48]

Although the formal contract of *stipulatio* was highly flexible, it had a number of disadvantages, including the fact that routine terms had to be spelled out and formally promised in each contract; that any discrepancy in the formal terms of the contract, however slight, between what the promisor and promisee said would nullify the contract; and that the parties had to meet in person (or have their agents meet in person) to commit themselves to the contract orally. These disadvantages were overcome in the consensual contract of sale, which was governed by standardized terms and was crucial to the development of commerce on a large scale and, more generally, to the development of a society in which it gradually became the norm for rights and obligations to be created and transferred via consensual transactions.

The differences between these two types of contract highlight a significant feature of the way in which consent has operated in western thought and practice. One of the central and perennial issues that arose once the transaction based on individual consent emerged as a major factor in the organization of human affairs concerns the range of matters that should be subject to this kind of transaction. At one end of a broad spectrum lies the view that all significant roles, obligations, and entitlements should fall onto individuals without regard to their consent, either by being ascribed to them by custom or by being assigned to them by law or by the wisest members of society (the last of these views, of course, is Plato's). At the opposite end we find the claim that all roles should be chosen by the individuals who fill them and all obligations assumed by consent of the individuals on whom they fall, insofar as it is possible to achieve this ideal.[49] The first view seeks to minimize the role of individual consent in human affairs, the latter claim to maximize it.

It is sometimes supposed that the role of consent will be maximized, and individual freedom protected, if individuals are free to reach agreements with one another about any matters and on any terms they choose. In terms that became familiar in the nineteenth century, the supposition is that a consent-based society must be one that allows complete freedom of contract subject only to the limitation that contracts to perform illegal actions will not be enforceable. In practice, however, this supposition is incorrect. The fact is that terms that are standardized by law and are therefore *not* subject to bargaining or negotiation by individual parties to an agreement often enable a society to attain a higher level of transactional activity than is possible when individuals are free to negotiate on any terms they choose. Standardized terms provide guarantees and efficiencies that commonly result in increases in the extent to which social relations are based on individual consent.

In antiquity, then, societies emerged in which individual consent played a large role in shaping social relations, and that role was reflected amply in the writings and legal systems of the ancients, especially the Greeks and Romans. It is nonetheless important to note that the role of consent in human affairs was limited sharply by the fact that many human beings were not regarded as capable of or entitled to give consent or to engage in consensual transactions. In all ancient societies that have contributed significantly to the history of western thought, women were regarded as less capable of consenting than men, and their rights to engage in consensual transactions were curtailed. All these ancient societies incorporated the institution of slavery in some form, and slaves were generally considered incapable of engaging in transactions requiring consent except when their owners authorized them to act as their agents, and even then only within limits. They were known to be human beings, but were not recognized as persons, either legally or socially. Many other forms of subordinate status that resulted in diminution or deprivation of the legal capacity to engage in consensual transactions existed. Ancient societies developed robust systems of social relations based on individual consent, but only for those—usually a relative few—who were accorded the highest status and the most extensive rights.

The Romans' conquest of extensive territories helped to ensure the wide dissemination of the norms and legal provisions that underpinned the Roman system of economic and social relations based largely on consensual transactions among individuals. After the collapse of the Western Empire in the fifth century, however, that system entered a lengthy period of gradual decline. While Roman law never vanished from Europe entirely, it was gradually integrated into and adapted to the provisions of the customary laws of the Visigoths, the Franks, and other "barbarians."[50] In comparison with assumptions that were widespread in Greek and Roman thought, these barbarian laws and practices reflected diminished confidence in the capacities of human beings to understand the world and to make informed, rational decisions within it. Reliance on consensual private transactions as a means of maintaining order in the social world accordingly declined.

One development that illustrates the diminished importance of individual consent in medieval thought is the emergence of the concept of a just price. As we have seen, in Rome the consensual contract of sale (*emptio venditio*) became standardized to a point at which it was necessary for the parties to a sale to determine only the object to be sold and its price. If the parties involved in a sale wanted to reach an agreement on terms other than those provided in the *emptio venditio*, they could always turn to the formal contract of *stipulatio*, which would allow them to reach an agreement on any terms they might choose. In medieval legal practice the *stipulatio* disappeared. Indeed, many transactions of sale took place under conditions in which the price was determined by custom with little room for accommodation of the wills of the parties involved. It is true that the emergence and persistence of a customary practice was generally regarded as a reliable sign that the practice in question commanded the assent of those who engaged in it, and the practice of exchanging goods at a customary price was no different in this regard from any other customary practice. But the consent that was thought to stand behind the concept of a just price was a generalized, diffuse, and usually intergenerational notion, not the individualized consent that is more characteristic of a commercial society. Attempts to exchange goods on terms that deviated from that price were commonly deemed to be instances of wrongdoing.[51]

This and many other medieval practices–the use of the ordeal to settle legal disputes, which was widespread throughout much of the territory now known as Europe from about 800 to about 1200 is another prominent example[52]– reflected a sense of the impotence of human beings in the face of a world whose order and workings appeared knowable only to God. As early as the late tenth century, however, we can detect some early signs of a gradual recovery of confidence in the capacities of humans to understand and to bring order to their world. At least two intellectual factors contributed to this resurgence: the recovery of Greek philosophy and the study of Roman law. At the outset of the Middle Ages Boethius (c. 480–524) had conceived the ambition to present Greek learning to a Latin world that had come very much under siege. Boethius achieved only a small part of his aim, but he did succeed in making available in Latin the main outlines of Aristotle's system of logic. Some five centuries after Boethius' birth, the scholar Gerbert, who settled in Rheims in 972, began lecturing systematically on Boethius' logical treatises, and from Gerbert's time until the early twelfth century Boethius was the conduit through whom scholars became acquainted with Aristotle's logical thought. About the same time scholars and practitioners were moving to develop a uniform system of canon law, and they repeatedly turned for guidance to the study of Roman law, which provided many of the methods that became standard in the work of the canonists. The impacts of Aristotelian logic and Roman law converged to demonstrate that it is possible through human devices to discern and to impose order on a world that otherwise appeared chaotic to human eyes. The basis had been laid for a renewal of confidence in the powers of the human mind—and in individual consent as an agency through which it is possible to achieve order in human affairs.[53]

The effects of this renewal of confidence were apparent in numerous steps, small and large, over the next several centuries. In 1215, for example, the Lateran Council forbade priests to take part in the administration of the ordeal, effectively undercutting the practice and forcing those involved in legal proceedings to turn from the apparent certainties of divine judgment to the probabilities that can be arrived at by human agency. The shift in values that resulted was crystallized three centuries later in the writings of the Protestant reformers, especially Martin Luther.[54] In contrast to the prevailing teachings and practices of the Catholic Church, Luther rejected the most expansive claims of clerical authority and insisted that Christianity is primarily a matter of faith based on a direct relationship between the individual and God. Luther, of course, was a believer in the power of human faith, not human reason. He had no greater interest in the niceties of Aristotelian logic or the orderliness of Roman law than his antagonists. Yet he inherited from these traditions of thought an expansive confidence in the capacities of human individuals to ascertain truth. His principal difference with Catholic orthodoxy lay in his insistence that each individual Christian should grasp and believe in the truth of Christianity rather than trusting to intermediaries for spiritual guidance.

Luther's thinking led to the notion that nothing can be more important to a person than freedom of conscience and, by extension, the freedom to shape his or her own life in accordance with his or her beliefs. To him, of course, it was imperative that those beliefs be the one and only true ones, and he was confident that Christians would arrive at these true beliefs if only they were allowed to free themselves from the corrupting influences of common clerical practices. The course of the Reformation over the next century or more undercut the faith of Luther's successors in the unifying tendencies of unchained Christian faith. But his insistence on the importance of individual conscience was taken up by innumerable disciples and spread throughout Europe, signaling an enormous shift in values and priorities and heralding an era in which social relations were transformed by a newly acquired sense of the importance and, indeed, the sanctity of individual consent.

This revival of the idea of individual consent as a basis for social relations was accompanied by a major transformation in the way in which that idea was applied. In antiquity, the role of individual consent in human affairs was limited by the fact that many human beings were excluded from the right to give consent. In practice, most of the bases for exclusion that were in effect in the ancient world remained in force in the early modern era. Yet the early modern revival of individual consent took place in an ideological context that differed dramatically from the circumstances of antiquity. Europe was overwhelmingly Christian, and Christianity had from the outset adopted a universalistic stance toward human beings. Indeed, Christian doctrine is designed to appeal especially to the poor, the weak, and the downtrodden—that is, to those who were least likely to be considered entitled to give consent. The early modern revival of faith in individual consent as a means for the coordination of human actions was accompanied by a strong universalizing tendency that ultimately placed the burden of proof on those who would deny to some human beings the right to engage in consensual transactions and relationships.

A Consent-Based Ideal

The stage had now been set for the emergence of the idea that in an ideal society, all or virtually all entitlements and obligations, including those to which the members of society are subject by law, would arise out of the wills of individuals through agreements to which all had consented freely. No one in early modern Europe developed this idea further than Hobbes, despite his penchant for political absolutism and his attachment to the hierarchical structure of society that was familiar to him in England in the seventeenth century. As we have seen previously, Hobbes maintained that the only thing that can give political authority legitimacy is the consent of the governed. This idea had a long pedigree, extending back to the ancient Israelites, Greeks, and Romans. Unlike most earlier writers who had endorsed it, however, Hobbes insisted that the consent in question must be given by each member of the political association as an individual. His reasoning was based in part on the premise that human beings are natural equals. "The inequality that now is," he says, "has been introduced by the laws civil."[55] Inequality is a product of human conventions and institutions, not a fact of nature. It seemed to Hobbes to follow that no one is entitled to speak for anyone else without the latter's consent or authorization. Moreover, Hobbes extended the idea that individual consent is at the basis of all obligations into areas of social relations to which few others have applied it. It is commonly assumed, even by those who endorse a consent-based vision of society, that at least a few types of obligations, such as those children are supposed to have toward their parents, are rooted in natural facts rather than in consent. But in Hobbes's view, both the entitlement of a parent to govern his or her child's affairs and the obligation of the child to obey the parent are products of consent:

> The right of dominion . . . which the parent hath over his children . . . is not so derived from the generation, as if therefore the parent had dominion over his child because he begat him; but from the child's consent, either express, or by other sufficient arguments declared.[56]

All these observations must be tempered by acknowledgment of the fact that Hobbes accepted coerced consent as a valid form of individual consent. Still, Hobbes's radically individualistic conception of political and social relations provided a new kind of foundation on which more liberal arguments about the bases of obligations and entitlements could be built.

Space permits us to touch on only a few high points in the development of the consent-based ideal of society. Among theorists of social relations, no advocate of this ideal was more eloquent than Adam Smith. Smith argued with great clarity that human beings are essentially one another's equals:

> The difference of natural talents in different men is, in reality, much less than we are aware of; and the very different genius which appears to distinguish men of different professions, when grown up to maturity, is not upon many occasions so much the cause, as the effect of the division of labor. The difference between the most dissimilar characters, between a philosopher and a common street porter, for example, seems to arise not so much from nature, as from habit, custom, and education.[57]

Like Hobbes, Smith drew from this observation the conclusion that individual men[58] are like independent proprietors, each entitled to speak for himself and each capable of entering into contractual agreements on a basis of equality with others. Unlike Hobbes, however, Smith was loath to accept the view that human beings had by consent accepted conventions and institutions that divided them into social ranks of super- and subordinates. That view points toward a society based on relations of domination and submission, command and obedience, even as that society is legitimated by the idea that it is rooted in consent given by equal individuals. For Smith, the independence that belongs to human beings by nature ought to permeate their social relations as well, so that each would regard his fellows as equal and independent proprietors entitled to bestow or to withhold consent to any proposed agreement at will. He praised the spread of commerce and manu-facturing in part because he believed that it had helped to bring about

> the liberty and security of individuals, among the inhabitants of the country, who had before lived almost in a continual state of war with their neighbors, and of servile dependency upon their superiors.[59]

Hobbes had articulated a vision of a society that is legitimated on the ground of individual consent. Smith put flesh on this skeletal vision by insisting that the actual social relations in a laudable society be dominated by agreements among independent and freely consenting human beings rather than by hierarchies of domination and subordination.

Among writers who focus on the characteristics of persons as distinct from the social relations of a consent-based society, Immanuel Kant and John Stuart Mill are arguably the most significant. Writing at about the same time as Smith and drawing considerable inspiration from the works of Jean-Jacques Rousseau, Kant supposed that human beings possess two attributes, free will and rationality, and that these two attributes constitute our highest nature. On this basis Kant constructed a moral theory and a theory of justice. The primary subject of his moral theory is what he calls inner freedom, while external freedom is the primary subject of his theory of justice. For Kant, human beings achieve inner freedom insofar as their aims are in conformity with what he calls the categorical imperative, a moral principle that can be expressed, among other ways, by the principle of universal law: "Act only on that maxim through which you can at the same time will that it should become a universal law."[60] Human beings achieve external freedom insofar as they act within a framework of external restrictions—laws and rules—that are based on this same principle and that they endorse freely.

For Kant, there is no higher attainment in human affairs than freedom. An individual is free only when he or she consents to his or her relations with others. The opposite of freely given consent is compulsion. These notions underpin Kant's conceptions of political freedom (the freedom to play a role in political decisions by voting) and civil freedom (the freedom to pursue whatever ends one chooses as long as one's actions do not infringe the liberty of others to do likewise).[61] Another term for Kant's notion of the highest attainment in human life is autonomy, by which Kant means self-direction in accordance with the moral law.

Unlike the theories of Hobbes and Smith, Kant's theory incorporates and draws attention to the notion that freedom is an attainment—not only in the sense that institutions may or may not protect freedom, but also in the sense that individuals may to a greater or lesser extent attain the personal attributes that are necessary to be free. Some individuals may be highly autonomous, others only potentially so. This notion creates a large theoretical space between a conception of persons as they would be if they were fully rational and autonomous and a conception of people as they actually happen to be. And within that space in Kant's theory, we can find a gap between the concept of rational consent and the concept of empirical consent. In short, while Kant's theory stipulates that in principle all obligations should arise out of the wills of individuals through agreements to which all have consented freely, in practice the kind of consent Kant seems to have in mind is that which would be given by a fully rational, fully autonomous person rather than the kind of consent that is likely to be forthcoming from real, imperfectly rational human beings. Kant's vision of society is based on an idealized and hypothetical kind of consent, not on the real consent that may or may not be forthcoming from flesh-and-blood human beings.

Like Kant and indeed like many other thinkers who were products of the Enlightenment, John Stuart Mill took a great deal of interest in the perfectibility of human beings. Yet Mill developed a consent-based vision of society that was not contingent on attainment of that perfection. Mill contended that a good society will permit and encourage its members to make the important choices and decisions that shape their lives without waiting for them to develop into fully rational, autonomous persons, because it is only by exercising their capacity to make choices that human beings develop the attributes of autonomous persons.

> He who lets the world, or his own portion of it, choose his plan of life for him, has no need of any other faculty than the ape-like one of imitation. He who chooses his plan for himself, employs all his faculties . . . It really is of importance, not only what men do, but also what manner of men they are that do it. Among the works of man, which human life is rightly employed in perfecting and beautifying, the first in importance surely is man himself.[62]

The conclusion of this line of reasoning is Mill's famous "harm principle," namely

> That the sole end for which mankind are warranted, individually or collectively, in interfering with the liberty of action of any of their number, is self-protection. That the only purpose for which power can be rightfully exercised over any member of a civilized community, against his will, is to prevent harm to others. His own good, either physical or moral, is not a sufficient warrant.[63]

Mill's harm principle can rightly be regarded as the apotheosis of the idea that all entitlements and obligations should stem from the wills of individuals as expressed by their freely given consent.[64] His vision of society is as diametrically opposed to Plato's conception of a rightly ordered political association as anything we can imagine. Where Plato believed that human beings should be assigned all their important tasks and roles so that each will do that to which he is best suited as skillfully and as productively as possible, Mill argued that all human beings who have attained maturity (and who enjoy the good fortune of living in a relatively developed society) should make all the decisions that will affect their lives in important ways for themselves. Where Plato was an adamant opponent of the idea that government is legitimated by consent and an advocate of the view that the primary purpose of the political association is to instruct its members about their responsibilities and, for those who are capable of learning, about the relations of reciprocal domination and submission Plato deemed to be just, Mill was one of the principal architects of the modern theory of government by consent.[65] No thinker in the history of moral and political thought better represents the opposition to the ideas of government based on consent and social relations based on the freely given consent of individuals than Plato. Similarly, no thinker more faithfully represents the advocates for these ideas than Mill.

The publication of *On Liberty* in 1859 represents the high water mark of a movement that had originated many hundreds of years earlier, a movement that led western thought from a low estimate of the efficacy of human actions in the world and a low regard for the value of social relations based on individual consent to a vision of society in which virtually all such relations would stem from the wills of individuals through consensual agreements. Viewed retrospectively, it is easy to suppose that this movement was driven by inexorable forces, and many thinkers in the nineteenth and twentieth centuries, arguably including Mill, reached just this conclusion. Sir Henry Maine's observation, published just 2 years after *On Liberty*, that the entire history of the world's societies can be viewed as a long progression from status to contract is typical of the thinking of the period.[66] Indeed, a century and a half after Mill's work appeared, we remain within a long historical moment in which, in western societies, the notion that individuals should be subject only to those obligations to which they have freely given their consent retains enormous power, power that continues to be apparent in the resolutions of innumerable legal and social issues.

It is not clear how long this moment will last, nor how far we should want it to do so. On the one hand, no serious alternative to government by consent exists. Even those who share Plato's view that it would be best in principle if the few among us who are genuinely wise could subject the rest to their rule without the need for consent can appreciate the force of Lord Acton's famous observation that "power tends to corrupt and absolute power corrupts absolutely."[67] Governments that rule by consent are more attentive to the interests of the governed than governments that hold power by other means. We have reason to wish that the era of government by consent of the governed will last through the ages.

On the other hand, the case for the view that individual consent should be the only or nearly the only basis for individual obligations is not so evident. For one thing, some kinds of obligations can be squared with this principle only by straining credibility. Despite Hobbes's exceptional effort to reconcile the relations between children and their parents with his vision of a society in which individual consent is the basis of all social relations, it does not seem plausible to claim that a child's obligations toward his or her parents are the products of his or her consent to those parents' dominion. These obligations may not be "natural" in the strictest sense of the term, but they do not appear to result from an act of consent by the child, either.

A major argument for the view that all or nearly all entitlements and obligations should stem from the freely given consent of individuals rests on the claim that if people voluntarily consent to a transaction, then that transaction must be mutually advantageous. This argument is correct within its own narrow limits, but it neglects at least two important wider considerations. First, while a voluntary transaction may be advantageous to all those who are parties to it, such transactions are often disadvantageous to others, because many transactions impose what economists call externalities. Pollution is a prime example of a (costly or "negative") externality. A factory that discharges pollutants into water or air—all as a result of voluntary transactions among factory owners, workers, suppliers of raw materials, and purchasers of the commodities the factory produces—imposes costs on those affected by the pollutants, many of whom may have had no part in the transactions at all. Second, for the most part, only those who can offer something of value to others can themselves benefit from the obligations those others assume voluntarily. Usually, people are willing to take on obligations because they expect to receive something of benefit to themselves in return. Some people, however—the disabled, the very young, and the very old, for example—may have little of value they can offer to others. In a world in which obligations can arise only from the freely given consent of individuals, these people would generally be neglected, and many would probably die of deprivation.

The idea that all entitlements and obligations should stem from individual consent is rooted in a point of view that focuses on particularized transactions rather than the institutional and social contexts that determine what transactions are conceivable and feasible in a given historical place and time. There is much to be said for the claim that many important decisions, including decisions that result in the creation or reallocation of entitlements and obligations, should be made by the individuals who are likely to be most directly and significantly affected by those decisions, even when those decisions, taken collectively, can be expected to have major social consequences. Decentralization makes it possible to draw upon vast amounts of dispersed information as well as to take more fully into account individual values than centralized decision-making processes generally allow. Yet radically decentralized decision making—decision making devolved entirely to individuals acting as independent proprietors—is liable to result in a kind of social myopia in which the course of events is determined by people whose vision is confined to the narrow limits of their own lives and individual imaginations. Many desirable social objectives, including objectives that are beneficial to the members of a society as individuals, can be achieved, or even imagined, only through collective action put into motion by the power of societies taken as a whole— action that will from time to time result in the imposition of both obligations and entitlements that are not the results of acts of individual consent.

Notes

1. I should like to thank Alan Wertheimer, Frank Miller, Julian Franklin, Michael Ravvin, Wendy Johnston, Nadia Urbinati, Jean Cohen, Charles Beitz, Philip Pettit, James Zetzel, Daniel Lee, and Ira Katznelson for their many insightful comments and suggestions, reserving responsibility for the remaining faults in this chapter to myself.

2. For the etymology see Alfred Ernout and A. Meillet, *Dictionnaire etymologique de la langue latine, histoire des mots,* 4th ed., 2 vols., Paris, C. Klincksieck, 1959–1960, vol. 1:353.

3. Hugo Grotius, *The Rights of War and Peace,* ed. J. Barbeyrac, trans. Anon. (London, 1738). For a discussion see Richard Tuck, *Natural Rights Theories: Their Origin and Development* (Cambridge: Cambridge University Press, 1979), ch. 3.

4. Samuel Beer, "The Rule of the Wise and Holy: Hierarchy in the Thomistic System," *Political Theory* 14 (August 1986):391–422, at 391.

5. *Exodus* 19:5-6, in *The New English Bible: The Old Testament* (Cambridge: Oxford University Press and Cambridge University Press, 1970).

6. *Exodus* 19:8.

7. *Isaiah* 55:3, in *New English Bible: The Old Testament.*

8. *Isaiah* 62:5.

9. Plato, *Republic*, trans. G.M.A. Grube, rev. C.D.C. Reeve (Indianapolis: Hackett, 1992) 358e–359a.

10. Plato, *Republic* 540d–541a.

11. For a fuller discussion, see David Johnston, *A Brief History of Justice* (Oxford: Blackwell, 2010), ch. 2.

12. "If a constitution is to survive, all the elements of the state must join in willing its existence and its continuance." Aristotle, *Politics*, trans. Ernest Barker (Oxford: Clarendon Press, 1960), Book II, ch. 9, sec. 22 (1270b). See also passages at Book IV, ch. 9, sec. 10 (1294b), Book IV, ch. 12, sec. 1 (1296b), and Book V, ch. 9, sec. 5 (1309b).

13. Gaius, *Institutes of Roman Law*, with translation and commentary by Edward Post, 4th. ed. (London: Oxford University Press, 1925) I. 3.

14. In *The Digest of Justinian*, trans. ed. Alan Watson (Philadelphia: University of Pennsylvania Press, 1998), vol. 1, Book I, sec. 3.

15. See Charles Howard McIlwain, *Constitutionalism: Ancient and Modern*, rev. ed. (Ithaca, NY: Cornell University Press, 1947):44.

16. For discussion, see Herbert A. Deane, *The Political and Social Ideas of St. Augustine* (New York and London: Columbia University Press, 1963), ch. 4.

17. St. Thomas Aquinas, *On Princely Government*, in *Aquinas: Selected Political Writings*, trans. J. G. Dawson, ed. A. P. D'Entrèves (Oxford: Blackwell, 1974):3–83.

18. Duns Scotus, *Opus Oxeniense* in *Opera Omnia* (Paris: L. Vives, 1891–1895), 18:266, trans. by Brian Tierney in "Hierarchy, Consent, and the 'Western Tradition,'" *Political Theory* 15 (November 1987):649.

19. Herveus Natalis, *De Iurisdictione*, ed. L. Hödl (Munich: M. Hueber, 1959):15–16.

20. To be sure, Marsilius does discuss the qualities rulers should possess. But he insists that it is election, not personal qualities as such, that confers legitimacy. See Marsilius of Padua, *Defensor Pacis*, trans. Alan Gewirth (Toronto: University of Toronto Press, 1980), Discourse I, ch. 14.

21. *The Treatise on the Laws and Customs of the Realm of England Commonly Called Glanvill*, ed. and trans. G. D. G. Hall (Oxford: Clarendon Press, 1993).

22. Henry de Bracton, *Bracton on the Laws and Customs of England*, trans. Samuel E. Thorne (Cambridge, MA: Harvard University Press in association with the Selden Society, 1977), vol. 2:21.

23. For a detailed and nuanced discussion of this point up to the time of Edward I, see Gaines Post, *Studies in Medieval Legal Thought: Public Law and the State, 1100–1322* (Princeton: Princeton University Press, 1964), chs. 3 and 4.

24. Wentworth and Coke are quoted in McIlwain, *Constitutionalism*:114–115.

25. Thomas Hobbes, *Leviathan*, ed. Richard Flathman and David Johnston (New York: Norton, 1997), Review and Conclusion:255 (emphasis added).

26. Hobbes, *Leviathan*, ch. 17:95.

27. John Locke, *The Second Treatise of Government*, in *Political Writings of John Locke*, ed. David Wootton (New York: Mentor Books, 1993) and Jean-Jacques Rousseau, *On the Social Contract*, in *The Basic Political Writings*, trans. Donald A. Cress (Indianapolis: Hackett, 1987). For an excellent discussion of the development of the idea of popular sovereignty in the English-speaking world, see Edmund S. Morgan, *Inventing the People: The Rise of Popular Sovereignty in England and America* (New York and London: Norton, 1988).

28. See generally Tuck, *Natural Rights Theories.*

29. One of the most prominent dissenters is David Hume, who argues that political obligations are "natural" in the same sense as familial obligations and that almost "all the governments which exist . . . have been founded originally either on usurpation or conquest or both, without any pretence of a fair consent or voluntary subjection of the people." See "Of the Original Contract" in *Hume's Moral and Political Philosophy*, ed. Henry D. Aiken (New York: Hafner Press, 1948):356–372, at 362.

30. *Genesis* 3:1-19, in *New English Bible: The Old Testament.*

31. *Genesis* 17.

32. *Exodus* 19:5–8 (cited above, p. 27).

33. *Genesis* 12:10–20.

34. *Genesis* 29.

35. Homer, *The Iliad*, trans. Robert Fitzgerald (Garden City, NY: Doubleday, 1974).

36. *Genesis* 18:16–33, 19:1–29.

37. *Ezekiel* 18:2, 19–20, in *New English Bible: The Old Testament.*

38. Quoted by Arthur W. H. Adkins, *Merit and Responsibility: A Study in Greek Values* (Oxford: Oxford University Press, 1960):78.

39. Aristotle, *Nicomachean Ethics*, trans. Martin Ostwald (Indianapolis: Bobbs-Merrill, 1962), Book V, ch. 1 (1129b29).

40. See the discussion in Adkins, *Merit and Responsibility*, ch. 4.

41. Plato, *Republic* 561c–e.

42. Plato, *Republic* 370a–c.

43. Plato, *Republic* 374b–c.

44. Adam Smith, *An Inquiry into the Nature and Causes of the Wealth of Nations*, ed. Edwin Cannan (New York: Random House [Modern Library], 1937), esp. Book I chs. 7, 10 and Book II ch. 2.

45. See Plato, *Republic* 425c–e.

46. Aristotle, *Nicomachean Ethics*, Book V, ch. 5 (1132b20–1134a16). For a discussion see David Johnston, *A Brief History of Justice*, ch. 3.

47. Aristotle, *Nicomachean Ethics*, Book III ch. 1 (1110b30–35) and Book V ch. 9 (1136a10–1136b14).

48. For a brief discussion, see David Johnston, *Roman Law in Context* (Cambridge: Cambridge University Press, 1999), ch. 5, sec. 1.

49. For classic statements see John Stuart Mill, *On Liberty*, ed. David Spitz (New York: Norton, 1975)(discussed below) and Herbert Spencer, *The Principles of Ethics*, 2 vols. (London, 1891). For a more recent statement, see Joseph Raz, *The Morality of Freedom* (Oxford: Oxford University Press, 1986).

50. See the brief but valuable account in Paul Vinogradoff, *Roman Law in Medieval Europe*, 2nd ed. (Oxford: Clarendon Press, 1929).

51. See Aquinas' discussion in *Summa Theologica* II-II, Question 77, Article 1, in *The Political Ideas of St. Thomas Aquinas*, ed. Dino Bigongiari (New York: Hafner, 1953):143–146.

52. For an excellent succinct discussion, see Robert Bartless, *Trial by Fire and Water: The Medieval Judicial Ordeal* (Oxford: Clarendon Press, 1986).

53. For a superb discussion of these themes in this period, see R. W. Southern, *The Making of the Middle Ages* (New Haven and London: Yale University Press, 1953), esp. ch. 4.

54. For a selection of Luther's writings in English translation, see *The Protestant Reformation*, ed. Hans J. Hillerbrand (New York: Harper & Row, 1968), Part I.

55. Hobbes, *Leviathan* ch. 15:84.

56. Hobbes, *Leviathan* ch. 20:110.

57. Smith, *Wealth of Nations* Book I, ch. 2:15.

58. Note, however, that unlike Hobbes, Smith did *not* make it clear that he regarded women as equally entitled to speak for themselves.

59. Smith, *Wealth of Nations* Book III, ch. 4:385.

60. Immanuel Kant, *Groundwork of the Metaphysics of Morals*, trans. H. J. Paton (New York: Harper & Row, 1964):88.

61. For a clear and cogent discussion, see Allen D. Rosen, *Kant's Theory of Justice* (Ithaca and London: Cornell University Press, 1993).

62. Mill, *On Liberty*:56.

63. Mill, *On Liberty*:10-11. Notoriously, Mill hastens to add that the harm principle does not apply to "those backward states of society in which the race itself may be considered as in its nonage."

64. Herbert Spencer's *Principles of Ethics* is an equally worthy candidate for this label.

65. Through his *Considerations on Representative Government* (Buffalo, NY: Prometheus Books, 1991).

66. Sir Henry Sumner Maine, *Ancient Law* (1861; reprint, Dorset Press, 1986).

67. Credited to Acton in a letter to Bishop Mandell Creighton of April 5, 1887 in *Bartlett's Familiar Quotations*, ed. John Bartlett, 14th ed. (Boston and Toronto: Little, Brown, 1968):750.

3

Autonomy and Consent

Tom L. Beauchamp

In biomedical ethics the language of "consent" has been framed almost entirely as "*informed* consent." This has had the effect of skewing our understanding of consent toward providing information and being informed. In law, this conception has carried an emphasis on the supreme importance of disclosure of information to patients and subjects. However, disclosure is not a necessary condition of informed consent and is only remotely connected to consent per se. An undue emphasis on disclosure and its intended target, understanding by patients and subjects, has led to the relative neglect of "voluntary consent." Voluntariness is almost certainly the most neglected dimension of consent in contexts of medical practice and research.

I will argue that autonomous choice and voluntariness are central to the notion of consent. I start by analyzing consent in terms of its normative features, its basic elements, and its senses. I then move to the nature of consent as autonomous and discuss whether requirements to obtain informed consent are justified in terms of the principle of respect for autonomy. I then turn to theories of autonomy, starting with split-level theories. I propose a different theory of autonomy, which features conditions of intentionality, understanding, and voluntariness. This theory is used to develop an account of degrees of autonomy. Finally, I consider the problem of constraining situations, which presents moral issues of undue influence and of the exploitation of research subjects.

I. Normative and Non-Normative Concepts of Consent

"Consent," "the obligation to obtain consent," and "the right to consent" are strikingly different notions. Likewise, "autonomy," "respect for autonomy," and "rights of autonomy" should be distinguished. "The obligation to obtain consent" and "the right to consent" as well as "respect for autonomy" and "rights of autonomy" are moral notions, but "autonomy" and "consent" are not obviously moral notions. It seems a matter of fact (or perhaps of metaphysics or the philosophy of mind), not a matter of ethics or value, whether one acts autonomously or consents.

This distinction between the factual and the moral is vital, but it may foster precarious claims such as: (1) analysis of consent and autonomy are conceptual and empirical tasks, not moral ones; and (2) a theory of consent and a theory of autonomy should not be grounded in moral notions, but on a theory of mind, self, or person. I will assess these claims with the objective of determining the nature of consent and autonomy. I will also examine what constitutes a consent, what sort of consent is valid, who qualifies as autonomous, and what sort of autonomy merits respect. I will argue that moral notions—in particular, the obligation to obtain consent and the obligation to respect autonomy—should affect how we construct theories of consent, theories of autonomous action, and theories of the autonomous person. At the same time, theories of consent and autonomy should not be understood as moral theories only; they require inquiry into the nature of mind and action.

II. The Elements of Informed Consent

A widely acknowledged approach to informed consent is analysis of the concept in terms of its basic elements, the most generic of which are *information* and *consent*. The information component refers to the disclosure of information and to the comprehension of what is disclosed. The consent component refers to a voluntary decision and an authorization to proceed. Legal, regulatory, philosophical, medical, and psychological literatures often propose the following five elements as the analytical components of these two generic units of informed consent[1]: (1) competence, (2) disclosure, (3) understanding, (4) voluntariness, and (5) consent. Some writers present these elements as the building blocks of a definition of *informed consent.* One gives an informed consent to an intervention if (and perhaps only if, but this claim is questionable) one is competent to act, receives a thorough disclosure, comprehends the disclosure, chooses voluntarily, and consents to the intervention.

I will accept these elements (though not the proposed definition) and pare them down in three respects. First, competence is a threshold element, precondition, or presupposition of informed consent. It is not part of the process of informed consent. Second, disclosure is not a necessary condition of informed consent. If a patient or subject already possesses the relevant information, a disclosure is not needed to give an informed consent. Disclosure has had a prominent position in the literature of informed consent because informed consent has its roots in contexts of legal liability for nondisclosure, but the important matter for understanding informed consent is having the relevant information. Third, I said earlier that "the consent component refers to a voluntary decision and an authorization to proceed." The language of "consent" covers both a *decision in favor* of a proposed course of action and an *authorization*. Authorization is a permission-giving act. It could be performed even if the consent were not informed. Accordingly, informed consent cannot be reduced entirely to permission giving.

In summary, the notion of informed consent should be chiefly understood in terms of central elements of understanding, voluntariness, and consent. Consent itself should be analyzed in terms of a favorable decision and an authorization. I will hereafter emphasize these elements, saying little about disclosure and competence.

III. Two Senses of "Informed Consent"[2]

Two different meanings of "informed consent" appear in current literature and contexts of medical practice and research. The distinction is critical for the argument developed in this chapter.

In the first sense, the notion of autonomous choice is central: An informed consent is an individual's *autonomous authorization* of a medical intervention or of participation in research. A person must do more than express agreement or comply with a proposal. He or she must *authorize* through an act of informed and voluntary consent. An informed consent occurs if and only if a patient or subject, with substantial understanding, and in the absence of substantial control by others, intentionally authorizes a professional to do something. This definition is preferable to the definition formulated in terms of *elements* in the previous section.

In the second sense, informed consent is analyzable in terms of *the social rules of consent* that determine legally or institutionally valid consent. Informed consents are not necessarily autonomous acts. Informed consent, in this sense, refers to an institutionally or legally effective authorization, as determined by prevailing social rules. For example, if a mature minor cannot *legally* authorize or consent to a medical procedure, he or she still may *autonomously* authorize the procedure. Thus, a patient or subject can autonomously authorize an intervention, and so give an informed consent in the first sense, without effectively authorizing the intervention, and thus without giving an informed consent in the second sense.

Institutional rules of informed consent (the second sense) often have not been judged by the more demanding standard of autonomous authorization (the first sense). As a result, institutions, laws, or courts may impose on physicians and hospitals nothing more than an obligation to disclose risks of proposed interventions and receive a signed consent form. "Consent" under these circumstances is not bona fide informed consent in the first sense.[3] Physicians who obtain consent under institutional criteria can fail— and often do fail—to meet the more rigorous standards of an autonomy-based model.

It is easy to criticize institutional rules as superficial, but it would be unreasonable to demand that health care professionals always obtain a consent that satisfies the demands of rigorous autonomy-protecting rules. Autonomy-protective standards may turn out to be excessively difficult or impossible to implement. We should evaluate institutional rules not only in terms of whether they lead to truly autonomous choices but also in terms of the probable consequences of imposing burdensome requirements on institutions and professionals. Policies of consent may legitimately take account of what is fair and reasonable to require in circumstances of practice. Nevertheless, I take it as axiomatic that the model of autonomous choice, following the first sense of "informed consent," ought to serve as the benchmark for the moral adequacy of institutional rules.

IV. Autonomy at the Foundation

But why should autonomy occupy such a central place in the analysis of informed consent? Is there an adequate justification for the claim that rules of informed consent are ultimately justified in terms of the principle of respect for autonomous choice?

I approach this subject through the early history of concern about research subjects in U.S. federal policy, which is roughly datable to the 1960s. Consent requirements had previously been adopted as a means to the minimization of the potential for harm to research subjects. In the 1940s, the Nuremberg Code presented a forceful insistence on voluntary consent in research but had not distinguished clearly between appeals to autonomy and appeals to nonmaleficence ("do no harm") as the justificatory basis of consent requirements. The Nuremberg Code served as a background model for early professional and governmental codes and set the stage for the continued blurring of the justifications for consent in harm prevention or autonomy, or both. The blurry lines continued for roughly a quarter of a century as informed consent requirements and our understanding of them evolved.[4]

In the early 1970s this unclarity was altered in the course of work on 17 volumes of research ethics published by the National Commission for the Protection of Human Subjects. This commission stated emphatically that the purpose of consent provisions is the protection of autonomy and personal dignity, including the personal dignity of incompetent persons incapable of acting autonomously. As the commission's *Belmont Report* put it, the purpose and justification of consent provisions (by contrast to other provisions in research ethics) is autonomy for autonomous subjects and protection from harm only in a situation of incompetence when a surrogate's consent must be given.[5]

In recent years various complaints have arisen in bioethics about the undue prominence of justifications based on autonomy. Despite these concerns, the view taken by the National Commission has remained dominant, at least in North America, since circa 1980. This is not to say that the view is without ambiguities, or that it has not been subjected to influential and constructive criticism. A number of responsible critics of the overextension of autonomy have emerged in recent biomedical ethics. The most carefully stated objections have come from Onora O'Neill, who has argued explicitly against the view that informed consent protections are justified in terms of respect for personal autonomy.[6]

O'Neill is concerned that several different conceptions and theories of autonomy abound in the literature that finds informed consent to be justified in terms of autonomy. Accordingly, she finds what is to be protected confusing: "the general agreement that informed consent is required for the sake of autonomy, and that autonomy is a basic ethical value, is more apparent than real, since there is substantive and persistent disagreement both about conceptions of autonomy, and about their importance in biomedicine."[7]

She argues that a better reason for supporting rules and practices of consent is that these rules assure patients and others that they will not be *deceived* or *coerced* and thereby wronged. The practice of informed consent, she says, should function so that it "provides reasonable assurance that a patient (research subject, tissue donor) has not been deceived or coerced."[8] In a more general formulation focused on wrongdoing, she says, "Consent matters because it can be used to protect research subjects and patients against grave wrongs."[9] In another formulation, she says, "Consent is a way of ensuring that those subjected to invasive interventions are not abused, manipulated or undermined, or wronged in comparably serious ways."[10] For these reasons, rules and practices of consent should be designed to give patients and research subjects control over the information they receive and an opportunity to refuse to participate at any point after their initial consent.

O'Neill's views need to be placed in the context of the claims that have been made about autonomy in bioethics literature. Three points deserve notice. First, protection against coercion and deception has been and should be conceived as grounded in the principle of respect for autonomy. O'Neill is right that the theory of autonomy needs to be improved, but the same can be said about the literature on her preferred notions of protection against deception, manipulation, and coercion.

Second, rules of informed consent help patients and subjects improve their level of understanding and the quality of their decision making, which is a matter of fostering autonomous choice (in a properly conceived theory of autonomy). The rules also protect against forms of ignorance and the control of information that constitute offenses against the principle of respect for autonomy (see sections VII and IX later, where manipulation and coercion are discussed and connected to autonomous choice).

Third, O'Neill is worried that the notion of autonomy is too unclear to express adequately what we want to protect through practices of consent, but often she herself understands autonomy at such a high level of individuality and deliberative choice that protection of autonomy is virtually impossible in biomedical contexts. In her interpretation of the relevant literature on autonomy, she says, "The principal source for most conceptions of *rational autonomy* is . . . not Kant, but John Stuart Mill's *On Liberty*."[11] She is right that the connection to Mill is firmer than to Kant, but if Mill's theory of individuality is the model (as it often seems to be in O'Neill's writings), this model is not what autonomy has meant or should ever come to mean in the literature on either autonomy or informed consent. Mill's theory is too demanding for reasons I discuss in the next section.[12] Moreover, as O'Neill seems to acknowledge, an adequate account of autonomy joined with a theory of what is to be respected by the principle of autonomy would go a long way toward alleviating her concerns.

O'Neill notes that her "intention is not to deny [the] importance [of informed consent], . . . but to take it sufficiently seriously to identify some of its limitations as well as its strengths."[13] There are problems in our practices of consent, and O'Neill appropriately points to many of them. Nonetheless, her arguments do not displace protection of autonomous choice as the primary justification of rules and practices of informed consent. There remains little doubt that the protection of autonomous choice is fundamental to the justification of rules of informed consent, even if these rules serve other functions as well. (I engage O'Neill's concerns about unclarity in the concept of autonomy in sections V–VII, especially VII.)

V. Theories of Autonomy

Attention thus far has centered on informed consent and its relationship to autonomous choice. I will now focus entirely on the theory of autonomy. Just as I earlier analyzed informed consent in terms of its elements and its two senses, I will here treat autonomy in terms of its conditions and meanings.

Self-governance is the conceptual root of autonomy for virtually all theories of autonomy. Two basic conditions of autonomy, from this perspective, are *liberty* in the sense of independence from controlling influences and *agency* in the sense of intentional action. These conditions are essential to autonomy. However, after this consensus starting point, disagreement emerges over how to analyze these conditions and over whether additional conditions are needed.[14] I begin with a distinction that helps explain why there is some conceptual confusion and disagreement.

Autonomous Persons and Autonomous Actions

Some theories of autonomy feature traits of the *autonomous person*, whereas others focus on *autonomous action*. Theories of the autonomous person are theories of a kind of agent. In discussions of informed consent, the autonomous person is the competent person—that is, one who is competent to consent. The autonomous person is portrayed in some general theories as independent, in command, impervious to authoritarian control, and the source of his or her basic values and beliefs. My account of autonomy to follow will not focus on such traits of the person, but instead on actions—in particular, making decisions and authorizing interventions. Because of my focus on acts of consent, I will not discuss general capacities of self-governance. I will assume, rather than argue, that autonomous persons sometimes fail, in particular circumstances, to act autonomously because of temporary constraints caused by illness or depression, circumstantial ignorance, coercion, or other such restrictive conditions. An autonomous person who signs a consent form without understanding the document and without intending to agree to its conditions is qualified to act autonomously, but fails to do so in this particular case. Similarly, persons who have rightly been judged incompetent to control their general affairs may nonetheless make some adequately autonomous choices.

The Role of the Principle of Respect for Autonomy in a Theory of Autonomy

A theory of autonomy should be consistent with the nature of autonomy presumed in the normative principle of respect for autonomy—a principle forged from common moral experience rather than philosophical theory. This principle requires that we respect an autonomous agent's right to control his or her affairs in accordance with personal values and beliefs.

Some theories of autonomy—including the most influential contemporary theory, which I discuss in section VI—do not consider whether the principle of respect for autonomy has any connection to the theory of autonomy. They do not mention the principle or attempt to conform the theory to its contexts and uses. However, a theory that distinguishes nonautonomous acts from autonomous acts implicitly teaches which actions we are to respect, opening up the possibility of legitimately not respecting certain choices that are of the most penetrating importance to persons, on grounds that these choices are nonautonomous.

Any theory that classifies acts as nonautonomous when these acts are well understood, intentional, and not controlled by others is a conceptually dubious theory of autonomy. It would be especially dubious, and morally dangerous, if the acts deemed nonautonomous are of the greatest importance to us in the basic governance of our affairs. For example, a theory might consider the acts of generally competent persons to be nonautonomous when they decide to see a doctor, consent for an x-ray for their children, or refuse a surgical procedure. In rendering such actions nonautonomous, the theory implies that another person may legitimately serve as guardian and decision maker. As O'Neill has cautioned in her work, it is extremely important in practical contexts not to set standards of autonomy so high that we cannot live up to them. She rightly argues that such high standards will have the devastating effect of inappropriately classifying "a far larger proportion of the patient population as lacking competence."[15]

An instructive example of the moral perils that a theory of autonomy can pose is found in the work of Julian Savulescu on decisions to limit choices for or against life-sustaining treatments. Savulescu realizes that he must set out the conditions of autonomy in the right way to obtain morally justified outcomes. If he fails in this account, the choices of patients may be inappropriately limited or reversed. Savulescu distinguishes autonomous and non-autonomous acts through a distinction between *mere desires* and *rational desires*. Autonomous actions are performed from rational desires. Accordingly, health care professionals and guardians are only required to respect the actions of a patient that arise from rational desire. A merely *expressed desire* is insufficient. Savulescu argues that many choices—for example, a Jehovah's Witness's decision to refuse a blood transfusion—can and should be judged not rational, and therefore not autonomous and lacking in moral weight in a critical setting of medical decision making.[16]

Various theories of autonomy seem to support the proposition that a Jehovah's Witness is not acting autonomously on grounds that his or her beliefs are unreflective assumptions instilled by authoritarian dogma, or what Savulescu calls irrational desires. I agree that such an individual might not be acting autonomously, but the issue is whether we have a compelling reason to declare the person nonautonomous. The fact that a person adopts beliefs and principles deriving from forms of institutional authority is not a sufficient reason for a finding of inadequate autonomy. The beliefs can still be that person's most cherished beliefs and principles. Individuals autonomously form beliefs that derive from many forms of cultural tradition and institutional authority. If the Witness's decision can be legitimately invalidated on grounds that he or she is not acting autonomously, so may a great many choices be invalidated that are of central importance to persons. A theory of autonomy that conflicts with this assumption I hypothesize to be a morally unacceptable and conceptually problematic theory.

VI. Split-Level Theories of Autonomy[17]

Perhaps the most widely discussed type of theory of autonomy today is problematic in this way. I shall refer to these theories as split-level theories. They maintain that autonomy consists of the capacity to control and identify with one's first-order desires or preferences by means of higher-level (second-order) desires or preferences through processes of deliberation, reflection, or volition. Harry Frankfurt's theory of the freedom of persons and Gerald Dworkin's theory of autonomy are prominent examples of split-level theories.[18]

An autonomous person, in this theory, is one who has the capacity to accept, identify with, or repudiate a lower-order desire or preference, showing the capacity to change (or maintain) one's preference structure or one's configuration of the will. All and only autonomous persons possess an appropriately distanced self-reflection in which second-order mental states have first-order mental states as their intentional objects and in which considered preferences are formed about first-order preferences and beliefs. For example, a long-distance runner may have a first-order desire to run several hours a day, but also may have a higher-order desire to decrease the running time to 1 hour. If he wants, at any given moment, to run several hours, then he wants at that moment what he does not authentically want. Action from a first-order desire that is not endorsed by a second-order volition is not autonomous and is typical of animal behavior.

Frankfurt argues that it is essential to being a person that the second-order desires or volitions be such that the individual "wants a certain desire to be his will."[19] He calls these second-order desires or volitions "second-order volitions." Since they are essential to being a person, any individual lacking these volitions is not a person. Dworkin somewhat similarly offers a "content-free" definition of autonomy as a "second-order capacity of persons to reflect critically upon their first-order preferences, desires, wishes, and so forth and the capacity to accept or attempt to change these in the light of higher-order preferences and values."[20] The language of "capacity" suggests that the theory is one of autonomous persons rather than autonomous actions.

This theory is problematic. Nothing prevents a reflective acceptance, preference, or volition at the second level from being caused and assured by the strength of a first-order desire. The individual's second-level acceptance of, or identification with, the first-order desire would then be the causal result of an already formed structure of preferences. For example, the alcoholic with a passion for red wine who identifies with drinking is not acting autonomously if his second-level volition or desire to drink red wine is causally determined by a first-level desire. Suppose the alcoholic forms, as a result of the force of first-order desire, a second-order volition to satisfy his strongest first-order desire. We say about such a person that he "needs help," because he cannot help himself. An alcoholic can reflect at ever-higher levels on lower-level desires without achieving self-control over his choices if identification at all levels is causally determined by initial desires.[21] A split-level theory of autonomy needs the supplementary condition that there must be no influences or desires that rob an individual of voluntariness by controlling the choice, even if the person identifies with the choice and intends the action(s).[22] Intentional actions are not autonomous if they are controlled by causes the agent does not control.

Frankfurt argues that "truly autonomous choices" require "being satisfied with a certain desire" and having preexisting "stable volitional tendencies."[23]

However, this analysis does not rescue the split-level theory. Anomalous actions sometimes arise from choices that are out of character as a result of surrounding events that are unprecedented in the actor's experience, such as serious disease. These acts can be well planned, intentional, and free from the control of other persons. The actors may be unaware of the motivational or conditioning history that underlies and prompts their actions and may have made no reflective identification with the origins of their actions. This is no reason to declare such actions nonvoluntary or nonautonomous.

This theory also runs afoul of the criterion of coherence with the principle of respect for autonomy, as mentioned earlier. If reflective identification with one's desires or second-order volitions is a necessary condition of autonomous action, then many ordinary actions that are almost universally considered autonomous, such as cheating on one's spouse, when one truly wishes not to be such a person, or selecting tasty snack foods while grocery shopping, when one has never reflected on one's desires for snack foods), would be rendered *non*autonomous in this theory. Requiring reflective identification and stable volitional patterns unduly narrows the scope of actions protected by a principle of respect for autonomy.

Depending on how "reflection," "volition," and the like are analyzed in this theory in practical contexts of competence and consent, surprisingly few choosers and choices will turn out to be autonomous.[24] Agents will often not have reflected on whether they wish to accept or identify with the motivational structures that underlie such actions. Actors may be unaware of their motivational or conditioning histories. Actions such as walking while lecturing, lying to one's physician about what one eats, and hiding one's income from a government agency might, in this theory, turn out to be nonautonomous. If so, individuals who have not reflected on their desires and preferences at a higher level deserve no respect for their choices even when they derive from their most deep-seated commitments, desires, and preferences.[25]

VII. A Concise Theory of Autonomous Action

I now turn to an account of autonomous choice that I have defended elsewhere and that I believe to be compatible with the constraints on theory outlined thus far.[26] This account of autonomy is specifically designed to be coherent with the premise that the everyday choices of generally competent persons are autonomous. The account is based on analysis of autonomous action in terms of normal choosers who act (1) intentionally, (2) with understanding, and (3) without controlling influences.

The Condition of Intentionality

Intentional actions require plans in the form of representations of the series of events proposed for the execution of an action. For an act to be intentional, it must correspond to the actor's conception of the act in question, although a planned outcome might not materialize as projected.[27] Imagine that Professor X intends to read a paper that he has written on a toxic chemical, and intends thereby to win first prize at a convention. His paper is on toxic chemical A. Professor X's plan entails executing a sequence of actions, chief of which is a particular set of arguments about A that he believes will be well received by this audience. However, in preparing to travel to the convention, Professor X accidentally packs the wrong paper, which is on the subject of toxic chemical B. The professor is absent-minded and does not realize when he reads his paper at the convention that it is the wrong paper. Despite this lapse, he wins first prize for the best paper. Professor X in this way read a paper on a toxic chemical and won first prize, which he intended, yet Professor X did not do so intentionally in the way the action was performed. His action did not correspond to how he planned to do it. His reception by the audience and his winning the prize were, as it turns out, accidental.

In a theory of autonomy (and of informed consent), we need to decide whether special kinds of wants or desires are necessary conditions of intentional action. It might be thought that foreseen acts that the actor does not want and does not desire to perform are not intentional. Alvin Goldman uses the following example in an attempt to prove that agents do not intend merely foreseen effects.[28] Imagine that Mr. G takes a driver's test to prove competence. He comes to an intersection that requires a right turn and extends his arm to signal for a turn, although he knows it is raining and that he will get his hand wet. According to Goldman, Mr. G's signaling for a turn is an intentional act. By contrast, his wet hand is an unintended effect, or "incidental by-product," of his hand-signaling. However, as I see it, getting the hand wet *is* part of an intentional action. It is willed in accordance with a plan and is neither accidental, inadvertent, nor habitual. There is nothing about the nature of intentional acts, as opposed to accidental occurrences, that rules out aversions. One's motivation for getting one's hand wet may reflect *conflicting* wants and desires, and clearly the driver does not want a wet hand, but this fact does not render the act of getting the hand wet less than intentional or autonomous.

Some intentional acts are wanted or desired for their own sake, and not for the sake of something else. For example, someone who loves to swim may want to swim for the sake of swimming, as may not be the case for another person who swims for the sake of a tanned or fit body. The desire to perform an act for its own sake is *intrinsic* wanting. Wanting for the sake of something else is *instrumental* wanting. When a surgeon cuts into the body of the patient, the patient has consented to the cutting and the cutting is part of the plan, but it is for the sake of better function or health. In such cases, the actor believes the action is the means to a goal wanted in the primary sense. Goldman would only consider an act intentional if at least one of these two forms of wanting is involved.

However, other intentional acts are not wanted in either of these two senses. An actor may view these acts as *ceteris paribus*, altogether undesirable or unwanted. They are performed only because they are entailed in the doing of other acts that are wanted. Such acts are foreseen and wanted acts in the sense that the actor wants to perform them in the circumstances more than he or she wants not to perform them. It is suitable in the kinds of examples just discussed to discard the language of "wanting" and to say that foreseen but not desired effects are "tolerated."[29] These effects are not so undesirable that the actor would choose not to perform the act in the first place. The actor includes them as a part of his or her plan of intentional action.

Accordingly, I use a model of intentionality based on what is *willed* rather than what is *wanted*. Intentional actions include any action and any effect specifically willed in accordance with a plan, including merely tolerated effects.[30] In this conception a physician can desire not to do what he intends to do, in the same way that one can be willing to do something but reluctant to do it, or even detest doing it. Consider Mr. X, who has become convinced that there is no meaningful way that he can consent to facial surgery but refuse the scarring involved. After considering the alternative of refusing surgery, Mr. X intentionally consents to *surgery*, and in so doing he intentionally consents to *being scarred* by surgery. Although his consenting to a facial scar is a toleration of and not a desire for the scarring, the intentional act of consenting to the scarring is no less Mr. X's *own* act than is his consenting to surgery. Mr. X, then, intentionally consents to being scarred by surgery.

Under this conception, the distinction between what agents do intentionally and what they merely foresee in a planned action is not viable.[31] For example, if a man enters a room and flips a switch that he knows turns on both a light and a fan, but desires only to activate the light, he cannot say that he activates the fan unintentionally. Even if the fan made an obnoxious whirring sound that he does not want, it would be incorrect to state that he unintentionally brought about the obnoxious sound by flipping the switch. Here, and in the other examples mentioned previously, one might introduce a distinction between what an agent intends and an intentional action.

Perhaps the agent does not intend the effect of a screeching fan and does not intend it as the goal of his action even though it is an intentional action. Likewise, one might be said to intentionally consent to being scarred in surgery, while not intending to be scarred. In short, what it means for an act to be intentional need not be equated with what the agent of the action intends.

The Condition of Understanding

Understanding is the second condition of autonomous action. An action is not autonomous if the actor lacks an appropriate understanding of it. Here the first question to ask is, "Do you understand what you are doing?" At a minimum, persons understand only if they have acquired pertinent information and have relevant beliefs about the nature and consequences of their actions. Their understanding need not be *complete*, because a grasp of the *material* facts is generally sufficient, but in some cases a person's lack of awareness of even a single risk or missing fact can deprive him or her of adequate understanding.

There are several reasons why limited understanding can occur in a process of deliberative choice and consent. Some patients and subjects are calm, attentive, and eager for dialogue, whereas others are nervous or distracted in ways that impair or block understanding. Conditions that limit their understanding include illness, irrationality, and immaturity. Deficiencies in the communication process also often hamper understanding. A breakdown in a person's ability to accept information as true or untainted, even if he or she adequately comprehends the information, can compromise decision making. For example, a seriously ill patient who has been properly informed about the nature of the illness and has been asked to make a treatment decision might refuse under the false belief that he or she is not ill. Even if the physician recognizes the patient's false belief and adduces conclusive evidence to prove to the patient that the belief is mistaken, and the patient comprehends the information provided, the patient still may go on believing that what has been (truthfully) reported is false.

The so-called "therapeutic misconception" occurs when subjects in research fail to distinguish between clinical care and research and fail to understand the purpose and aim of research, misconceiving their participation as therapeutic in nature.[32] Such a therapeutic misconception may invalidate the subject's consent to research. Some participants understand that they are involved in research, and not clinical care, but overestimate the therapeutic possibilities and probabilities, that is, the odds that a participant will benefit.[33] This overestimation may render a choice insufficiently autonomous and invalidate a consent. However, a therapeutic misconception will not in every circumstance invalidate consent, for reasons Franklin Miller discusses elsewhere in this volume.

The Condition of Noncontrol, or Voluntariness

The third of the three conditions of autonomous action is that a person be free of controls exerted either by external sources or by internal states that rob the person of self-directedness. Influence and resistance to influence are basic concepts for this analysis. Not all influences exerted on another person are controlling. Many influences are resistible, and some are welcomed. The category of influence includes acts of love, threats, education, lies, manipulative suggestions, and emotional appeals, all of which can vary dramatically in their impact on persons. My analysis will focus on three categories of influence: persuasion, coercion, and manipulation.[34]

Persuasion is here understood as rational persuasion. A person comes to believe something through the merit of reasons another person advances. This is the paradigm of an influence that is not controlling and also warranted. If a physician presents reasons that persuade the patient to undergo a procedure when the patient is reluctant to do so, then the physician's actions influence, but do not control. In health care settings, there is often a problem of distinguishing emotional responses from cognitive responses and of determining whether the cognitive or the emotional is the primary factor in a decision. Some informational approaches that rationally persuade one patient overwhelm another whose fear or panic short-circuits reason.

Coercion occurs if and only if one person intentionally uses a credible and severe threat of harm or force to control another.[35] If a physician orders a reluctant patient to undergo a diagnostic examination and coerces the patient into compliance through a threat of abandonment, the physician's influence controls the patient. The threat of force used by some police, courts, and hospitals in acts of involuntary commitment for psychiatric treatment is coercive. Some threats will coerce virtually all persons (for example, a credible threat to imprison a person), whereas others might succeed in coercing only a few persons (for example, a parent's threat to cut off funding for a son in college unless the son consents to the donation of one of his kidneys to his sister).

Compliance merely because a person *feels* threatened, when no threat has been issued, is not coercion. Coercion occurs only if a credible and intended threat disrupts and reorders a person's self-directed course of action. Under these coercive conditions, even intentional and well-informed actions can be nonvoluntary. Handing over one's wallet to a thief with a gun is both intentional and well informed, though nonvoluntary. Being coerced does not entail that the person coerced lacks voluntary decision-making capacity in complying with a threat. It also does not entail that the person did not choose to perform the action or that the coercion involved always invalidates consent. The point is only that the action was not voluntary.

Manipulation is a term for several forms of influence that are neither persuasive nor coercive. It involves getting people to do what the manipulator wants through a nonpersuasive means that alters a person's understanding of a situation and motivates the person to do what the agent of influence intends. In health care and research the most likely forms of manipulation are informational manipulation that nonpersuasively alters a person's understanding and offers of rewards or potential benefits. Critics of various recruiting practices in biomedical research have suggested that there is often informational manipulation through withholding critical information about risks together with a misleading exaggeration of benefits. Other critics have said that offers of compensation and health care are manipulative when made excessively attractive.

Nevertheless, it is easy to inflate the threat of control by manipulation beyond its actual significance in health care. We typically make decisions in a context of competing influences such as familial constraints, legal obligations, offers of rewards, and institutional pressures. These influences usually do not control decisions to a morally questionable degree. In biomedical ethics we need only establish general criteria for the point at which influence threatens autonomous choice, while recognizing that in many cases no sharp boundary separates controlling and noncontrolling influences.

I have concentrated in this section on *external* controlling influences—usually influences of one person on another. No less important are *internal* influences on the person, such as those caused by mental illness. These conditions can also be voluntariness depriving. However, I will not here pursue the vexing problems of lack of internal control. I simply stipulate that an adequate theory of voluntariness must take account of both internal and external controlling influences.

VIII. Degrees of Autonomy

The first of the conditions of autonomy in the theory just sketched—intentionality—is not a matter of degree: Acts are either intentional or nonintentional. By contrast, acts can satisfy both the conditions of understanding and the absence of controlling influence to a greater or lesser extent. For example, threats can be more or less severe; understanding can be more or less complete; and mental illness can be more or less controlling of action. Actions are autonomous by degrees, as a function of satisfying these conditions to different degrees. A continuum of both understanding and noncontrol runs from full understanding and being entirely noncontrolled to full understanding and being fully in control. Cut-off points on these continua are required for the classification of an action as either autonomous or nonautonomous. The line between what is an adequate degree of understanding and noncontrol must be determined in light of specific objectives of decision making such as deciding about surgery, choosing a university to attend, and hiring a new employee. Any theory of autonomy that demands a high threshold of decision-making capacity and a robust personal history of reflective identification with one's personal values may render nonautonomous or questionably autonomous many individuals normally regarded as autonomous. By contrast, if a theory demands only a low threshold of decision-making skills and ability to resist influence, many individuals who are normally regarded as nonautonomous will be rendered autonomous.

IX. Constraining Situations[36]

The conditions under which an influence controls a person's choices and the reason why those choices lack moral justification may be clear in the abstract, as formulations of a theory of autonomy, but they have a way of being less clear in concrete situations. In this section I will focus on noncoercive situations in which research subjects and surrogates report feeling pressured to enroll in clinical trials even though enrollment, by the book, is classified as voluntary.[37] These individuals might be in desperate need of medication, or it might be that participation in research is a vital source of income. Attractive offers such as free medication, in-clinic housing, and money can leave a person with a sense of having no meaningful choice other than participation in research. Influences of a sort that persons ordinarily find resistible in their lives can control abnormally weak and dependent patients and subjects.[38]

Difficult choices for a patient or surrogate have sometimes been said to be "coerced" if the patient is forced by circumstances to participate in a clinical trial. However, there is no coercion if no one has *intentionally* issued a threat in order to gain compliance. A *perception* of coercion by a decision maker is not sufficient to constitute coercion. The problem is that many patients and potential subjects feel acutely pressured to make a decision they wish to avoid and see as admitting of only one choice. For example, the prospect for a homeless person of another night on the streets or another day without food constrains him or her to accept an offer of shelter and payment as a research subject, just as such conditions could constrain a person to accept a job cleaning up hazardous chemicals or sewers that the person would otherwise not accept. Such persons appropriately report feeling that they had no choice and that it was unthinkable to refuse the offer. This perceived absence of options does not render a choice nonvoluntary. However, these constraining situations are in need of moral attention for related reasons.

Payment, Undue Influence, and Undue Profit

In constraining situations, monetary payments and offers such as shelter or food give rise to moral questions of both *undue influence* and *undue profit*. Monetary payments to research subjects seem unproblematic if the payments are welcome offers and the risks are at the level of everyday risks. The offer of research involvement is, in effect, an offer of a job or contract in which mutual benefit can and should occur.[39] However, inducements become increasingly problematic (1) as risks are increased, (2) as more attractive inducements are introduced, and, in some cases, (3) as the subjects' economic disadvantage or lack of available alternatives or resources is increased. As risks, inducements, or disadvantage is elevated, "exploitation" looms larger. The heart of the moral problem of exploitation and related problems about psychological voluntariness is whether persons offered participation in research are disadvantaged and without viable alternatives, whether they feel compelled to accept attractive offers that they otherwise would not accept, and whether they assume increased risk in their lives. As these conditions are mitigated, problems of exploitation and voluntariness diminish; as these conditions increase, problems of exploitation and involuntariness increase.

The condition of an irresistibly attractive offer is a necessary condition of "undue inducement," but this condition is not by itself sufficient to make an inducement *undue*. In addition, there must be a risk of harm of sufficient seriousness that the person's welfare interest is negatively affected by assuming it, and it must be a risk the person would not ordinarily assume. I will not try to pinpoint a precise threshold of risk, but it would presumably need to be above the level of such common job risks as those of unskilled construction work. Inducements are not undue unless they are above the level of standard risk (hence "excessive" in risk) and irresistibly attractive (hence "excessive" in payment or attractiveness) in light of a constraining situation. Although these offers are not coercive, because no threat is involved, the offer can be manipulative.

Undue inducements should be distinguished from *undue profits*, which arise from too small a payment, rather than an irresistibly attractive, large payment. In circumstances of undue profit in research, the subject receives an unfair payment and the sponsor receives more than can be justified. This is what critics of pharmaceutical research often seem to be maintaining: The subjects are in a poor bargaining position, constrained by their poverty, and are given a minor compensation and an unjust share of the benefits, while companies reap unseemly profits from the research.

How, then, should we handle these two moral problems of exploitation—undue inducement (unduly large and irresistible payments to subjects) and undue profit (unduly small and unfair payments to subjects)? One strategy is that if research involves exceptional, and therefore excessive, risk (that is, risk with more than a minor increment above minimal risk), it should be prohibited for healthy subjects, even if a good oversight system is in place and regardless of the form of consent involved. This answer is appealing, but it leaves us with the problem of delineating a threshold of excessive risk, irresistibly attractive payment, unjust underpayment, and constraining situations—all difficult problems commonly ignored in literature on the subject.

The argument thus far suggests that exploitation occurs not because persons are not shown respect for their autonomy, but because there is undue profit (offering too little for services) or an undue influence (offering too much for services). The most straightforward way to avoid such exploitation is to strike a balance between a rate of payment high enough that it does not exploit subjects by underpayment and one low enough that it does not exploit by undue inducement. If this strategy is the best available, there still is no a priori way to set a proper level of payment—for example, at the level of unskilled labor—because that level might not satisfy the golden-mean standard. Payment at the level of unskilled labor rates might themselves be exploitative, either by creating an undue influence or generating an undue profit. The general objective should be that the sponsor of the research pay a fair wage at the golden mean for moderate-risk studies and not increase the wage in order to entice subjects to studies with higher levels of risk.[40] If this mean is unattainable, all research offers will be exploitative: There will be either an undue profit by underpayment or an undue influence by overpayment.

I cannot here pursue this conclusion. I will mention only one point about the danger of altogether prohibiting research or calling on investigators to pull out of communities in which constraining situations might be a significant presence. Even if the degree of voluntariness is judged to be lower in persons who are in such circumstances, to deny them the right to make choices about participation in biomedical research on grounds that the choice itself is nonvoluntary is morally suspect. To deny them the opportunity of research participation can be paternalistic, demeaning, and economically distressing.

X. Conclusion

I have noted that vagueness surrounds both the ordinary concept of autonomy and philosophical theories of autonomy. These theories make for compelling reading, but the practical implications of the theories for informed-consent settings deserve as much attention as the features of mind pointed to in the theories. In the future, as we develop and assess new work on autonomy, we should be mindful not to stray from our pretheoretical judgments about what deserves respect in human choices. The moral value of respect for autonomy precedes and should ground the theory of autonomy.

Notes

1. See the following early and influential sources on this subject: Alan Meisel and Loren Roth, "What We Do and Do Not Know about Informed Consent," *Journal of the American Medical Association* 246 (1981): 2473–77; President's Commission for the Study of Ethical Problems in Medicine and Biomedical and Behavioral Research, *Making Health Care Decisions*, vol. II (Washington, DC: Government Printing Office, 1983), 317–410, esp. 318, and vol. I, ch. 1, esp. 38–39; National Commission for the Protection of Human Subjects of Biomedical and Behavioral Research, *The Belmont Report* (Washington, DC: DHEW Publication OS 78-0012, 1978), 10.
2. The account of two senses in this section derives from the treatment in Ruth R. Faden and Tom L. Beauchamp, *A History and Theory of Informed Consent* (New York: Oxford University Press, 1986), ch. 8.
3. See Jay Katz, "Disclosure and Consent," in *Genetics and the Law II*, ed. A. Milunsky and G. Annas (New York: Plenum Press, 1980), 122, 128.
4. See the reprinting of the Nuremberg Code in Jay Katz, ed. *Experimentation with Human Beings* (New York: Russell Sage Foundation, 1972), 305 (Principle One). See, further, A.C. Ivy, "The History and Ethics of the Use of Human Subjects in Medical Experiments," *Science* 108 (July 2, 1948): 1–5; Henry K. Beecher, *Research and the Individual: Human Studies* (Boston: Little, Brown and Co., 1970); Joseph V. Brady and Albert R. Jonsen, "The Evolution of Regulatory Influences on Research with Human Subjects," in Robert Greenwald, Mary Kay Ryan, and James E. Mulvihill, eds., *Human Subjects Research* (New York: Plenum

Press, 1982); Robert J. Levine, *Ethics and Regulation of Clinical Research* (Baltimore: Urban & Schwarzenberg, 1981): 287–89. These authors were all close to and involved in some of the historical events of the period mentioned.

5. National Research Act, July 12, 1974. Public Law 93-348; National Commission for the Protection of Human Subjects of Biomedical and Behavioral Research, *The Belmont Report: Ethical Principles and Guidelines for the Protection of Human Subjects of Research* (Washington, DC: DHEW Publication OS 78-0012, 1978); National Commission for the Protection of Human Subjects of Biomedical and Behavioral Research. Archived Materials 1974–78. "Transcript of the Meeting Proceedings" (for discussion of the Belmont Paper at the following meetings: February 11–13, 1977; July 8–9, 1977; April 14–15, 1978; and June 9–10, 1978). All archived material is at the Kennedy Institute Library, storage facility, Georgetown University. See also James F. Childress, Eric M. Meslin, and Harold T. Shapiro, eds., *Belmont Revisited* (Washington, DC: Georgetown University Press, 2005).

6. Her views are expressed in O'Neill, "Some Limits of Informed Consent," *Journal of Medical Ethics* 29 (2003): 4–7; Neil C. Manson and Onora O'Neill, *Rethinking Informed Consent in Bioethics* (Cambridge: Cambridge University Press, 2007); O'Neill, *Autonomy and Trust in Bioethics* (Cambridge: Cambridge University Press, 2002); O'Neill, "Autonomy: The Emperor's New Clothes," *Proceedings of the Aristotelian Society*, supp. vol. 77 (2003): 1–21. Jim Childress and Dana Kelly each pointed me to several instructive passages in O'Neill's work.

7. O'Neill, *Rethinking Informed Consent in Bioethics*, 17. Compare her earlier expression of this view in *Autonomy and Trust in Bioethics*, 21–27.

8. O'Neill, "Some Limits of Informed Consent," 5.

9. O'Neill, *Rethinking Informed Consent in Bioethics*, 17 (in her section entitled "Improving Justification: The Quest for Autonomy").

10. O'Neill, *Rethinking Informed Consent in Bioethics*, 82.

11. O'Neill, "Autonomy: The Emperor's New Clothes," 3. Similar views are expressed very clearly in *Autonomy and Trust in Bioethics*, 29–34, 45.

12. I there discuss the theory of Harry Frankfurt, as does O'Neill, immediately following the material just quoted. We are clearly thinking about the same author(s) in contemporary literature on autonomy.

13. O'Neill, "Some Limits of Informed Consent," 4.

14. Compare, for example, the diverse treatments of autonomy in Joel Feinberg, *Harm to Self*, vol. III, in *The Moral Limits of the Criminal Law* (New York: Oxford University Press, 1986), chs. 18–19; Gerald Dworkin, *The Theory and Practice of Autonomy* (Cambridge: Cambridge University Press, 1988); Rebecca Kukla, "Conscientious Autonomy: Displacing Decisions in Health Care," *Hastings Center Report* 35 (March–April 2005): 34–44; and Thomas E. Hill,

Jr., *Autonomy and Self-Respect* (Cambridge: Cambridge University Press, 1991), chs. 1–4.

15. O'Neill, *Rethinking Informed Consent in Bioethics*, 25, 189. See also her *Autonomy and Trust in Bioethics*, sect. 7.6, 154–60.

16. Julian Savulescu, "Rational Desires and the Limitation of Life-Sustaining Treatment," *Bioethics* 8 (1994): 191–222.

17. This section draws from my "Who Deserves Autonomy and Whose Autonomy Deserves Respect?" in *Personal Autonomy*, ed. Taylor, 310–29.

18. Dworkin, *The Theory and Practice of Autonomy*, chs. 1-4; Harry G. Frankfurt, "Freedom of the Will and the Concept of a Person," *Journal of Philosophy* 68 (1971): 5–20, as reprinted in *The Importance of What We Care About* (Cambridge: Cambridge University Press, 1988), 11–25. Frankfurt may not have a theory of autonomy; but see his uses of the language of "autonomy" in *Necessity, Volition, and Love* (Cambridge: Cambridge University Press, 1999), chs. 9, 11. Frankfurt's early work was on *persons* and *freedom of the will*. In his later work, he seems to regard the earlier work as providing an account of autonomy, which is a reasonable estimate even if it involves some creative reconstruction.

19. Frankfurt, "Freedom of the Will and the Concept of a Person," in *The Importance of What We Care About*, 16. Frankfurt modified his earlier theory of identification in his later philosophy. See his "The Faintest Passion," in *Necessity, Volition, and Love*, 95–107, esp. 105–6.

20. Dworkin, *The Theory and Practice of Autonomy*, 20.

21. Frankfurt apparently addresses this problem as follows: "whether a person identifies himself with [his or her] passions, or whether they occur as alien forces that remain outside the boundaries of his volitional identity, depends upon what he himself wants his will to be." "Autonomy, Necessity, and Love," in *Necessity, Volition, and Love*, 137.

22. Problems of this sort were first called to my attention by Irving Thalberg, "Hierarchical Analyses of Unfree Action," *Canadian Journal of Philosophy* 8 (1978): 211–26. Personal discussion with Thalberg influenced my early thinking on the subject.

23. "The Faintest Passion" and "On the Necessity of Ideals," in *Necessity, Volition, and Love*, esp. 105, 110.

24. O'Neill similarly suggests that such a theory sets "a higher hurdle for cognitively adequate consent, so shrink[ing] the range of cases in medical and research practice for which informed consent could be required." *Rethinking Informed Consent in Bioethics*, 21.

25. There are still more demanding theories than these second-order theories. They require extremely rigorous standards in order to be autonomous or to be persons. For

example, they demand that the autonomous individual be authentic, consistent, independent, in command, resistant to control by authorities, and the original source of values, beliefs, rational desires, and life plans. O'Neill sometimes seems to assume such a theory of autonomy. For early and influential theories that suggest this view, see Stanley Benn, "Freedom, Autonomy and the Concept of a Person," *Proceedings of the Aristotelian Society* 76 (1976): 123–30, and *A Theory of Freedom* (Cambridge: Cambridge University Press, 1988): 3–6, 155f, 175–83; R. S. Downie and Elizabeth Telfer, "Autonomy," *Philosophy* 46 (1971): 296–301; Christopher McMahon, "Autonomy and Authority," *Philosophy and Public Affairs* 16 (1987): 303–28.

26. See my "Whose Autonomy," in Taylor. See also Faden and Beauchamp, *A History and Theory of Informed Consent*, ch. 7; and Beauchamp and James Childress, *Principles of Biomedical Ethics*, 6th ed. (New York: Oxford University Press, 2009), ch. 4.

27. For a "planning theory" and its relation to theories of autonomy, see Michael Bratman, "Planning Agency, Autonomous Agency," in Taylor, *Personal Autonomy*, 33–57.

28. Alvin I. Goldman, *A Theory of Human Action* (Englewood Cliffs, NJ: Prentice-Hall, 1970), 49–85.

29. Hector-Neri Castañeda, "Intensionality and Identity in Human Action and Philosophical Method," *Nous* 13 (1979): 235–60, esp. 255.

30. This analysis draws from Faden and Beauchamp, *A History and Theory of Informed Consent*, ch. 7.

31. I follow John Searle in thinking that we cannot reliably distinguish, in many situations, among acts, effects, consequences, and events. Searle, "The Intentionality of Intention and Action," *Cognitive Science* 4 (1980): esp. 65.

32. This now widely used label seems to have been coined by Paul S. Appelbaum, Loren Roth, and Charles W. Lidz in "The Therapeutic Misconception: Informed Consent in Psychiatric Research," *International Journal of Law and Psychiatry* 5 (1982): 319–29. For evidence that the misconception is still widespread, see Appelbaum, Lidz, and Thomas Grisso, "Therapeutic Misconception in Clinical Research: Frequency and Risk Factors," *IRB: Ethics and Human Research* 26 (2004): 1–8. See, further, W. Glannon, "Phase I Oncology Trials: Why the Therapeutic Misconception Will Not Go Away," *Journal of Medical Ethics* 32 (2006): 252–55.

33. See Sam Horng and Christine Grady, "Misunderstanding in Clinical Research: Distinguishing Therapeutic Misconception, Therapeutic Misestimation, & Therapeutic Optimism," *IRB: Ethics and Human Research* 25 (January–February 2003): 11–16.

34. See the original formulation of this view in Faden and Beauchamp, *A History and Theory of Informed Consent*, ch. 10.

35. This formulation is indebted to Robert Nozick, "Coercion," in *Philosophy, Science and Method: Essays in Honor of Ernest Nagel*, ed. Sidney Morgenbesser, Patrick

Suppes, and Morton White (New York: St. Martin's Press, 1969), 440–72; and Bernard Gert, "Coercion and Freedom," in *Coercion: Nomos XIV*, ed. J. Roland Pennock and John W. Chapman (Chicago: Aldine, Atherton Inc. 1972), 36–37. See also Alan Wertheimer, *Coercion* (Princeton, NJ: Princeton University Press, 1987).

36. This section is indebted to my "The Exploitation of the Economically Disadvantaged in Pharmaceutical Research," in *The Intersection of Bioethics and Business Ethics*, ed. Denis Arnold (Cambridge: Cambridge University Press, 2009).

37. See Sarah E. Hewlett, "Is Consent to Participate in Research Voluntary?" *Arthritis Care and Research* 9 (1996): 400–04; Hewlett, "Consent to Clinical Research—Adequately Voluntary of Substantially Influenced?" *Journal of Medical Ethics* 22 (1996): 232–36; and Robert M. Nelson and Jon F. Merz, "Voluntariness of Consent for Research: An Empirical and Conceptual Review," *Medical Care* 40 (2002): suppl., V69–80.

38. See Charles W. Lidz et al., *Informed Consent: A Study of Decision Making in Psychiatry* (New York: Guilford Press, 1984), ch. 7, esp. 110–11, 117–23.

39. The justification of monetary inducement in terms of mutual benefit is defended by Martin Wilkinson and Andrew Moore, "Inducement in Research," *Bioethics* 11 (1997): 373–89; and Wilkinson and Moore, "Inducements Revisited," *Bioethics* 13 (1999): 114–30. See also Christine Grady, "Money for Research Participation: Does It Jeopardize Informed Consent?" *American Journal of Bioethics* 1 (2001): 40–44.

40. Compare the different conditions proposed by Leonardo D. de Castro, "Exploitation in the Use of Human Subject for Medical Experimentation: A Re-Examination of Basic Issues," *Bioethics* 9 (1995): 259–68, esp. 264; Tom L. Beauchamp, Bruce Jennings, Eleanor Kinney, and Robert Levine, "Pharmaceutical Research Involving the Homeless," *Journal of Medicine and Philosophy* (2002): 547–64; and Toby L. Schonfeld, Joseph S. Brown, Meaghann Weniger, and Bruce Gordon, "Research Involving the Homeless," *IRB* 25 (Sept./Oct. 2003): 17–20.

4

Preface to a Theory of Consent Transactions: Beyond Valid Consent

Franklin G. Miller and Alan Wertheimer

In moral theory, as elsewhere, necessity is the mother of invention. As we struggled with several issues raised by the principle of informed consent in medical research, we found that we had to widen our angle of vision to consider other contexts in which consent is morally transformative. This chapter reports the highlights of our inquiry into general characteristics of consent transactions by virtue of which they are morally transformative—that is, they make it permissible for A to act with respect to B in a way that would be impermissible absent valid consent. Ultimately, we have come to the view that whereas "valid consent" captures much of what is important and is an eminently serviceable notion for most purposes, it is not quite right. In our view, the central question is whether a consent *transaction* between A and B is morally transformative and, in particular, whether a consent transaction renders it permissible for A to proceed. To answer this question it is necessary to go beyond valid consent.

We need a wide-angle lens as well as a microscope. Because bioethics has been in the grip of a specific historical legacy and an associated set of canonical statements and legal doctrines, it has adopted a parochial view of consent; it has failed to locate its own principle of informed consent within the more general terrain of contexts in which people alter their moral and legal status by consent. As soon as one looks at other social contexts, one realizes that the principle of informed consent so familiar to bioethics is actually quite special.

Indeed, the very idea that morally transformative consent must be *informed* is virtually unique to the medical context. With some exceptions (such as the sale of a house, where disclosure of known defects is required), we speak of consent—not informed consent—in most of the other realms in which people make mundane decisions, such as ordering meals and authorizing car repairs, as well as life-changing decisions, such as sexual relations, contracts, jobs, and marriage. In our view, a theory of informed consent should be rooted in a theory that is adequate for the full range of consent contexts.

Standardly, a consent transaction is an interaction between two persons in which B tokens consent to A to do X. In many cases A and B will mutually consent to an interaction, making them both consenters and recipients of consent. We contend that a theory of consent transactions must account for both standard consent transactions and flawed consent transactions, in which it is reasonable and fair for A to believe that B has tokened consent despite the fact that B has not actually given consent.

We title this chapter "A *Preface* to a Theory of Consent Transactions." Although we seek to change the angle of vision, we do not provide many details of the altered landscape. First, we seek to change the focus from the characteristics of a party's mental states to a focus on the *bilateral transaction* between the consenter and the recipient of consent. The crucial question is not whether the consenter gives "valid consent," but whether the consent *transaction* renders it permissible for the (putative) recipient of consent to proceed, even when a full accounting of the transaction would reveal that valid consent has not been given. Interestingly, we shall also argue that there are contexts in which a consent transaction may not be morally transformative even when valid consent has been given. In general, "valid consent" and moral transformation or permissibility to proceed go hand in hand. But when they do not, we argue that it is moral transformation and not valid consent that is of fundamental moral importance.

There are, of course, many contexts in which A is permitted to proceed *without* B's consent, as when A (a physician) administers medical treatment to an unconscious B. In those cases, there is permissibility without a transformation. Here we are concerned with contexts in which it is generally thought that consent is necessary. In those contexts, the prevailing theory of consent can be described as *the lock-and-key/autonomous authorization* model (LK/AA) of consent transactions. LK has two parts: (1) the claim that valid consent is necessary and sufficient for moral transformation and (2) a conception of valid consent. LK holds that valid consent is the key that opens the lock of moral transformation. Although there is room for argument as to what constitutes "valid consent," the prevailing theory, best developed by Faden and Beauchamp, is that valid consent is defined by the concept of autonomous authorization.[1] In other words, A is permitted to proceed in doing X in response to B's consent token if, and only if, B has autonomously authorized A to do X. The general outlines of AA are quite familiar. On AA, B's consent is valid if and only if B's consent reflects her autonomous will, that is, only if it is substantially voluntary, only if B is competent to make such choices, only if B is suitably informed and understands that to which she is consenting, and so forth. It is not necessary here to spell out precisely what AA requires. The main point is that AA emphasizes the authenticity of B's choice or what T.M. Scanlon has called the "quality of will."[2] In principle, the lock-and-key model of moral transformation could be combined with different (non-AA) criteria of valid consent that are sensitive to context. Although we once favored that approach, we found that even if the criteria of valid consent are relaxed, LK will still prove implausible. And so we were driven to look elsewhere.

We will argue that the LK/AA model of consent suffers from serious practical and theoretical difficulties. As an alternative, we develop a *fair transaction* model (FT) of consent transactions. Simply put, FT claims that A is morally permitted to proceed on the basis of a consent transaction if A has treated B fairly and responds in a reasonable manner to B's token or expression of consent or what A reasonably believes is B's token or expression of consent.

It is important to forestall a possible misunderstanding of FT. It might be thought that LK/AA represents the best "ideal" conception of informed consent against which the ethics of consent transactions "in the real world" needs to be assessed, even though strict adherence to LK/AA is impractical in various contexts. That is not our view. We argue that FT is a superior moral conception or paradigm of consent transactions. In our view, by tying morally transformative consent to the consenter's autonomous choice, LK/AA presumes an excessively narrow conception of the values at stake. In particular, a morally defensible theory of consent transactions needs to account for the interests both of the consenter and of those who solicit consent (and society at large) in having clear, practicable, and fair standards by which recipients can determine when they are entitled to proceed with cooperative or transactional activities. Approaches that place "valid consent" at the center fail to do justice to the *bilateral* nature of consent transactions.

Our Plan

A relatively complete theory of consent transactions should elucidate a number of related elements. We will first examine the logic of consent transactions and describe some of the ways in which consent can be morally transformative. We will then examine the values that underlie consent transactions. We will argue that consent transactions serve to protect and promote the consenter's well-being (or interests) as well as autonomy. We will also argue that consent transactions serve both to protect the consenter's negative autonomy or control over herself and, quite crucially, to serve her positive autonomy by facilitating mutually beneficial and altruistic interactions with others. Transactional fairness also serves the interests and autonomy of recipients of consent—their interest in being permitted to proceed in interactions with consenters and thus to achieve the purposes of cooperative activities. We then consider the "ontology" of consent. Is consent a mental state or an action (or performative) or a hybrid of these components?

We then turn to the criteria of moral transformation (CMT). When does a consent transaction between A and B render it permissible for A to proceed? We examine CMT in a range of contexts, such as sexual consent, commercial consent, employment, and the like. We will argue that CMT will have different implications in different contexts. Consider fairness. To be fair to one's opponents in golf is to penalize oneself for unobserved infractions (such as inadvertently moving the ball), whereas a flagrant foul may be unfair in basketball, but one is hardly expected to call a foul on oneself. Similarly, fairness in negotiating a business deal may not be identical to fairness in seeking a sexual encounter. With that discussion in hand, we then argue that FT provides a better account of moral transformation and consider some objections to it. Finally, we briefly consider two applications of FT.

The Logic of Consent Transactions

The purpose of consent is to produce moral transformation in the relationship between people. As John Kleinig argues in Chapter 1, there are several ways in which B's consent can be morally transformative. B's consent may give A permission to do X if it would otherwise be wrong for A to do X. In some contexts, we may say that B's consent authorizes A to do X. In still other contexts, B's consent may constitute a promise and give rise to an obligation to A. B's consent can also generate a transfer of ownership of some resource to another person.

We will be primarily interested in consent that renders it morally permissible to proceed. Two clarifications are in order. First, the phrase "permissible to proceed" can be understood in at least two ways: (1) it is morally permissible for A to proceed and (2) it (morally) should be permissible for A to proceed under some set of legal or institutional rules and regulations. Although this distinction can be of considerable importance, we mostly ignore it here. Second, the transformative powers of consent are somewhat limited. To say that B's consent renders A's action morally permissible is to say, among other things, that A does not violate B's rights if she performs the proposed action. It may also entail that third parties are not entitled to interfere with A's doing X to B. That said, even if B's consent renders it *permissible* for A to do X, B's consent is not sufficient to generate a positive moral assessment of A's action. For example, it may be permissible for A to engage in casual sex with B if B gives morally transformative consent, but it does not follow that such relations have positive moral value.

The Value of Consent Transactions

Roughly speaking, consent and consent transactions seem to serve two primary values: (1) well-being or the agent's interests and (2) autonomy or self-determination. Although most commentators tend to see the value of consent in terms of autonomy and respect for persons, consent also protects and advances the agent's interests or well-being. After all, a person's well-being at least partly depends on "the particular aims and values of that person."[3] Moreover, even with respect to those dimensions of well-being that are objective or universal, competent persons are often better positioned than others to know what will best serve those ends and are also more motivated to pursue them. In addition, people typically want to make decisions for themselves and the satisfaction of this desire is also a component of their well-being apart from the intrinsic value of making decisions for oneself.

Second, consent serves the noninstrumental value in self-determination or autonomy or rights. It is commonly thought that we have reason to respect a person's decisions or acknowledge her right to autonomy, even when doing so does not maximize her well-being. Being regarded as an autonomous person is also integral to one's self-respect. The problem, of course, is that although consent serves to protect an agent's autonomy and to advance her well-being, those values appear to sometimes conflict. An agent may refuse to consent to an intervention or transaction that would advance her well-being and may consent to an intervention or transaction that does not. That said, we think that the tension between these values is overstated. The value we ascribe to autonomy is strongly tied to the agent's well-being. If human beings consistently made choices that did not advance their interests, it is hard to imagine that we would come to value what we call their autonomy or their right to make such decisions. Moreover, it cannot be entirely coincidental that the very conditions that are thought to render an agent less than fully autonomous—coercion, deception, incompetence—are also conditions that reduce the likelihood that her decisions advance her well-being. If an infirm widow were to sign a contract to sell a $100,000 farm for $10,000, we would not say, "Ah, this doesn't advance her interests, but we need to respect her autonomous choice." Rather, we would say, "This likely wasn't an autonomous choice; she probably didn't know what she was doing."

As indicated above, it is important to recognize that the morally transformative power of consent transactions serves the values of autonomy and well-being through a protective or negative function and a facilitative or positive function. We violate a person's negative autonomy when we intervene without her consent. We fail to respect a person's positive autonomy when we do not allow her to trigger an intervention to which she consents. Given that a consent transaction serves both negative and positive autonomy, it is not clear what we should do when an agent's decision is less than robustly autonomous or rational, say, because the subject is not fully informed or competent. To emphasize the protective function of consent by not allowing a person to enter into transactions unless her consent is robustly autonomous or authentic is, in effect, to compromise the facilitative function of consent transactions by disabling her from entering into transactions and relationships that she seeks.

The Ontology of Consent

There are two principal questions that we can ask about consent transactions: (1) Does B token consent (at all)? (2) If so, is B's token of consent morally transformative? The first is a question about the ontology of consent; the second is a moral question. Roughly speaking, there are three principal accounts of what constitutes what we might call the "ontology" of consent. A subjective view argues that consent is a psychological phenomenon: B consents if and only if she has the relevant mental state. A behavioral view defines consent in terms of observable behavior: B consents if and only if she tokens or expresses consent in a conventionally appropriate way. A hybrid view maintains that the appropriate mental state and the appropriate behavior are both requirements of consent.

The present issue is not linguistic. Rather, the issue is which understanding of the ontology of consent explains how a consent transaction between B and A could render it permissible for A to do what would otherwise be impermissible for A to do. From this perspective, it is hard to see how B's mental state—by itself—can do the job. We readily grant that tokens of consent are morally significant precisely because they are generally reliable indicators of the consenter's desires, intentions, choices, and the like. But if the point of consent is to actually alter one's normative relations with others, then some observable indication of one's will is required.

If morally transformative consent requires a behavioral component, there is room for disagreement as to what constitutes B's tokening consent to A's doing X. Does one consent to pay the bill for one's meal simply by ordering? Does one consent to sex by silently not resisting or even responding positively to another's advances? Consider these cases.

> *Auction.* It is general practice that nodding one's head in response to the auctioneer's query indicates a willingness to pay the specified amount ("Will anyone give me $1,000?"). As the auctioneer made his query, C asks B a question. B nods her head. The auctioneer believes that B has agreed to pay.

> *Department Meeting.* A, a department chair, says, "I'm going to appoint C to our new position unless anyone objects." B is daydreaming, and says nothing. A assumes that B has authorized him to appoint C.

We do not think that B has actively tokened consent in these cases. But the question remains: Is the *consent transaction* morally transformative? Although it is unlikely that B is obligated to pay in *Auction*, it is certainly arguable that B's silence renders it permissible for A to proceed in *Department Meeting,* not because B has actually consented, but because it is reasonable for A to act as if he did. Note that *Department Meeting* is not a genuine case of tacit consent, where the parties understand that silence constitutes consent.[4] But if we are right, *Department Meeting* exemplifies our claim that a consent transaction in which it is reasonable for A to believe that B has tokened consent can be morally transformative even without valid consent, particularly when the absence of (valid) consent results from a "flawed consent process."

If B is to consent to A's doing X, it seems that B must consent to A's doing X as opposed to some other action that A might perform.

> *Lawn Blower.* A asks B whether he can borrow B's lawn blower, about which (unbeknownst to A) B is quite proprietary. B mistakenly thinks that A has asked to borrow his lawn mower, about

which he is not proprietary. B says, "Sure, it's in my garage; help yourself when you need it."

In *Lawn Blower*, B understands that she is consenting to allow A to borrow something (as opposed, say, to being kissed), but is mistaken about that which A seeks to borrow. Linguistic intuitions go both ways about these sorts of mistakes and misunderstandings. B might say: (1) "I didn't realize I was agreeing to let you take the lawn blower but I guess I did" or (2) "I didn't agree to let you take the lawn blower, but, given the misunderstanding, you didn't do anything wrong." In our view, the important moral question is not whether (1) or (2) is linguistically correct, but whether A is justified in taking B's lawn blower. And, we will argue, that is a question that is better answered by FT than LK/AA.

Criteria of Moral Transformation

In most contexts, we assume that "no means no"—period. If a person refuses to token consent to an intervention that is rendered permissible only with (valid) consent, then the other party is not entitled proceed even if the refusal to consent is nonautonomous. By contrast, we do not always assume that "yes means yes." We might well say, "B was drunk when she agreed to have sex with A, and so A should disregard B's yes." And so assuming that B tokens consent, we must still determine if B's token of consent is morally transformative. Some put this point in terms of the distinction between a (mere) token of consent and valid consent. Peter Westen distinguishes between "descriptive consent" and "prescriptive consent."[5] But however the distinction is put, what we call the criteria of moral transformation is the site of the most important theoretical action about consent transactions. To see some of the difficulties, consider these cases.[6]

> *Condom.* Elizabeth Wilson was awakened at 3:00 a.m. by Joel Valdez, who was approaching her with a knife. He ordered her to take off his pants. Ms. Wilson, fearing that Valdez would stab her if she resisted and that he would infect her with HIV if she submitted, agreed to submit to sexual intercourse with Valdez if he put on a condom.

> *Biopsy.* A mammogram reveals suspicious areas in B's breast. A tells B that he wants to do a biopsy under general anesthesia and, if positive, perform a lumpectomy. B listens, but her anxiety overwhelms her thought processes. A asks her to sign a consent form authorizing both

procedures (if necessary). B reads the form but does not process its content. B thinks that A will only be doing a biopsy. She signs.

Illiterate Contractor. A presents B a contract to sign. Because B is embarrassed that he cannot read, he pretends to read the contract and signs.

Infatuated Patient. B is infatuated with her psychotherapist, A. She proposes that they have sexual relations. A accepts.

Leaky Roof. B is proposing to buy A's home. B does not ask about the condition of the roof, but A's disclosure form fails to note that the roof leaks. B signs a contract to purchase.

Single. A and B meet in a night class, and have several dates. B makes it clear that she refuses to have sex with married men. When asked, A lies and says that he is single.

Rental Car Speeding. B rents a car from A's company. The fine print of the rental contract contains a clause stating that vehicles driven in excess of the 75 miles per hour will be charged $150 per occurrence and that this will be billed to the renter's credit card. A uses a GPS system to track B's driving. The system finds that B is driving over 80 miles per hour and charges $150 to B's credit card.

Trust. A tells B that she needs surgery for breast cancer. As A begins to explain the options, B says, "I trust you; do whatever you think is best."

Dinner. A invites B to dinner, asking for a firm commitment. A does not disclose the other invitees and B does not ask. B accepts.

Inhibitions. A and B have dated. B has said that she is not ready for sex. Without thinking much about it, B consumes several drinks at a party. When A proposes that they have sex, she feels much less inhibited than usual and says, "There has to be a first time."

Although B has tokened consent in all of these cases, B has certainly not given morally transformative consent in *Condom* or *Leaky Roof* on both LK/ AA and FT. But some cases illustrate the contrast between AA/LK and FT. On AA/LK, A may not be permitted to proceed in cases such as *Biopsy, Illiterate Contractor,* and *Rental Car Speeding* or acquire an obligation in a case such as *Dinner.* On FT, however, it is an open question as to whether B's consent is morally transformative. To resolve that question definitively requires a more complete theory of fair transactions than we are prepared to offer here. We are, however, inclined to think that it is permissible for A to proceed in *Trust* and that B has made a morally binding commitment in *Dinner*, even though neither consent was fully informed. Why? Because B has tokened consent in a context in which A has treated B fairly and because a contrary view would be unfair to A. Although the existing law and prevalent moral beliefs may not reflect the best moral view, when we look at the range of contexts of consent transactions, we often find that we require nothing approximating AA consent as necessary for moral transformation. It will prove useful to begin with a very brief survey of some of these contexts.

Consent to Sexual Relations

Unlike informed consent to receive invasive medical procedures and to participate in research, where we require written disclosures of pertinent information and tokens of consent, one can token consent to sexual relations verbally or by one's behavior, without any disclosure of information. Some think that the sexual arena is packed with cases in which there are genuine misunderstandings as to whether B has tokened consent. But assuming an adequate token of consent, there is still the question as to when B's token of consent renders it permissible for A to proceed. There is no lack of clarity as to whether B tokens consent in *Single* or *Infatuated Patient*. The question is whether B's consent is morally transformative.

As we have noted, the standard view is that morally transformative consent must be voluntary, informed, and competent. This is fine as far as it goes, but each of these general criteria must be interpreted, as what they require varies considerably depending on the context. (These issues are considered in some detail in Chapter 8) For present purposes, it is worth noting that the informational requirements for consent to sex are comparatively low. Physicians must provide patients with far more information regarding the risks of surgery than we require of prospective sexual partners regarding the risks of sexual intercourse. Presumably, this reflects the idea that most people, as a matter of common knowledge, have sufficient understanding of the latter but not of the former. Moreover, we have generally been quite permissive with respect to outright deception in sexual relations. A commits no crime in *Single*, and we have found that people differ as to whether A's lie is seriously wrong.

With respect to competence, we allow people to have sex at younger ages than we allow them to drive, sign contracts, or authorize medical procedures. We also allow people to grant permission to others to have sex with them after they have become quite intoxicated, as in *Inhibitions*. *Infatuated Patient* demonstrates another form of compromised competence. We treat the patient's consent as invalid because it is believed that the process of psychotherapy can systematically distort a patient's judgment and a sexual relationship is likely to be harmful in ways that the patient may not anticipate. Consent by the mentally retarded exhibits the tension between the negative or protective and positive or facilitative functions of consent. We could protect the mentally retarded from sexual predators by claiming that they are simply not capable of giving valid consent to sexual relations, but doing so would come at the price of disabling them participating in an important dimension of human life.

Commerce

Consent in the commercial context ranges over a wide range of activities, and there is no univocal standard as to what counts as giving the sort of consent that results in a valid agreement. Many agreements require a token in writing, but one can agree to pay for a meal simply by ordering it (even if one is not told the price), and one can authorize an auto repair ("You need a new transmission") or the sale of stocks over the phone. Although many states now require the seller of a home to disclose known defects in writing, this is not true of most goods. We no longer endorse *caveat emptor*, because we do frown on fraud, but with the exception of some products, there is no assumption that a seller must provide a prospective purchaser with information about the risks of a product. Think of a bicycle, for example.

Contracts can be regarded as valid or binding even when made in the face of considerable pressure. If McDonald's threatens one of its suppliers to take its business elsewhere unless the supplier agrees to a reduction in price, the agreement would certainly be regarded as valid. Commerce is a context in which very hard bargaining is thought to be consistent with morally transformative consent.

Although people typically know to what they are agreeing when they consent to sex (even if they may not understand all of its consequences), this is not always so in commercial contexts. A and B may lack "convergent intentions." What then? If B believes he is agreeing to X (say, teach three courses per year) but signs an agreement to do Y (say, teach four courses per year), the law does *not* rely on a version of AA/LK. It does not say, "B is not bound by the contract because he was mistaken about the terms of the agreement." No, the law will make a judgment as to who should bear the liability for the mistake. And depending on the circumstances, the law may well decide to treat B's consent to do Y as binding. If A was not acting unfairly and if B had a fair opportunity to understand the terms of the agreement, the law may side with A. On the other hand, if A was trying to sneak something by B, or if the penalties are regarded as excessive, perhaps as in *Rental Car Speeding*, the law might side with B.

Gambling

Gambling is an interesting example for a theory of consent, for the risks can be considerable. The person who makes a wager is, in effect, consenting to allow the other party to keep her money if she loses the wager. There are typically few, if any, requirements with respect to disclosure of information. We allow people to gamble who have no understanding of the actual odds of winning, and whereas we worry as to whether the "therapeutic misconception" (the belief of patient-subjects that treatments and research procedures they receive in randomized clinical trials are aimed at promoting their medical best interests) compromises the validity of consent to research, we do not worry about those who suffer from the "gambler's fallacy" (the belief that the odds for something with a fixed probability increase or decrease depending on recent occurrences—"It's been red four times in a row, so black is more likely to come up now.")

   With respect to competence to gamble, the tests are also quite minimal. There are minimal age requirements, but that's about all. We allow people to make significant wagers—risking their economic well-being—while severely intoxicated. We take no position here as to whether we should regard the intoxicated assumption of risk by gamblers as legally valid or morally permissible. We are simply noting that, as a matter of fact, we impose very low standards for legal if not moral transformation in this context.

Jobs

We allow people to consent to employment under considerable strain and on the basis of relatively little information about the responsibilities and risks involved. Employers do not typically have an obligation to inform prospective employees of the risks of employment. Some such risks are reasonably transparent. People understand that timber cutting, coal mining, and military service (in time of war) are risky, although they may not understand the level of risk or may discount future harms (black lung disease) inappropriately. But some occupational risks are much less transparent. Do 7–11 clerks understand the risks of being victimized by armed robbery?

Of course, morally transformative consent to employment must also be voluntary. Note that we do not say that people are coerced into taking jobs because they would otherwise be poor or unemployed. Moreover, whereas many worry as to whether financial incentives somehow compromise the consent to participate in research, we obviously have no such worries with respect to ordinary employment.

Marriage

The point here is simple. The decision to marry is one of life's momentous choices, but the standards of morally transformative consent are not particularly high. We do set minimal age standards (generally 18), although, as with assent to participation in research, one can marry at a younger age if one's parents consent. More important, one can give legally valid consent to marry on the basis of relatively little information about the other party and with minimal competence to understand the long-term implications of one's decision.

Gifts and Donations

Unlike most other consent contexts, where B believes that a transaction will advance his or her interests, consent also underlies altruistic behavior. We allow people to give small and large amounts of their resources to charity on the basis of very little information. Charities are under no positive obligation to disclose the uses to which their money will be put or their efficacy in using its funds. In addition, we make no effort to assess the competence of the donor. Moreover, we allow the potential recipients of such donations to manipulatively appeal to the emotions of the prospective donors in ways that we would not dream of permitting in other contexts such as medical research.

Medical Care

Here we want to make two points. First, the explicitness of consent to treatment varies considerably with the nature of the treatment and is premised on the assumption that physicians have a fiduciary obligation to promote the interests of their patients. Physicians need not explain the risks and benefits of taking a patient's blood pressure or the insertion of a device into the vagina. It may be thought that in agreeing to be treated by a physician, patients give a form of *ex ante* consent to whatever minimally risky procedures the physician thinks necessary, but that is far from clear. Second, virtually all of the concern with consent to treatment focuses on information rather than voluntariness. In particular, we do not regard the pressure exerted by illness itself as under-mining the voluntariness of the patient's consent to treatment. Here lurks a crucial point about the criteria of moral transformation. Although a patient may face a choice between death and consenting to surgery, we do *not* say that it is impossible to make a morally transformative choice because there is only one reasonable option for the patient to choose. For if we did say that morally transformative consent were impossible under these conditions, then the physician would not be permitted to proceed.

The lack of concern with the pressure exerted by illness is hard although perhaps not impossible to explain on LK/AA. It is relatively easy to explain on FT. On FT, the gunman's proposal ("Your money or your life") robs consent of its transformative power not because the target has only one reasonable alternative, for that is also true in cases of severe illness, but because the gunman unfairly (to say the least!) proposes to violate the target's rights if she does not acquiesce. By contrast, the patient's consent is morally transforma-tive because the physician treats the patient fairly within the framework of B's background conditions even though B has no other reasonable alternatives.

What have We Learned?

We are not attempting to derive an ought from an is. We have seen that—as a factual claim—the practically operative criteria of morally transformative consent vary significantly from context to context. It surely does not follow that the criteria *should* vary in that way. It is theoretically possible that a strong version of LK/AA would be the preferred moral view in all of the contexts we have considered. Possible, but not likely. Even if some revision in our criteria of moral transformation is to be preferred, we should first look for an account of those criteria that can accommodate and justify the differences that we have noted.

We have argued that the CMT for each context of consent must be sensitive to a wide range of moral considerations. From that perspective, there are several reasons to think that LK/AA should be rejected as a general model of moral transformation, although we may want to approximate its demands in some contexts. First, any acceptable moral principle must be responsive to the basic facts about human beings and social life. Our competence, information, and knowledge are always imperfect. Second, we don't want insistence on autonomous authorization to undermine the object of choice. We don't insist on informational disclosure and written consent for sexual relations because, among other things, it would thoroughly distort the activity to which consent is being given. Third, a prospective consenter may have an interest in foregoing information or the effort to understand that information even though it is relevant to the decision at hand. The acquisition and understanding of information is costly in terms of time, mental energy, psychic stress, and money. Moreover, if, as in most cases of medical treatment, a prospective subject can have confidence that the authorized intervention is in her interest, then it is perfectly rational—from her perspective—to think that the benefits from the acquisition of further information and comprehension may not justify the costs of its acquisition or the effort comprehension would require.

Fourth, LK/AA is one-sided insofar as it privileges negative autonomy, that is, protecting people from interventions to which they have not given autonomous authorization. We need a conception of moral transformation that is sensitive to the agent's interest in being able to facilitate interventions she desires even when her decision is less than fully autonomous. To be sure, in some cases, it is reasonable not to worry excessively that we may wrongly preclude a moral transformation. If we do not allow a 14-year-old to render it permissible for a 30-year-old man to have sex with her, no great harm has been done, whereas the costs of wrongly permitting such a transformation can be grave. Other situations are more difficult. Permitting assisted suicide or active euthanasia risks ending the lives of people with reduced cognitive functioning and when their choices, driven by suffering or despair, are not fully autonomous. On the other hand, if we do not permit a person to authorize the removal of life support because we think the decision is not fully autonomous, then we may compel her to live with intolerable suffering.

Or consider consent that is a given under desperate background conditions. Although we may think that we are offering agents protection of their (negative) autonomy when we refuse to treat their consent as transformative, to prohibit them from entering into (otherwise) consensual transactions is to prevent them from moving from a very bad state of affairs to a less (but still) bad state of affairs, and this is inconsistent with the fundamental values that consent is meant to serve. When we evaluate the criteria of moral transformation from the prospective consenter's own perspective, we see that strict adherence to LK/AA does not represent a compelling moral vision.

Finally, the criteria of moral transformation must also reflect the choice among potential decision makers. Someone has to make decisions. If we are worried about B's ability to make an autonomous decision, before we decide that we should not recognize B's consent as morally transformative, we might need to conclude that someone else is better positioned to consent or to refuse to consent on B's behalf. And that will frequently not be so.

The Fair Transaction View

The fair transaction view states that a consent transaction between B and A is morally transformative if B tokens consent under conditions in which A has acted fairly toward B or, in the case of a flawed or unsuccessful consent transaction, that A is permitted to proceed in the absence of B's consent if it is fair for A to do so. On this view, the transformative power of B's consent (or behavior) is a function of the transactional circumstances under which B chooses (including the behavior of A) rather than the specific mental states that characterize or motivate B's choice. Although FT acknowledges that minimal comprehension and intention are necessary for valid consent, it rejects the LK linkage between valid consent and moral transformation. For example, FT maintains that it may be permissible for A to proceed in cases such as *Lawn Blower* or *Department Meeting* where it is arguable that B does not consent to A's doing X (much less give valid consent), so long as A has not unfairly sought to take advantage of B's mistake.

One advantage of the fair transaction approach is that it offers a theoretically attractive unifying account of the various criteria of morally transformative consent—voluntariness, information, and competence—that is consistent with our intuitions about moral transformation across a range of contexts and that avoids some of the difficulties associated with LK/AA. If A threatens to harm B unless B agrees to some transaction or interaction, then A has obviously not acted fairly toward B and thus B's consent token is not morally transformative. If, as a general rule, it is unfair to deceive another in seeking to gain her consent, then the resulting consent is not morally transformative. Interestingly, however, there are cases in which consent *is* morally transformative in the face of deception, and one advantage of FT is that it can explain why that is so. If A and B are negotiating the sale of a home, and A falsely states that he will not pay more than $400,000 (he would actually pay $425,000), then B's consent to sell at $400,000 is morally transformative if, as is commonly thought, fairness in negotiations does not require that one be truthful about one's reservation price.

If outright deception is sometimes compatible with fairness, it is also true that fairness sometimes requires more than nondeception. FT may require that A provide B with certain information if the consent transaction is to be morally transformative. When is that so? If the information is relatively accessible to all, then the consenter has a fair opportunity to make an informed decision at an acceptable cost without the recipient's assistance, whether or not her decision is autonomous. If the information is deeply asymmetrical, as in medical treatment or research or the sale of a house, then fairness may require that the more knowledgeable party make the information available to the less knowledgeable party. Interestingly, there are some contexts of asymmetrical information in which the more knowledgeable party is not required to share his information with the less knowledgeable party and FT may also show why this is so.

> *Art.* A has spent years studying art history. A estimates that a painting owned by B has a market value of $100,000. A offers to buy the painting from B for $50,000. B accepts.

If A has made significant investments in acquiring general knowledge about art and particular information about B's painting, then fairness may not require that he share such information with B and B's consent might be morally transformative even given this asymmetry.

Defects in competence are a bit trickier but here, too, we believe that FT has advantages over LK/AA. There is no large gap between LK/AA and FT with respect to permanent deficiencies in competence. The (relatively) permanent noncompetent are not capable of autonomous authorization and do not have a fair opportunity to avoid transactions that set back their interests. By contrast, LK/AA and FT may have different implications with respect to temporary self-inflicted deficiencies in competence. Recall *Inhibitions.* Although it is arguable that AA must treat intoxication as invalidating consent, the transformative power of B's consent remains an open question on FT. Here we can distinguish FT from a closely related view. On what we will call the *fair opportunity* view, B's consent is morally transformative if B has had a *fair opportunity* (FO) to make an autonomous choice even if B does not use that opportunity to make an autonomous choice. Although FO and FT converge in most cases, we believe that FT is the superior account. On FO, B's consent is clearly morally transformative in *Inhibitions,* given that she had a fair opportunity not to become intoxicated. Even so, it may still be unfair for A to take advantage of B's self-inflicted incompetence, and, if so, B's consent token would not render it morally permissible for A to proceed on FT.

A principal virtue of FT is that it explicitly acknowledges that there are at least two parties to a consensual transaction. It is, of course, important that B is able to make a decision that reflects her preferences and aims. But it is also of moral importance that A is able to know whether he can proceed with the transaction or interaction. Fairness is bilateral. It's not so much that B must be fair to A, although that is true. Rather, it is crucial that the moral and legal regime in which transactions occur must be fair to A in determining whether it is permissible for him to proceed given B's token of consent.

Consider the problem of mistakes again.

> *Rock Star.* B consents to sexual relations with A because she believes A to be a rock star, although A has made no such representation and has no reason to think that this is what motivates B's consent.

Assuming that A has acted in good faith, it would be unfair to A to refuse to treat B's consent token as morally transformative. On the other hand—and this is worth stressing—if A believes that B consents to sex with him because she confuses him with a rock star, then A has not acted fairly toward B and we think it is not *morally* permissible for him to proceed, although we might also endorse a legal regime in which A would not be guilty of a crime.

Another advantage of FT is that it also accommodates cases in which B's background conditions or circumstances are unfair or desperate, but where A has acted fairly toward B within the framework of those conditions. Some have analogized desperate background conditions to coercion and thus think this establishes that such consent is not transformative. But if we are careful to analogize such pressures to *third-party* coercion, we think the analogy may work but that it does not support the supposed conclusion.

> *Pimp.* C tells B that he will beat her up unless she earns $500 this evening. B proposes to A that they have sexual relations for $100. A accepts.

Now whatever else we might want to say about prostitution, the present question is whether B's consent is morally transformative. Has A engaged in "nonconsensual" sexual relations with B? It might be thought that B's consent *cannot* be transformative if B is coerced into having sex, but that seems much too quick. The standard cases of coercion are those in which the coercer is also the recipient of consent. Here, B is coerced by C, not A, and whatever else we might think of A, we do not think A is guilty of rape. Here the difference between FT and FO reappears. Although B does not have a fair opportunity to avoid transacting with A, FT's conception of fairness is *bilateral* or transaction specific, not global. And in the small corner of the world in which A and B transact, there is no reason to assume that A has treated B unfairly. Indeed, there is no reason to think that *B* thinks that A has treated B unfairly. After all, B solicits A. It might be objected that the transformative power of B's consent turns on whether A knows (or should believe) that B is coerced by C. We think not. Given B's objective condition—that she will be beaten by C if she does not earn enough—B wants A to accept her proposal. Now we might well say that A should reject B's proposal because acceptance would make him *complicit* in C's coercion of B and, perhaps, because it gives the pimps of the world more reason to engage in such coercion. But even if that is so, B's consent remains morally transformative in the case at hand. If we are right about this case, it is difficult to see how the moral transformation can be explained in terms of AA.

If third-party coercion (as between C and B) does not necessarily negate the transformative power of B's consent, then, *a fortiori*, the general background unfairness of B's situation does not necessarily undermine the transformative power of B's consent. Consider the following cases.

> *Unjust Firing.* C has unjustly fired B from her previous job as a well-paid lawyer. B accepts A's offer to teach business law at the local community college at a much lower salary than she had been receiving.

> *Battery.* C has intentionally injured B. B seeks medical care from A and authorizes A to perform a procedure and agrees to pay A's fee.

In these cases, B would not transact with A but for her unfair and pressing circumstances. Nonetheless, her consent to take a job or to authorize A to perform a medical procedure (for a fee) is morally transformative. Why? Because A has acted fairly toward B within the framework of those unfair conditions. To regard B's consent as not transformative is doubly unfair. It is unfair to A, assuming that A has no obligation to rectify conditions for which he is not responsible. Moreover, to regard B's consent as not transformative is unfair to B. If we say that B can give valid morally transformative consent only when her background conditions are "globally" fair, then to treat B's consent as nontransformative is to deprive B of the opportunity to improve her condition by transacting with A.

We have argued that FT provides an attractive and reasonably comprehensive explanation of moral transformation across a range of contexts. We have not attempted to justify FT from the ground up, as it were. The criteria of morally transformative consent are the output of moral theorizing. Consequently, the question as to whether LK/AA or FT or some other view provides the best account of moral transformation will depend on the question as to what constitutes the best moral theory. Not surprisingly, we hardly have the answer to that question. Nonetheless, we believe that FT is attractive on its face, is compatible with our intuitions, and is also consistent with two major nonconsequentialist approaches to moral theory that might be used to generate a theory of consent, and this gives us more confidence that we are on the right track. Although the consideration of these nonconsequentialist theories does not constitute a positive argument for FT, we would have less confidence in FT if it were clearly incompatible with a plausible moral theory. We think it is not.

Why *non*consequentialist? If consequentialism is the right moral view, then the correct view about morally transformative consent is, in principle, an empirical matter: What view of moral transformation has the best consequences? A consequentialist outlook would no doubt require some stable and predictable criteria by which the parties (and others) can judge whether a transaction is morally transformative. The precise content of that regime is up for grabs, although we suspect that regime would be closer to FT than to LK/AA, particularly given that FT is more concerned with the welfare-advancing value of consent.

If we set consequentialism aside, we can first note that FT is consistent with a deontological commitment to respect for persons and autonomy. It might be thought that a Kantian version of a deontological approach would require autonomous authorization for moral transformation. We think not. We show respect by refusing to hold persons accountable for choices that they did not have a fair opportunity to avoid, but we also show respect for them— including their choice to decide carelessly or imprudently—when we hold people responsible for those choices made under reasonably favorable conditions. Moreover, A does not violate the deontological principle that one should not treat another merely as a means when A responds to what she— in good faith—regards as B's autonomous consent, even when she is mistaken about this. In addition, a deontological commitment to respect for persons would have to be sensitive to the rights and obligations of *both* parties to a consent transaction, and this tells in favor of FT. After all, deontologists cannot be silent as to whether A acts wrongly in *Lawn Blower*.

One could also argue for FT from a contractualist perspective. Along Rawlsian lines, we could think of the criteria of moral transformation as those that individuals would chose *ex ante* in an original position from behind the veil of ignorance, where the criteria they choose would have to take account of cases involving less than fully autonomous decisions, failed consent transactions, and the like. From that perspective, it is more likely that they would opt for a perspective that is sensitive to the interests of *both* parties to a consent transaction rather than focusing exclusively on the authenticity of the consenter's decision. T.M. Scanlon's version of contractualism argues that we can think of the principles of morality as those that "no one could reasonably reject as a basis for informed, unforced general agreement."[7] Although Scanlon does not endorse FT in so many words, he specifically rejects what he calls the "quality of will" approach that underlies LK/AA. Rather, "the fact that an outcome resulted from a person's choice under good conditions shows that he was given the choice and provided with good conditions for making it, and it is these facts which make it the case that he alone is responsible."[8] And so a consideration of contractualism gives us no reason to think we are on the wrong track. In sum, although we have not argued that these various nonconsequentialist theories would support FT over AA/LK, we believe we have shown that FT is not obviously problematic from those perspectives.[9]

Validity, Permissibility, and Moral Transformation

We have suggested that FT holds that a consent transaction can be morally transformative even if B does not intend to give consent at all or is mistaken as to what she is consenting. Recall *Department Meeting*. If B is completely unaware that his silence is generally understood as indicating agreement to A's proposal, it is difficult to claim that B is actually consenting to A's proposal, much less that B gives valid consent. Nonetheless, on the assumption that it is reasonable for others to construe B's silence as a token of consent, it is arguably reasonable for A to proceed and to let the burden of B's daydreaming fall on B rather than A. If, however, A is aware that B is likely to reject his proposal and is attempting to take advantage of B's propensity to daydream, then it is arguable that it is not justifiable for A to proceed. FT seems to give the right answer.

Monica Cowart would disagree. Cowart argues that a "speech act" analysis of consent can help to resolve moral disputes about consent. And, she suggests, "Consenting can only occur if both participants in the conversation understand what X is. When [A] proposes X to [B], [A] must have the same understanding as [B] of what X is."[10] We have two responses. First, and as a matter of ordinary expression, we believe that people can say that they unwittingly consented to X: "I didn't think I was agreeing to let you take my lawn blower, but I guess I did. My error." Second, and more important, the speech act analysis does nothing to resolve the moral issue. Assuming for the sake of argument that B has not consented to A's taking her lawn blower, we still have to decide whether A has acted unjustifiably or impermissibly. And it seems highly dubious to insist that A has acted wrongly when he innocently acts on what he reasonably believes is B's consent.

Interestingly, although FT holds that it may be permissible for A to proceed even though B has not given valid (AA) consent, it also holds that it may sometimes be *im*permissible for A to proceed to do X even though B *has* given valid AA consent to A's doing X. Consider the following case.

> *Nondisclosure.* A intentionally fails to disclose information about the risks of a surgical procedure because he fears that B will wrongly overestimate the importance of those risks. Unbeknownst to A, B has consulted with another physician and has a full grasp of the risks. B signs the consent form because she wants A to perform the surgery.

Because A has not treated B fairly and because A does not *know* that B's consent is fully informed, we believe that A is not permitted to proceed even though B's consent is fully informed and thus compatible with LK/AA. Once again, this case demonstrates that B's mental state is not the key to morally transformative consent: The consent transaction between A and B must be fair.

To see how moral transformation does not always track valid consent, consider the table below, which includes two cases we have discussed and two additional cases.

> *Business Bluffing.* A tells B that he will not accept less than $25,000 for the car that B wishes to purchase. A is actually prepared to accept $24,000. B agrees to pay $25,000.

> *MRI.* B has been experiencing back pain. A (B's physician) recommends an MRI because he profits from each procedure. A does not actually believe that an MRI is necessary. B agrees to have an MRI.

	Valid Consent	Moral Transformation
Business Bluffing	(?)	Y
MRI	N	N
Lawn Blower	N	Y
Nondisclosure	Y	N

In *Lawn Blower*, we have moral transformation without valid consent. In *Nondisclosure*, we have valid consent without moral transformation. The table also illustrates the contextual nature of moral transformation. *Business Bluffing* is a tricky case on LK/AA, because it is not clear whether B's consent is valid. Nonetheless, it seems that the deception in *Business Bluffing* is compatible with moral transformation, whereas this is not the case in *MRI* because this sort of deception is arguably fair in business but not in medicine. The main point is that the moral transformation column is the site of the important moral action, not the valid consent column.

Now, in saying that it is permissible for A to proceed in cases of "mistaken" (or non-) consent, such as *Lawn Blower* and *Department Meeting*, it may be argued that we have confused two claims: (1) A is justified in proceeding and (2) A is not justified in taking B's lawn blower (without B's valid consent), but A's action can be *excused*, given that A has a reasonable belief that B has given consent. Although we think that (1) is more accurate, we do not think much turns on the distinction between (1) *excuse* and (2) *justification* in the present context. If, as seems evident, the truth of (2) turns on the *reasonableness* of A's belief rather than the belief itself, then we are making a decidedly moral judgment about the propriety of A's action in (2) as well as (1). This is, perhaps, clearer in *Department Meeting*. There it seems odd to say that A is not justified in proceeding (given that B was simply daydreaming) but that he is excused. If we are correct that A is permitted to proceed in *Lawn Blower* and *Department Meeting*, then the interesting theoretical conclusion follows that valid consent is not a necessary condition for moral transformation. Likewise, our account of *Nondisclosure* suggests that valid consent is not sufficient for moral transformation. Rather, we need to focus on the fairness of the bilateral consent transaction.

We have argued that whereas a morally transformative consent transaction is typically triggered by valid consent, it is the moral transformation that matters ultimately, not the presence of valid consent. Does this mean that the canon should be revised? Does this mean that we should remove "informed consent" as a requirement of ethical medicine and research and put moral transformation in its place? We think not. Although we think the deeper ethical truth is that it is moral transformation that matters, the framework of valid consent or informed consent (where that is the coin of the realm) is well entrenched and serves the relevant values reasonably well. We do not seek to be linguistic reformers. We aim to develop a theory that can help us resolve the difficult questions about consent.

Two Applications

Although developing and applying FT is a long-term project, here we want to sketch how it can shed light on two controversies—a practical controversy relating to research ethics and a theoretical controversy relating to the relationship between exploitation and morally transformative consent.

Therapeutic Misconception

As we noted above, bioethicists have debated whether a participant can give valid informed consent if he or she is in the grips of a therapeutic misconception (TM) and thereby confuses personalized medical care with participation in a randomized clinical trial. (See Chapter 15 for an extended discussion of the therapeutic misconception.) On our view, the question is not whether participants can give "valid consent" if they are in the grip of TM, but whether they can give morally transformative consent.

Our view should now be clear, as should the relevance of our discussion of mistakes, such as *Lawn Blower*. Although bioethicists seem to treat the therapeutic misconception as an issue that is special to research, the failure to comprehend the content or meaning of a transaction is a potential problem for a wide range of consent contexts. FT provides an attractive solution. In some cases, such as *Lawn Blower*, A is probably not obligated to do more than speak clearly. In the case of clinical research, FT would endorse an affirmative obligation of investigators to disclose pertinent information to prospective subjects, because the asymmetry of information about risks and benefits makes it fairer to assign the informational burden to investigators than to prospective subjects. Still, and as in *Lawn Blower*, FT does not require comprehension as a sine qua non of moral transformation, even in medical research. First, any observation of the subject or test of comprehension will not be fail-safe. Second, and more important, even if prospective subjects comprehended the information on a cognitive level, they may fail to appreciate its meaning for them. Denial and (excessive) optimism can be powerful forces.

Consider LK/AA from the subjects' perspective. Somewhat ironically, a requirement of comprehension places a greater burden on subjects than they may reasonably desire. The comprehension requirement unduly restricts the freedom of choice of prospective subjects when research offers them a personally favorable risk–benefit ratio or presents no more than minimal risks. A stringent comprehension requirement would exclude people who do not comprehend accurately what research participation involves even though they have had a fair opportunity to understand.

We also worry that LK/AA would place excessive obligations on researchers. FT may well require that investigators take affirmative steps to counteract therapeutic misconceptions by clarifying the differences between research participation and medical care in their disclosures to prospective subjects, by avoiding language that conflates these two activities, by taking appropriate steps to ascertain whether key features of the research have been understood, and perhaps by signaling the distinction between research by paying patient-subjects (at least) a nominal fee for volunteering as a symbol that they are undertaking an activity different from medical care (in which the patient pays the doctor). All that is fair. But while the steps required by FT may be rather extensive, they do not go so far as to require that the information actually is understood. To require comprehension is not only impossible and impractical but also unfair.

Exploitation

The FT model gives rise to the following theoretical question: If a transaction is morally transformative only if A treats B fairly, can B give morally transformative consent to a transaction in which A exploits B? Let us set aside those cases of patently nonconsensual exploitation in which A coerces or deceives B or in which B is suffering from a deficiency of information or competence. Rather, we focus on cases where consent seems to be morally transformative *apart* from worries about exploitation.

> *Rescue.* B's car slides off a snow-covered road into a ditch late at night. A comes by and proposes to pull B out for $200 with his four-wheel-drive pick-up truck and a chain and says it will take 5 minutes. B believes that it would be hours before another person were to come by or before AAA could help. B agrees to pay.

In an earlier work, one of the authors describes this as a case of consensual and mutually advantageous exploitation.[11] It is consensual because there is a consent token, because B understands that to which she is consenting, and because it is rational for B to consent. Moreover, A's proposal is not coercive because A does not propose to violate B's rights if she declines (assuming that he has no obligation to help). It is true that B may feel that she has no other option but to accept A's proposal, but, as we have argued, that is no more true in this case than if B consented to surgery in order to avoid death, and we have established that such consent is not coerced.

The transaction is mutually advantageous because it is better for B to be rescued for $200 than not to be rescued at all.

Now determining whether a transaction constitutes exploitation is more difficult than is often supposed. If an entrepreneurial A roams the highway every night, offering his services to those in distress, $200 may not be excessive.

For all we know, his average pay may be less than $25 per hour. But if A is an opportunistic passerby in *Rescue,* then we believe this is a paradigm case of wrongful exploitation.

But is B's consent morally transformative? Does it render A's action permissible? On LK/AA, the transformative quality of B's consent *cannot* turn on whether the transaction is exploitative. To see why, suppose, on the one hand, that AA holds that B's decision satisfies the mental state conditions for AA consent because B's plight is a "background circumstance" for which A bears no responsibility. Faden and Beauchamp would say that B does not act freely, because she may have "no meaningful choice," but they quickly add that "this loss of freedom cannot be equated with a loss of autonomy."[12] If so, B's consent in *Rescue* is morally transformative on AA, the exploitation notwithstanding. On the other hand, if the pressures of background circumstances undermine the transformative quality of B's consent on AA, then this cannot turn on whether A's proposal is *exploitative.* Whether A proposes to rescue B for $5 or $200, B's background circumstances are such that she has no alternative but to pay. In either case, the exploitativeness of the transaction has no bearing on whether B's consent is morally transformative.

Things are different with FT. If we examine *Rescue* through the lens of FT, it would seem that B's consent is not morally transformative given that A has not treated B fairly. But that might be too quick. The case may involve multiple moral transformations. Consider two questions: (*1*) Does B's consent give A permission to tow B's car? (*2*) If B promises to pay A $200, is B obligated to pay the full amount? We believe that the answer to (*1*) may be yes, but that the answer to (*2*) may be no. Assuming that this is right, it is not clear why this is so. We might distinguish between procedural fairness and substantive fairness. It may turn out that procedural fairness is sufficient to render it permissible for A to proceed (tow the car) but that it is not sufficient to generate an obligation for B. For that, something like substantive fairness may be required. As we said, this is a *preface* to a theory of consent transactions. Details will have to wait.

Conclusion

The development of the fair transaction model of consent has been motivated by two considerations: (*1*) there are cases of flawed consent transactions in which it is reasonable to judge that moral transformation has occurred without valid consent and (*2*) there are areas of conduct in which widely accepted standards of morally transformative consent do not appear to conform with autonomous authorization. On our view, this makes the prevailing LK/AA model deficient as a theory of consent. By contrast, we have argued that FT can accommodate both (1) and (2). Typically, moral transformation will depend on valid consent; however, we have argued that it is unfair to recipients of consent to insist that moral transformation *always* depends on valid consent. More important, in view of the values served by consent, it is unfair to consenters to insist on autonomous authorization as necessary to effect moral transformation. In sum, the FT model has the merit of emphasizing the bilateral nature of consent transactions (in contrast to the emphasis on the mental state of the consenter in the prevailing model), and it gives due recognition to individuals' interest in facilitating cooperative activities by consent tokens that fall short of robust AA.

Notes

1. Ruth Faden and Tom Beauchamp, *A History and Theory of Informed Consent* (New York: Oxford University Press, 1986).
2. T.M. Scanlon, "The Significance of Choice," in *Tanner Lectures on Human Values* Vol. 8 (Salt Lake City, UT: University of Utah Press, 1989).
3. Allen Buchanan and Dan Brock, *Deciding for Others* (Cambridge, MA: Cambridge University Press, 1989), 37.
4. See Chapter 11 for a discussion of tacit consent and political obligation.
5. Peter Westen, *The Logic of Consent* (Burlington, VT: Ashgate Publishing Co, 2004).
6. Many of these cases are borrowed from Alan Wertheimer, *Consent to Sexual Relations* (Cambridge, MA: Cambridge University Press, 2003).
7. T.M. Scanlon, *What We Owe to Each Other* (Cambridge, MA: Harvard University Press, 1998).
8. Ibid., 184.
9. We thank Connie Rosati for helping us to formulate this point.
10. Monica Cowart, "Understanding Acts of Consent: Using Speech Act Theory to Help Resolve Moral Dilemmas and Legal Disputes," *Law and Philosophy* 23 (2004): 495–525, 509.
11. Alan Wertheimer, *Exploitation* (Princeton, NJ: Princeton University Press, 1996).
12. Faden and Beauchamp, *History and Theory,* p. 345.

5

Paternalism and Consent

Douglas Husak[*]

A Relatively Clear Case

I begin with an ordinary, everyday example from which I hope to generalize about the justifiability of paternalism and, to a lesser extent, about the difficulties of justifying paternalism in the criminal law. When permitted to eat anything he chooses, 4-year-old Billy skips his vegetables altogether and eats only his ice cream dessert. His father has tried to explain the reasons to eat a balanced diet, but Billy is unmoved, and has not changed his behavior. Suppose his father comes to you for advice about what to do at their next dinner. I stipulate that the father's only reason for seeking advice is to improve Billy's health and welfare by ensuring that he eats a more nutritious meal than if left to his own devices. It seems reasonable for you to recommend that Billy not be permitted to eat his ice cream unless and until he finishes his

[*] I would like to thank participants at the Criminal Theory Workshop at the International Congress of Political and Legal Philosophy at Krakow, Poland. I also received valuable help from members of the Department of Philosophy at Virginia Commonwealth University as well as from members of an NIH seminar at Georgetown University. Special thanks to Youngjae Lee, Frank Miller, Alec Walen, Peter Westen, and Alan Wertheimer, each of whom provided detailed written assistance on earlier drafts.

vegetables. Suppose his father decides to follow your advice. This example not only describes a situation in which Billy is treated paternalistically but also represents a relatively clear case in which the paternalistic treatment is justified.[1] In any event, I make these two assumptions about this case.

I stipulate that the father's only reason for withholding ice cream is to improve Billy's health and welfare because I construe paternalism to be a function of the *motives* for interfering in the liberty of another. Paternalism should not be defined in terms of its beneficial effects or consequences, but rather in terms of the reasons for which it is imposed. His father acts paternalistically even if he unwittingly worsens Billy's health or welfare. Because of this feature in my understanding of paternalism, few rules or laws are unambiguously paternalistic—that is, *purely* paternalistic.[2] Most (and perhaps all) rules or laws are promulgated by authorities or legislators whose motives for enacting the rule or law are a mixture of paternalistic and nonpaternalistic motivations. Laws requiring the wearing of seat belts, for example, probably are designed both to minimize the severity of automobile accidents and to reduce the insurance costs to all drivers. The case I have described, however, is a good candidate for an example of pure paternalism. It is hard to see what other reason his father might have for withholding ice cream from Billy. In any event, I stipulate that his only motive is paternalistic.

Why might you offer the aforementioned advice? Five criteria conspire to make this example a relatively clear case of justified paternalism. *First*, the intrusion is a fairly minor interference in Billy's liberty—as minimally intrusive as can be imagined to accomplish its objective. Billy is not beaten or deprived of something of great significance to induce him to change his behavior. *Second*, the objective sought by his father is obviously valuable. No one contests the importance of health. *Third*, the means chosen are likely to promote this objective. If Billy's desire for ice cream is sufficiently strong, he is likely to alter his behavior and eat his vegetables. And any competent nutritionist agrees that vegetables are an essential part of a healthy diet—more essential than ice cream. *Fourth*, Billy himself is not in a favorable position to make the right decision. Children have notorious cognitive and volitional deficiencies relative to competent adults that prevent them from recognizing their best interests, or from acting appropriately even when they do. *Fifth*, his father stands in an ideal relationship to Billy to treat him paternalistically. Parents have special duties to protect and enhance the welfare of their children. I believe that my example satisfies each of these five criteria.

If I have misapplied any of these conditions, I would have to withdraw my claim that Billy's case represents a clear instance of justified paternalism. Since I have a few reservations, I describe this case as *relatively* clear. It is surprisingly difficult to find uncontroversial examples of justified paternalism. In particular, the application of the third criterion to my case might be contested. Among other difficulties, the father's plan may backfire. Arguably, the paternalistic treatment to which children like Billy are subjected may induce them to eat more poorly in the long run, when they no longer remain under parental supervision. Applying criteria of when paternalism is justified will always raise controversies, some of which involve disputes about matters of fact. My main focus, however, is on the criteria themselves. With only a bit of ingenuity, I believe that most and perhaps all questions about the justifiability of any paternalistic interference can be raised within the parameters of these five criteria.

Four comments about these criteria are worth making. First, there are potential difficulties with my strategy of beginning with a relatively easy case, identifying what is easy about it, and applying these criteria to other examples. In particular, each of my criteria may not need to be satisfied to justify an instance of paternalism. Why, for example, must the subject be less than fully competent? Doesn't this criterion automatically preclude what Joel Feinberg calls "hard paternalism"?[3] In order to avoid such questions, I do not insist that these criteria must be satisfied before an instance of paternalism is justified. Instead, each criterion merely contributes to the judgment that a case is easy. Whatever else may be said about instances of hard paternalism, they surely are more difficult to justify than cases of paternalism in which the subject is less than fully competent. I take no firm position on what we should ultimately say about a case in which it is dubious whether one or more of these conditions are satisfied. I hold only that it progressively becomes less clearly justified, and eventually is clearly unjustified.

Second, conditions one and three are the most important of several reasons why *criminal* paternalism is so difficult to justify. Consider the first condition. A paternalistic interference becomes harder to defend when the means required to attain its objective involve a greater hardship or deprivation of liberty. The criminal law, by definition, subjects persons to state *punishment.* If the state must punish someone to protect his interests and well-being, we have reason to suspect that the cure is worse than the disease. It may be bad for persons to use drugs, for example, but it may be even worse to punish them to try to get them to stop. When punishments are severe, their gains typically will not be worth their costs for the persons on whom they are inflicted. But when punishments are not severe, they rarely will create adequate incentives for compliance and thus will fail to improve the behavior of the persons coerced. An acceptable set of constraints to limit the imposition of the criminal sanction will require that criminal laws must be reasonably

effective in attaining their objectives.[4] A criminal law motivated by a paternalistic end will fail to satisfy this condition if it does not alter conduct or
actually makes the subject worse off, all things considered. I doubt that
paternalistic reasons will justify state punishment in more than a handful of
cases.

Criminal paternalism also is jeopardized by the third condition. To be
justified qua paternalism, the interference must actually benefit the person
coerced. Laws are general, however, and apply to a great many persons in a
variety of circumstances. Statutes requiring persons to buckle their seat belts
or activate their air bags, for example, protect the vast majority of drivers, but
actually increase the risk of harm for a minority. Persons who plunge into
water, for example, are more likely to drown if they are wearing seat belts.
In addition, drivers who are unusually short are much more likely to be
injured by air bags than persons whose height is close to average. In principle,
of course, criminal laws can create exceptions for given kinds of circumstances, either by allowing a defense or by including an exceptive clause in the
offense itself. In practice, however, it is nearly inevitable that rules will be
overinclusive and persons will be criminally liable despite the fact that they act
in circumstances in which compliance with the law would not have benefited
them. In a one-on-one confrontation, such as that involving Billy and his
father, we need be less worried that the generality of a rule motivated by a
paternalistic objective will actually operate to the detriment of some of the
persons coerced.

Third, most proposals to treat competent adults paternalistically are
rendered problematic by the fourth criterion. A diet consisting solely of ice
cream is probably no less unhealthy for middle-age individuals than for Billy,
but sane adults rarely suffer from the deficiencies of typical 4-year-olds.
Of course, age is simply a crude proxy for what is relevant: the state of
cognitive and volitional capacities characteristic of sane adults. An adult
who is cognitively and volitionally comparable to a child is an equally
plausible candidate for paternalistic intervention. Unfortunately, some such
adults exist. Thus, I see no reason to suppose that the paternalistic treatment
of adults is never permissible.

Fourth, the final criterion is the most questionable in the set. Suppose
that someone who does not stand in a special relationship to Billy has an
opportunity to treat him in exactly the same way for exactly the same reason as
his father, withholding ice cream until he finishes his vegetables in order to
enhance his health by improving his diet. May he do so as well? We might
disapprove of his tendency to meddle, but should we conclude that his
interference would be unjustified? In a genuine emergency, I am sure that

the fifth condition becomes totally irrelevant. If a child is playing in the road in the path of an oncoming bus, the identity of the person who snatches him away is immaterial. But what should we say about less extreme cases, like that of Billy? I am unsure how this question should be answered, and it provides the main basis for the misgiving I will express near the end of this chapter. In any event, the importance of the remaining criteria seems more secure. Suppose that the child is quite a bit older and more competent, the end that is sought is less clearly valuable than health, the interference is less likely to attain its objective, and/or the means employed involve a greater deprivation of liberty. For example, 13-year-old Jimmy might be prevented from playing with his friends until he finishes practicing the bassoon. Clearly, this instance of paternalism is far more difficult to justify. As these examples suggest, each of these criteria involves a matter of degree. As I have indicated, at some point on a continuum what is otherwise a clear case of justified paternalism becomes less clear, and eventually is not justified at all. Reasonable minds will differ about the precise point along this spectrum—or, indeed, along the several spectra—at which a particular instance of paternalism crosses this elusive threshold and becomes unjustified.

The foregoing is helpful in introducing my central thesis. Suppose we are given one additional piece of information about the ordinary, everyday case of justified paternalism with which I began. Imagine we are told that Billy does not consent to the treatment I have proposed. He strongly objects to what his father does, and protests loudly when his ice cream is withheld until he finishes his vegetables. I trust that no one who agreed with my initial verdict about this case would change his opinion in light of this new information. In fact, it seems odd to describe this piece of information as *new*; most readers would have assumed it to be true in their initial reflections about the case. In any event, it would be remarkable to suppose that Billy's lack of consent to his treatment is material to whether the act of paternalism is justified. When one person *A* treats another person *B* paternalistically and is justified in so doing, *B's* lack of consent is irrelevant. Much of the point of the example is to show that his father is justified in treating Billy paternalistically, even though his son does not consent to being treated in this way.

In fact, Billy's consent almost certainly would entail that the case no longer qualifies as an example of paternalism at all, quite apart from whether it is justified.[5] Suppose his father threatens to withhold ice cream, and Billy, an exceptionally precocious child, replies that the threat is unnecessary to ensure his compliance. His past behavior notwithstanding, he now has come to understand the importance of health and the instrumental value of a good diet. He resolves not to eat his dessert before finishing his vegetables, and proceeds to act accordingly. In such an event, I would say that his father threatened to treat Billy paternalistically, but did not actually have to do so, since Billy complied without the need for interference—that is, without the need for his father to make good his threat.[6] Billy has been persuaded, not coerced. The clearest cases of paternalism involve *coercion,* or an *interference* with liberty.[7] If I am correct, persons are not treated paternalistically when they consent to their treatment.

But not all cases are clear, and philosophers have challenged my claim that paternalism involves an interference in liberty and that the absence of consent is irrelevant to its justification. Much of this paper is designed to respond to this challenge. So-called *libertarian paternalism* poses a possible complication for my claim that paternalism involves an interference in liberty.[8] Libertarian paternalism works primarily by designing default rules to correct for well-known cognitive biases and volitional lapses, thereby minimizing the likelihood that persons will make decisions that are contrary to their own interest. Consider the following two examples. Rather than explicitly choosing to participate in an efficient company health plan, employees might be enrolled automatically unless they opt out. Seat belts might be constructed to buckle immediately upon closing a car door, although occupants would be able to unbuckle them if they chose to do so.[9] Might consent be crucial to the justification of libertarian paternalism? Perhaps. But are these provisions really paternalistic? If persons can change the impact of these rules, it is doubtful we should say that an *interference* with choice has occurred. Notice that it might be true that individuals "can" alter the default rule in two senses. First, persons who elect not to participate in the company health plan face no legal penalty. Second, opting out is not onerous, requiring a mere stroke of a pen or click of a switch. When these two conditions are satisfied, it seems more appropriate to construe these rules as designed merely to *influence* persons to pursue their self-interest.[10]

Admittedly, some provisions appear paternalistic even though they actually expand choice. The Federal Trade Commission, for example, mandates a 3-day cooling-off period for door-to-door sales. It seems facetious to characterize this rule as interfering with the options of a buyer—unless we suppose that the state has interfered with his choice to make a spontaneous purchase that is irrevocable.[11] Instead of construing these provisions as paternalistic, I believe they are better understood as assisting persons in satisfying their preferences rather than as interfering with their liberty. But I do not *insist* that any of these devices cannot be conceptualized as paternalistic; they embody what might be called the *spirit* of paternalism. When the effort required to change the operation of a default rule becomes overly burdensome—

involving reams of paperwork, for example—we may be tempted to think that an interference with choice has taken place. I see no reason to suppose that there always must be a "right answer" to how paternalism should be defined, or how the definition should be applied to particular examples. Apart from my claim that the presence of consent would disqualify the case as an instance of paternalism, I make little further effort to offer a definition. At some point or another, theorists must resort to stipulation, and further quibbles about the exact nature of paternalism become fruitless. I hope my failure to provide a precise definition does not undermine any of the points I will defend. What is controversial is whether and how any or all of these devices can be justified, not whether they "really" qualify as instances of paternalism.

On the topic of paternalism and consent, I believe that not much more needs to be said. Although many difficult questions surround consent— whether it is a mental state or a performative, under what conditions it is voluntary, whether it should be a defense for serious inflictions of injury, and the like—none of these issues need concern the paternalist.[12] Hard cases notwithstanding, lack of consent on the part of the person treated paternalistically simply is not relevant to whether the interference is justified.[13] If all cases were as clear as my example of Billy and his father, the topic of paternalism and consent would be straightforward and uninteresting.

Alas, matters are not so simple. Consent seemingly becomes controversial in justifying paternalism because many examples deviate from the ordinary case I have described. In the kinds of cases I will discuss, consent to a given treatment is *noncontemporaneous;* that is, consent is withheld at the moment the paternalistic treatment takes place, even though it is given at some other time. Despite the complexities about noncontemporaneous consent I will examine, however, I believe that my thesis remains basically correct: The absence of consent is irrelevant to whether a case of paternalism is justified. I will, however, express a misgiving about my thesis—a misgiving that leads me to describe my thesis as tentative. If consent is relevant to whether paternalism is justified, it is material to my fifth and final criterion: to the issue of *who* is entitled to treat another paternalistically. Ultimately, however, I am unsure whether this fifth criterion should be retained.

Apart from my reservation, it might be thought that consent is implicitly involved in the preceding case after all. I have simply assumed that his father is justified in treating Billy paternalistically. Even if my assumption is granted, we still may disagree about *why* his action is justified. According to Gerald Dworkin's pioneering article, consent plays a crucial role in answering this question. He alleges that what he calls "future-oriented consent" is the key to justifying paternalism. Dworkin writes: "Paternalism may be thought of as a wager by the parent on the child's subsequent recognition of the wisdom of the restrictions. There is an emphasis on what could be called future-oriented consent—on what the child will come to welcome rather than on what he does welcome."[14] Dworkin's proposal, as I construe it, is that the paternalistic intervention is justified if Billy subsequently comes to appreciate it, but is unjustified if he does not. If Dworkin is correct, my stipulation that the father is justified in withholding ice cream implies that Billy eventually will consent to the restriction.

Elsewhere, I have contended that this rationale fails for two related but distinct reasons.[15] First, criteria are needed to justify paternalism *ex ante*, when the parent must decide whether to impose it. We do not offer helpful advice to Billy's father if we inform him that no one can tell whether his proposed interference is justified until some future moment when Billy will decide whether or not to welcome what his father once did. And which of several possible future moments should we privilege? Billy may *vacillate*, changing his mind throughout his lifetime.[16] He might resist the interference for a short while, welcome it subsequently, only to resent it again later. As this possibility suggests, the fundamental problem with Dworkin's proposal is that Billy's *ex post* opinion is irrelevant to whether his father is justified—even if we could accurately predict Billy's *ex post* judgment *ex ante*. We should not conclude that his father is unjustified in treating Billy paternalistically simply because Billy never actually consents. Billy may fail to appreciate the wisdom of the restriction because he grows up to be stubborn or stupid, or—in the most extreme case—because he does not grow up at all. Suppose that Billy is hit by a bus and killed before he is old enough to assess his father's decision. Surely we should not conclude that his father's treatment was unjustified. The decision was justified *whatever* may happen to Billy at a later time.

A third difficulty is that Dworkin is not really talking about consent at all. It is unlikely that consent *can* be retrospective.[17] Even if consent can be retrospective in some unusual circumstances, I certainly do not consent to everything I subsequently come to welcome. Often I am in a better position to assess how events affect my welfare long after they occur, but this superior perspective should not be mistaken for consent if I later come to realize that the treatment I disliked at the time operated to my benefit. Suppose my wife runs off with another man and breaks my heart, and the details of how our property is to be divided depend on whether I consented to the separation. Suppose further that I find and marry a woman I adore even more, and come to believe that I never really loved my first wife at all. Someone would seemingly rewrite history if he claimed that I now consent to having been abandoned. I would agree that my first wife did me a favor by leaving me, even though I did not realize it at the time. But I would not say that I consented to her departure. Surely my first wife could not argue that I gave my future-oriented consent to the separation, so our property should be divided accordingly.

If consent ("future-oriented" or otherwise) does not justify his father's treatment of Billy, what does? In my view, paternalism is justified when it is reasonable, and the father must make a judgment of whether his restriction qualifies.[18] Obviously, no formula will govern determinations of reasonableness. But when each of the five criteria I have described is satisfied to a significant degree, I believe that paternalism will clearly be justified. In other words, paternalism is justified when it is reasonable, and the criteria I have provided will help us decide when this is so. Of course, some contractarians explicate reasonableness in terms of hypothetical consent. What is reasonable *is* what rational persons would agree to under appropriate conditions of choice. I need not try to dissuade these philosophers. Perhaps rational persons under appropriate conditions of choice would agree that paternalism is justified when each of my five criteria is satisfied to a significant degree. In any event, hypothetical consent simply is not *actual* consent, and my conclusion is that the latter, whenever conveyed, is irrelevant to the justifiability of paternalism.

Prior Consent: Self-Exclusion Programs

It would be hasty, however, to conclude that the absence of consent never is relevant to any determinations of whether paternalism is justified. In an interesting subset of cases, the justification of paternalism *seems* to originate in the actual consent of the very subject treated paternalistically. Despite the consent of the person whose liberty is infringed, these cases still seem to qualify as genuine instances of paternalism. In the kinds of cases I have in mind, consent is real and given *ex ante*, not hypothetical or given *ex post*. Describing and assessing such cases will require a bit more effort than was involved in my previous example of Billy and his father.

Economists have come to appreciate that few of us are very proficient at maximizing our own happiness or utility.[19] This realization helps to justify a range of practices beyond the so-called libertarian paternalism I mentioned previously. Most of us recognize our own weaknesses and tendencies to perform acts that are bad for us and that we subsequently regret. If we are intelligent, we develop strategies to overcome these difficulties or to minimize the damage they cause. A number of prominent theorists, including Thomas Schelling,[20] Jon Elster,[21] George Ainslie,[22] and George Lowenstein,[23] have described several of these strategies in impressive detail. Suppose that painful experience leads Eric to understand his tendency to become intoxicated at parties. He may employ any number of *commitment strategies* to minimize the risk that he will suffer as a result of his behavior. For example, Eric may take a cab to the party so that he cannot drive home. These strategies involve what might be called *paternalism toward oneself*—a mode of paternalism that often is pure, not containing the mixture of paternalistic and nonpaternalistic motives so common for rules and laws imposed upon others. As far as I can discern, few interesting moral questions are presented when these commitment strategies do not enlist the assistance of others persons. These plans may be clever or dumb, effective or ineffective, but they rarely pose serious ethical issues. Moral difficulties arise, however, when a commitment strategy requires the cooperation of another party. These difficulties must be confronted because the second party may need to resort to coercion to ensure the success of the commitment strategy.

These moral issues are somewhat less acute (although not nonexistent) when a person specifically stipulates in advance how he wants to be treated when his contemporaneous consent cannot be given—because he will be unconscious, for example. Many individuals have executed "living wills" that specify their preferences if we are on life support and incapable of expressing our consent at the time a medical intervention is proposed. Moral problems are compounded, however, when we seek to provide in advance how we wish to be treated when we know that our contemporaneous consent *can* be given, but is likely to diverge from what we now believe will be in our best interest. Suppose that Eric drives to a party and entrusts his keys to his friend Jill, imploring her not to return them if he becomes drunk. Again, no difficulties are presented as long as he maintains his resolve. But moral problems must be confronted if Eric changes his mind and later decides that he no longer prefers to abide by the restrictions to which he had agreed. In this event, Jill must decide what she ought to do. Should she follow his earlier instructions and retain the keys, or comply with his present wishes and return them?

The first thing to notice about this kind of case is that it places Jill in an awkward position. On the one hand, Eric is likely to be angry with her today if she refuses to return his keys when he demands them. Jill will cite her earlier promise as her justification for noncompliance, but Eric (if he is sufficiently sober) will point out that promises ordinarily bind only as long as the promisee does not release the promisor from her promissory obligation. Both morality and law tend to privilege contemporaneous expressions of consent or nonconsent over prior conflicting preferences. Expressed in the simplest terms, persons generally are free to change their minds. On the other hand, Eric is likely to be angry with Jill tomorrow if she complies with his request to return his keys today. He will remind her that his sole reason for extracting her promise in the first place was to prevent him from changing his mind should this very contingency arise. Thus, he places Jill in a "lose-lose" predicament. One valuable lesson to be learned is that persons should be reluctant to make promises to cooperate with others who seek to attain paternalistic ends through a commitment strategy that enlists their assistance. Because we should be hesitant to place others in an uncomfortable moral position, we should make every effort to try to overcome our weaknesses without soliciting the help of others.

I propose to explore this sort of issue in the context of a fairly recent and fascinating phenomenon: *self-exclusion programs* that enable persons to voluntarily place themselves on a list to be barred from casinos. A majority of the 48 of 50 states that presently allow gambling have provided a device by which individuals can authorize casinos to eject them should they attempt to enter. The details of these programs vary enormously from one jurisdiction to another; generalizations are almost impossible to draw. New Jersey, for example, allows individuals to obtain forms by mail or over the Internet, but applicants must appear in person at a handful of designated locations to complete their enrollment.[24] Participants may request exclusion for a minimum of 1 year, for 5 years, or for life, and the exclusion is irrevocable throughout whatever period is elected. Casino personnel are instructed to refuse entry to persons on the list, or to prevent them from making wagers in the event they manage to gain admission. If participants in the program somehow gamble and win, their winnings are to be confiscated. If they lose, their losses are not to be returned. Participation in a self-exclusion program is an excellent example of a commitment strategy that requires the cooperation of another person. Individuals give their explicit consent to be excluded, but enlist the help of casino personnel to ensure that they maintain their resolve.

Like the previous examples I have discussed, no important ethical questions arise if the gambler conforms to his earlier position. No one need treat another paternalistically as long as the participant in the self-exclusion program does not attempt to gamble. In this event, these programs may be conceptualized as a helpful means to increase the probability that persons will attain objectives they recognize to be in their self-interest. Problems occur, of course, when the participant changes his mind. Suppose that Smith appears at a casino several years after having authorized a lifetime exclusion. He goes directly to the manager and explains that he has overcome the problems that led him to enroll in the program, and now wants to place a modest wager notwithstanding his prior request to be banned. The casino manager must decide whether to honor Smith's current preference or the preference he expressed in his distant past. In many respects, the manager's predicament resembles the uncomfortable position in which Eric placed his friend Jill when he sought her assistance in avoiding the consequences of his intoxication. The manager seeks advice from a moral philosopher. What advice should we offer?

The question I intend to raise might be construed somewhat differently. We want to know whether and under what circumstances a subject's prospective consent to a burden (which he undertakes for his own good) to which he subsequently objects remains *valid* or *effective* in morality—that is, whether his consent is sufficient in morality to permit the actor to impose the burden despite the subject's contemporaneous objection. Apart from the misgivings I describe later, my thesis is that consent does *not* make a difference to whether others are entitled to treat persons like Smith paternalistically. If it is permissible to treat him paternalistically, the ongoing validity of prior consent is not what does the justificatory work.

In assessing this thesis, notice how odd it would be to think that prior consent had any special significance when a given interference is motivated by a *non*paternalistic rationale. That is, the absence of consent gives us no reason to judge a deprivation to be impermissible when it is designed to prevent harm to others. Suppose Craig is painfully aware of his tendency to molest children, and requests city officials to escort him from a playground whenever he is found there. I stipulate that his sole reason for alerting the officials is to protect potential victims. Suppose that Craig appears at the playground, is asked to leave, and indicates that he withdraws his prior consent to depart. What should the official do? Whatever the answer to this question may be, I do not believe it differs from the answer the official should reach when confronted with Jason, whose tendency to molest children is known to be equally great but who has not issued an earlier request to be made to leave. Craig's prior consent is not effective in authorizing what would be impermissible in its absence. My tentative thesis about the irrelevance of consent entails that whatever is permissible to do to Craig is permissible to do to Jason. Later I will return to the issue of how the criteria to justify paternalistic interferences might be *un*like those that justify nonpaternalistic interferences. My present point is that these criteria do not appear to differ with respect to the relevance of prior consent.

Since paternalistic interferences are generally thought to be so much more difficult to justify than those grounded in a harm-to-others rationale, prior consent might appear far more significant in cases such as self-exclusion programs from casinos. The crucial test of my thesis is as follows. Imagine

Jones, a second gambler who is identical to Smith in all relevant respects except for the fact that he has not given his prior consent to be placed on the self-exclusion list. From a moral perspective, my thesis entails that the manager would be warranted in treating Jones similarly to Smith, since the criteria I have identified would be applied in exactly the same way to both persons. If Jones, who has not consented, should be treated exactly like Smith, who has consented, it follows that consent is irrelevant to whether paternalism is justified.[25]

My tentative thesis does not dictate how any of the persons in the examples I have presented *should* be treated. I am not confident how to answer the question of whether Smith or Jones should be admitted or excluded from the casino; I only conclude that they should be treated identically. More to the point, I contend that no general answer to this kind of question should be given. In other words, no one-size-fits-all solution is optimal for each of the Smiths and Joneses I have described thus far. Admittedly, the answer is relatively clear in some kinds of cases. One might think that the decisive factor in favor of honoring Eric's earlier preference rather than his later demand is that he was more competent at the time he formed it.[26] Eric is to be commended for anticipating his future impairment and for enlisting someone to protect him from the consequences of his subsequent behavior. If I am correct that consent is irrelevant to the justifiability of paternalism, however, one must appeal to factors other than his prior request to explain why this case is easy.[27] Indeed, Eric's case *is* easy, but differs from Smith's in several important respects—differences that make it hard to know whether to provide the same answer.

It may be true that Smith, like Eric, knew exactly what he was doing when he decided to place himself on the lifetime self-exclusion list. But why suppose that his original judgment must be respected for all time? Curiously, Feinberg seemingly believes not only that prior fully voluntary consent is relevant, but also that it is decisive. In fact, he would always privilege the earlier judgment. Feinberg claims

> "when the earlier self in a fully voluntary way renounces his right to revoke in the future (or during some specified future interval), or explicitly instructs another, as in the Odyssean example, not to accept contrary instructions from the future self, then the earlier choice, being the genuine choice of a sovereign being, free to dispose of his own lot in the future, must continue to govern."[28]

But this position pushes the idea of personal sovereignty too far. In addition, it is at odds with a wealth of empirical research. An abundance of data confirms that persons are notoriously poor in predicting what they will want at a later time under different circumstances. Young adults often proclaim that they would prefer to forego treatment and die rather than to live with a severe disability that would dramatically decrease the quality of their lives. When they actually suffer from the very condition they fear, however, they frequently cling to life. Why privilege their earlier judgment when they express a preference for a future contingency they can barely imagine?[29] Arguably, they are in a far better position to recognize their true preferences when they experience the very disability in question.

Someone may respond that gambling is different from an ordinary disability. Gambling is an addiction, all addictions compromise cognition or volition, and it is in the nature of addictions that no one can be cured.[30] This response, I think, involves more ideology than sound social science. Even if gambling qualifies as a genuine addiction, and addictions undermine voluntary choice, why suppose that someone who once was addicted will not be able to moderate his behavior in the future without relapsing into his prior addictive state?[31] As individuals mature, many learn to moderate their addictive behaviors. With hindsight, the decision to exclude oneself permanently from a casino seems a particularly rigid solution to an acknowledged gambling problem that might have been addressed more effectively by a commitment strategy that allows greater flexibility.

In addition, Smith need not have been an addict in the first place.[32] His earlier decision to enroll in the lifetime exclusion program may have been rash or the product of external pressure, reflecting less competence and cool deliberation than he now displays when requesting to be allowed to gamble. Perhaps his wife, morally opposed to gambling, threatened to leave him should he set foot in a casino, and Smith loved his wife more than he liked to gamble. Desperate to keep his wife, Smith may have enrolled in the self-exclusion program, even though he did not have a gambling problem at all. But imagine that his wife left him anyway, and Smith's second wife does not share her predecessor's moral aversion to gambling. The general point is that persons who oversee self-exclusion programs have no means to determine why applicants sought to exclude themselves; their own decisions in the matter are final and irrevocable. Moreover, unlike the case of Jill and Eric, the casino manager is not in an ideal position to observe whether Smith still is vulnerable to whatever compulsive tendencies he may have had. The manager cannot determine whether admission is likely to harm Smith—the third condition in my criteria of when paternalistic interferences are justified. Although mistakes always are possible, Jill is better able to detect whether Eric is intoxicated and should not be given his keys. Thus, even if compulsive gambling is an addiction, and addictions are an incurable disease, there is no good reason to infer that Smith ever was afflicted with it, is less rational today than when he made his irrevocable commitment, or would actually be harmed were he allowed to change his mind.

But didn't Smith make more than a vow or a pledge not to gamble? Didn't he make a promise—perhaps even a contract—not to enter a casino? Of course, the whole point of a promise or contract is to prevent persons from changing their minds by requiring them to pay damages in the event they default. If we think of Smith as having made a promise or a contract with the casino to treat him paternalistically, we may feel somewhat more comfortable about excluding him. For two reasons, however, we should not conceptualize these self-exclusion agreements as creating contractual obligations between Smith and the casino.[33] First, nearly all contracts are reciprocal and involve a bargain, conferring what each of the parties regards as a benefit. In this case, however, it is unclear how the casino gains from the agreement. In short, the absence of consideration is likely to render this so-called contract unenforceable.[34] More important, a contract model fails to explain why the casino manager would lack the power to release Smith from any promise he has made. Both contract law and the moral conventions surrounding the institution of promises allow parties to amend their agreements by mutual consent. Some theoreticians have proposed ingenious devices to preclude parties from subsequently modifying their prior agreement, but none has proved especially effective in law or appealing in morality. If an automatic preference for honoring the earlier judgment were desirable, one might reasonably anticipate that mechanisms in law and principles in morality would be available to ensure this result.[35]

As Peter Westen indicates, "nonreciprocal irrevocable commitments are sufficiently rare that the paradigm for it comes not from law but [from fiction]: from Homer's account of Odysseus' encounter with the Sirens."[36] The fictional Odysseus, however, resembles Eric more than Smith; the Sirens drove sailors mad, making them less competent than when their songs could not be heard. Even here, prior consent does no substantive work. If Odysseus had not issued his prior command to remain tied to the mast, his crew would have been equally justified in ignoring his subsequent pleas. Why heed the commands of a madman who instructs his sailors to steer to their doom? By contrast, Smith's competence does not clearly vary from one time to another.

Thus, I assume that the manager should not automatically defer to Smith's prior request to be excluded from the casino for life. It is even easier to show that Smith's later demand to be admitted is not automatically entitled to deference. Morality should not contain an absolute bar against enlisting the assistance of others in devising a commitment strategy. Without cooperation, we sometimes cannot design an effective means to protect ourselves from our own weaknesses and tendencies to perform acts that we recognize to be bad for us. Few respondents believe that Eric's later demand for his car keys (or Odysseus's pleas to be untied) must be honored because contemporaneous preferences invariably trump those expressed at an earlier time.

If the casino manager should automatically defer neither to Smith's earlier preference nor to his current decision, what should he do? It is important not to misconstrue the nature of this question or to confuse it with three others that might be posed. First, I am not concerned with the self-interest of the casino manager. Even from this perspective, the answer is uncertain. On the one hand, it is evident that casinos make money by admitting patrons, not by excluding them. Persons who are barred by self-exclusion programs probably represent a significant loss of revenue for casinos.[37] On the other hand, compliance with these programs may generate favorable publicity for a beleaguered industry. Casinos might prosper more in the long run by maintaining a policy of refusing admission to persons who admit their gambling problem. Second, I am not concerned with the applicable law. Special statutory provisions govern self-exclusion programs in the several states, and the hands of a manager may be tied by a particular law to which he is subject. He may incur liability in the event he makes the wrong decision—whatever that decision may be. Perhaps Smith can recover damages from the casino if it culpably admits him.[38] Or perhaps the casino must pay a fine to the state or risk the loss of its license.[39] But suppose that no statutes clearly specify what the manager is legally obligated to do. In this instance, it is doubtful that courts should impose liability on a casino manager who does not make whatever decisions we believe to be correct. His predicament is sufficiently difficult that we may want to protect him from liability for *either* choice he makes in good faith, even if we regard one outcome as better than the other. Finally, I am not concerned with the empirical question of whether this commitment strategy is effective.[40] Excluded gamblers may simply be displaced to other venues such as racetracks or state lotteries, where the odds of winning are even more remote than in casinos. Interesting though these three perspectives may be, I put each of them aside.

Instead, I want to inquire what the casino manager ought to do from the *moral* point of view. My central (but tentative) thesis in this chapter is that the absence of consent is irrelevant to the justification of paternalism, even when it is given explicitly in the past. If this thesis is correct, the casino manager should proceed in exactly the same way as Billy's father or Eric's friend Jill: He must determine what is reasonable. I have identified five criteria that I think should guide this determination. I do not pretend that the application of these criteria is simple: It is not nearly as easy as in Billy's or Eric's case. The following difficult issues must be addressed to make a decision. At what time was Smith more competent to assess his own interests and to make the better judgment? As I have indicated, this question is especially important in cases in which reasonable minds differ about whether the interference is really worth the costs to the person coerced. Smith appears to be an unimpaired adult who does not suffer from any of the obvious deficiencies of Billy or Eric, and I see no reason to suppose that there always is a particular time—in the past or in the present—when persons who want to gamble are better able to assess their own interests. Second, how important is Smith's liberty interest, and how severe is the interference with it? Unfortunately, we lack a convenient metric to evaluate the value of the many liberties we recognize. Intuitively, exclusion from a casino is a larger infringement of liberty than the denial of ice cream, especially when the ice cream is withheld temporarily rather than permanently. Still, the ability to gamble is not ranked especially high on most scales of liberties. The two states that ban gambling altogether—Hawaii and Utah—are not typically thought to violate significant liberties. Third, how valuable is the objective to be achieved? Preventing gambling addicts from losing large amounts of money can be a significant achievement, but I have already expressed reservations about whether persons on the list are addicts. Fourth, what is the likelihood that exclusion will be effective in preventing Smith from losing money? Empirical research is needed to shed light on this matter. Finally, is the casino manager in the appropriate position to treat Smith paternalistically? I will have more to say about this final condition in a moment. At the present time, I repeat my confidence about how these five factors should be balanced in Billy's or Eric's case, and my lack of certainty about how they should be balanced in Smith's case. We need far more information before we should be clear about our answer, and are likely to remain ambivalent even when all of the facts are known. My more modest goal, however, is not to resolve this difficult issue, but to examine the role consent plays within the framework in which the question should be addressed.

My tentative thesis is that consent does not enter into this moral frame- work at any point in the analysis. The fact that Smith gave his prior consent is not material to whether the manager should ban him for his own good.

Admittedly, this position seems somewhat counterintuitive—even to me. My own intuitions on this topic are frail and unstable. Can it really be true that prior consent plays no role whatever in the face of contemporaneous nonconsent? If so, why are so many philosophers inclined to believe otherwise? Three answers seem promising. First, consent may alter the burden of proof in determining whether or not paternalism is justified. It is almost never clear whether a particular instance of paternalism satisfies my test. Perhaps the burden of showing these criteria are *not* satisfied should be allocated to the person to be treated paternalistically when he has given his prior consent to the interference. A second point is closely related. We are entitled to try especially hard to persuade someone to act in his own interest when he has requested that we do so. Suppose, for example, that your friend urges you in the morning not to let him succumb to laziness if he fails to keep his promise to meet you in the gym later in the day. When he changes his mind and proposes to stay home, you are permitted to remind him forcefully of his previous request. If he continues to decline, however, I think we must respect his contemporaneous rather than his prior choice. Finally, and most obviously, consent appears to be important because it serves as *evidence* that some of my criteria are satisfied. In particular, it provides a reason to believe that Smith has a gambling problem he once thought to be sufficiently serious to warrant his permanent exclusion. In the absence of his earlier consent, the casino manager almost certainly will have more reason to believe that the ban protects Smith's interests more than those of Jones, the patron with the identical gambling problem. But I propose to put such epistemological considerations to one side. Suppose for the sake of argument that the casino manager happens to know just as much about Jones as he knows about Smith. As a matter of principle, I do not understand how consent should be a factor in our advice about whether either or both may be excluded. If I am correct, both Smith and Jones should be treated similarly, and the absence of consent is irrelevant to the question of whether their paternalistic treatment is justified.[41]

To bolster my thesis, we should notice that consent is equally irrelevant in deciding how Eric, the intoxicated but prudent guest, should be treated. Imagine that Jill finds the keys that Patricia, another guest, has misplaced at her party. Patricia is now as drunk as Eric, and demands that her keys be returned so she can drive home. Unlike Eric, Patricia has not voluntarily entrusted her keys to Jill should this very contingency arise. But if their circumstances are identical otherwise, it is hard to see why Jill should return Patricia's keys but withhold those of Eric. With the following caveat, each of my five criteria applies equally to both persons.

I confess to misgivings about denying an important (nonevidentiary) role to consent in the cases of Smith or Eric. Because of these misgivings, I have persistently qualified as tentative my thesis about the irrelevance of consent to the justifiability of paternalism. Arguably, Smith's prior consent has normative significance because it is material to the fifth criterion in my test of whether paternalistic interferences are reasonable and thus justifiable. Recall that parents stand in an ideal (or special) relationship to their children to treat them paternalistically. Biology and the duties conventionally attached to parents are not, however, the only source of special relationships. Smith's prior consent may create the special relationship between himself and the casino that entitles the manager to treat him paternalistically. Even though "special relationships" ordinarily are posited to justify the creation of *duties,* they also are capable of justifying the creation of privileges or permissions. In any event, no such relationship exists between Jones and the casino, or between Patricia and Jill. Is the existence of a special relationship needed before paternalism is justified? I am agnostic; my intuitions tug me in different directions.

But if my misgivings are sound, and the identity of the person who interferes is relevant to whether that interference is permissible, we have a possible basis for contrasting the justifiability of paternalism from that of nonpaternalism. Earlier, I suggested that Craig and Jason should be treated similarly if they have comparable tendencies to molest children. But it is hard to see why anyone would think that the identity of the individual who proposes to evict either Craig or Jason from a public playground should be a factor in determining whether the eviction is permissible. This fifth and final criterion in our test of when paternalism is reasonable has no clear analogue in cases in which the interference is motivated by nonpaternalistic considerations.

Suppose my misgivings are correct, and Smith's actual, prior consent is crucial to whether his paternalistic treatment is justified because it creates a special relationship with the casino manager. If so, we are left with an interesting result. Jones is (otherwise) identical to Smith. With respect to Jones, however, we would have a case of (otherwise) justifiable paternalism, with no one in an appropriate position to impose it. We could try to surmount this hurdle by multiplying the number of relationships we hold to be special. We might allege a relationship is special whenever one person is in a position to treat another paternalistically. Perhaps Jones's mere appearance in a casino creates a special relationship that would satisfy the fifth condition in my criteria. Maybe the act of hosting a party and finding Patricia's keys creates a special relationship that warrants paternalistic intervention. But this solution, though sensible in some contexts, has limits, and threatens to render my fifth criterion all but vacuous. Special relationships are *special*, after all. Unless the number of special relationships is multiplied beyond recognition, a plausible objection to a great deal of (otherwise) justifiable paternalism is that no one stands in a suitable relation to impose it on the person to be treated paternalistically.

If we hold the fifth criterion in my test of reasonableness to be important, we may have an additional reason to be skeptical of *criminal* paternalism—of laws that subject persons to punishment for their own good. Arguably, the state lacks an appropriate (or special) relation to its citizens to be eligible to treat them paternalistically. On some minimalist conceptions of the state, its only function is to prevent persons from harming others. Of course, a defense of this liberal (or libertarian), nonperfectionist political view requires nothing less than a theory of the state and a corresponding theory of criminalization— tasks well beyond the scope of this chapter.[42] Here I offer a single observation about why we should be reluctant to elevate my misgivings into a general opposition to all legal paternalism. Political philosophers who resist a perfectionist theory of the state will be hard-pressed to defend the probable implications of their views for the justifiability of so-called libertarian paternalism. If the state does not stand in a proper relation to its citizens to treat them paternalistically, it is unclear why it has good reason to design default rules to protect persons from the consequences of their own weaknesses. This conclusion strikes me as counterintuitive, even if we are skeptical of paternalism in the criminal domain. After all, the state must provide *some* content to default rules. On what other basis should they be formulated? *Ceteris paribus,* why should the state be precluded from designing default rules to influence citizens to pursue their own good? No abstract argument against perfectionism and in favor of a liberal (or libertarian) theory of the state is likely to provide a satisfactory answer to this question. Generally, we should find it easier to resist criminal paternalism than state actions in (what I have loosely called) the spirit of paternalism pursued through noncriminal means.

Earlier, I suggested that the final criterion in my 5-fold test of reasonableness is the most questionable. I conclude that insofar as we regard this fifth criterion as unimportant, we should not believe that Smith's previous decision to seek exclusion is relevant to how the casino manager should proceed. In this event, the case of Smith and Jones, as well as that of Eric and Patricia, stand or fall together. Moreover, their cases resemble that of Craig and Jason, whose liberty is deprived not for paternalistic reasons, but to prevent harm to others. Unless the final criterion in my test is retained, and the justifiability of paternalism depends partly on the identity of the person who imposes it, my thesis is that consent makes no difference to the criteria we should apply in deciding whether we are permitted to treat someone paternalistically.

Notes

1. I do not contend that this second assertion is beyond serious dispute. See *infra* p. 109. Fortunately, nothing of importance turns on any particular example; I need only to assume that *some* case of justified paternalism can be described, and that its justification depends on the criteria I provide.

2. Literally, rules or laws are not the kinds of thing that *can* be paternalistic. To say that a rule or law is paternalistic is best interpreted to mean that it is adopted or enacted largely from a paternalistic motive. Generally, see Douglas N. Husak, "Legal Paternalism," in *Oxford Handbook of Practical Ethics,* ed. Hugh LaFollette (New York: Oxford University Press, 2004), 387.

3. See Joel Feinberg, *Harm to Self* (New York: Oxford University Press, 1985).

4. See Douglas Husak, *Overcriminalization* (New York: Oxford University Press, 2008).

5. Perhaps this conclusion can be applied to all attempts to justify paternalism by reference to consent—even when consent is noncontemporaneous. See Thaddeus Mason Pope, "Monstrous Impersonation: A Critique of Consent-Based Justifications for Hard Paternalism," *University of Missouri-Kansas City Law Review* 73 (2005): 861.

6. It is not clear how a parent can *threaten* to treat someone paternalistically when paternalism is justified. Typically, threats are distinguished from offers because they make their recipients worse off. If Billy is indeed better off when treated paternalistically, as I have stipulated, his father's proposal is difficult to categorize as a threat.

7. Some philosophers contend that not all cases of paternalism involve interference. Presumably, a doctor may treat an unconscious patient paternalistically, although he could hardly interfere in a choice the patient is incapable of making. See Bernard Gert and George Culver, "Paternalistic Behaviors," *Philosophy & Public Affairs* 6 (1976): 46.

8. See Cass R. Sunstein and Richard H. Thaler, "Libertarian Paternalism Is Not an Oxymoron," *University of Chicago Law Review* 70 (2003): 1159.

9. See J.D. Trout: "Paternalism and Cognitive Bias," *Law and Philosophy* 24 (2005): 393.

10. Taxes designed to discourage people from engaging in activities that create risks of harm, such as using tobacco products, probably should be conceptualized

similarly. Unless rates of taxation become prohibitive, they should be thought to influence rather than to interfere with choice. Generally, see the discussion of the "robustness principle" in Jim Leitzel, *Regulating Vice: Misguided Prohibitions and Realistic Controls* (Cambridge: Cambridge University Press, 2008), esp.72–92.

11. See Colin Camerer et al.: "Regulation for Conservatives: Behavioral Economics and the Case for 'Asymmetric Paternalism,' " *University of Pennsylvania Law Review* 151 (2003): 1211. Complications arise if the price for the spontaneous and irrevocable purchase is lower than that for the revocable purchase.

12. For a nice discussion, see Peter Westen, *The Logic of Consent* (Burlington, VT: Ashgate Publishing Co., 2004).

13. Formulations of the consent defense in criminal law accord with this position. The Model Penal Code provides that consent is "ineffective" if "it is given by a person whose improvident consent is sought to be prevented by the law defining the offense." American Law Institute, *Model Penal Code* §2.11(3)(c) (1962).

14. Gerald Dworkin, "Paternalism," *Monist* 56 (1972): 64.

15. Douglas Husak, "Paternalism and Autonomy," *Philosophy and Public Affairs* 10 (1980): 27.

16. See Tziporah Kassachkoff, "Paternalism: Does Gratitude Make It Okay?" *Social Theory and Practice* 20 (1994): 1.

17. For serious consideration of the possibility that consent can be retrospective, see Westen, *Logic,* 254–61.

18. Elsewhere, I have suggested that paternalistic interferences are reasonable when they promote the conditions of personal autonomy. See Husak, "Legal Paternalism."

19. An enormous literature has grown around this topic. Generally, see Michael Bishop and J.D. Trout, *Epistemology and the Psychology of Human Judgment* (New York: Oxford University Press, 2005).

20. See Thomas C. Schelling, "Self-Command in Practice, in Policy, and in a Theory of Rational Choice," *American Economics Review* 74 (1984): 1. Schelling lists several self-regulatory strategies, including relinquishing authority to someone else, disabling oneself, removing resources, submitting to surveillance techniques, incarcerating oneself, arranging rewards and penalties, rescheduling one's life, avoiding precursors, arranging delays, using teams, and setting bright line rules.

21. Jon Elster, *Sour Grapes: Studies in the Subversion of Rationality* (Cambridge: Cambridge University Press, 1983).

22. George Ainslie, *Picoeconomics: The Strategic Interaction of Successive Motivational States within the Person* (Cambridge: Cambridge University Press, 1992).

23. George Lowenstein and Ted O'Donoghue, " 'We Can Do This the Easy Way or the Hard Way': Negative Emotions, Self-Regulation, and the Law," *University of Chicago Law Review* 73 (2006): 183.

24. Information and forms about this program are available at http://www. state.nj. us/casinos/forms/excludeform.pdf.

25. At least in this case. Admittedly, a factor that is irrelevant in one pair of cases need not be irrelevant in all such pairs. Generally, see the discussion of the "Principle of Contextual Interaction" in F.M. Kamm, *Intricate Ethics* (New York: Oxford University Press, 2007), 17.

26. According to Joel Feinberg, we should rely on the subject's most "voluntary" decision in cases of conflict. See *Self,* 83.

27. The time at which the person is more competent is not the only basis for privileging Eric's judgment, even if it is the most important. Suppose that Alan, who consented to cosmetic surgery in a sober moment, becomes terrified when the operation is about to be performed. Clearly, he may withdraw his consent at this later time, even though his judgment is likely to be impaired by his fear.

28. Feinberg, *Self,* 83.

29. Questions of advance directives that allegedly bind demented patients raise problems of personal identity that are not clearly replicated in my example of self-exclusion programs. See, for example, Allen Buchanan, "Advance Directives and the Personal Identity Problem," *Philosophy & Public Affairs* 17 (1988): 277.

30. See Constance Holden, " 'Behavioral' Addictions: Do They Exist?" *Science* 294 (2001): 980.

31. The debate about whether addictive behaviors can be moderated is waged most fiercely in the context of alcoholism. See Frederick Rotgers, Mark F. Kern, and Rudy Hoeltzel, *Responsible Drinking: A Moderation Management Approach for Problem Drinkers* (Oakland, CA: New Harbinger Publications, Inc., 2002).

32. Some commentators appear to assume that self-excluded gamblers must be addicts. See the otherwise informative contribution by Justin E. Bauer, "Self-Exclusion and the Compulsive Gambler: The House Shouldn't Always Win," *Northern Illinois Law Review* 27 (2006): 63.

33. Perhaps my conclusions can be avoided by supposing that the promise is made to (or the contract is made with) a party other than the casino—say, to the state agency that establishes the self-exclusion program. The same problem would arise, however, if Smith asked an agent of the state to release him from his promise (or contract).

34. Arguably, this technical problem could be overcome if Smith paid considera-tion—say, a sum of $10—in exchange for the casino manager's promise to exclude him.

35. See Kevin Davis, "The Demand for Immutable Contracts: Another Look at the Law and Economics of Contract Modifications," *New York University Law Review* 81 (2006): 487.

36. Westen, *Logic*, 253.

37. According to one study, compulsive gamblers provide between 30% and 52% of all casino revenues. See http://www.casinofreephila.org/research/gambling-revenues-compulsive-gamblers.

38. For a negative answer, see *Merrill v. Trump Indiana, Inc.*, 320 F.3d 729 (7th Cir. 2003).

39. For an affirmative answer, see id.

40. According to one study, 30% of the participants completely stopped gambling once enrolled in this kind of program. See Robert Ladouceur et al., "Brief Communications Analysis of a Casino's Self-Exclusion Program," *Journal of Gambling Studies* 16 (2000): 453.

41. This position resembles the controversial view Joseph Raz has defended in the context of analyzing political authority. According to Raz, "consent is a source of obligation only when some considerations, themselves independent of consent, vindicate its being such a source." Joseph Raz, "The Problem of Authority: Revisiting the Service Conception," *Minnesota Law Review* 90 (2006): 1003, 1038.

42. For further thoughts, see Husak, *Overcriminalization*.

6

Hypothetical Consent

Arthur Kuflik

I. Introduction

What *is* "hypothetical consent"? Though more a term of art in philosophical discussion than a familiar expression in everyday conversation, the phrase "hypothetical consent" does suggest a line of thought that is not altogether unfamiliar to us. There are many situations in which, although consent *has not actually been given*, it nevertheless seems reasonable to infer, and somehow relevant to insist, that if certain conditions (*1*) had obtained, (*2*) were to obtain, or (*3*) will yet obtain, then someone's consent (*1*) *would have been*, (*2*) *would be*, or (*3*) *will yet be* given.

Let's begin by taking a closer look at some of these contexts—contexts in which consent (or some suitably related idea) is typically hypothesized:

1. *"Substituted judgment" in medical ethics.* A person who previously had, but presently lacks, decision-making capacity is in a condition that raises questions about possible medical treatments—treatments that might (or might not) prolong life, improve health, prevent disability, and/or alleviate discomfort. It is hypothesized that if the individual in question were to regain decision-making capacity, and were to know and understand the prognosis, the treatment options, the prospective benefits, and associated risks, and so forth, then that individual *would authorize* family members and/or doctors to undertake (or to refrain from undertaking) certain measures.

2. *Benevolent paternalism and the hypothesis of future "consent":* A parent is concerned to have her beloved child vaccinated against a deadly and/or debilitating disease. As the child unhappily resists, the parent comforts herself (and perhaps even the child) with the thought that later on, if and when he is more mature, more thoughtful, and more adequately informed about health matters, the adult that the child becomes *will endorse* what the parent has done *and will consent* to comparable measures that might be needed to maintain and/or enhance the immunity thus established.

3. *Respect for those who have died:* Friends and relatives are trying to honor a recently deceased person by handling some of that person's posthumous affairs in a way that they believe that person *would have* wanted them to do *and* indeed *would have authorized* them to do, if only (or so they believe) the deceased had managed to anticipate and more explicitly address such matters with greater specificity. Knowing the deceased person's values and lifestyle commitments, they hypothesize that their beloved relative (or friend) would not have consented to a large funeral with lots of eulogies or to burial in an expensive casket. Knowing the great love he had for his niece and nephew and the genuine empathy with which he related to them, they hypothesize that he would have consented to transferring his butterfly collection to his nature-loving niece and his baseball card collection to his baseball-loving nephew.

4. *Interpreting legislative intent:* A court hears a case in which the literal application of an existing statute would provide an unexpected incentive to engage in behavior that other well-established statutes (for example, prohibiting and punishing murder) are clearly aimed at discouraging. To illustrate: A man has been murdered by his grandson who, having feared that he would soon be cut off from the grandfather's will, took deadly action to make sure that such changes not be made. The extant will, bequeathing a generous sum to the grandson, would be considered technically valid in light of the literal meaning of the statutes governing wills. But the (majority on the) court reasons differently. They *hypothesize* that if the legislators had managed to anticipate a circumstance such as the one that has now come before the court, they would surely have qualified the statute to make perfectly clear that a designated heir loses his right to inherit when he has sought to activate the execution of the will by committing a crime, such as murder, against the testator. Thus, their hypothesis about what the legislators would have agreed to had they only known about cases of this sort plays a critical role in their interpretation and application of the law actually legislated.[1]

5. *Not obtaining actual "consent" (even though it would have been perfectly possible to do so)*: Researchers set out to observe "subjects"; instead of soliciting the informed consent of those individuals, they contend that actual consent is unnecessary. They *hypothesize* that the research in question is sufficiently non-burdensome to the individuals thus observed, and that if they were to be asked, such individuals would surely give their consent anyway.[2]

6. *Ideal contract theory in moral and/or political philosophy:* A purely *imaginary* (and highly idealized) deliberation procedure is envisioned. Reasoning is then advanced to the effect that the parties to such a procedure (who in turn may be only constructs of our idealizing moral imagination) would (or would not) agree to certain *general principles* for regulating the design of society's most basic political and economic institutions.[3] The truth of this hypothesis is thought to lend significant support to the view that such principles do indeed specify what is most reasonable and just.

2. Challenging the Relevance of Hypothetical Consent?

So the notion of what would (or would not) be agreed to by persons (real or imagined) under circumstances that do not presently (and that may or may not ever) obtain does enter into a number of different conversations. But *what point*, if any, is thereby revealed or reinforced by this "hypothesis" of consent? Does the role played by the hypothesis *vary* along with the context in which it is put forward? Or, does the appeal to hypothetical consent *fail* to serve any valid moral purpose at all?

A significant challenge to the relevance of "hypothetical consent" can be found in the writings of the distinguished MIT philosopher Judith Jarvis Thomson.[4] Thomson considers two contexts: (1) a typical medical ethics scenario in which someone who is presently unconscious can only be saved from death if an invasive medical procedure is performed (for example, the amputation of a leg); and (2) the more abstract theoretical deployment of hypothetical consent by "contractarian" moral and political theorists such as T.M. Scanlon and John Rawls.[5]

1. In cases of the first sort, Thomson argues that the truth of the hypothesis that consent would (or would not) be given by a patient presently lacking decision-making capacity is neither a necessary nor a sufficient condition for determining whether medical personnel ought

to undertake the invasive procedure. From this she seems to infer that hypothetical consent is basically irrelevant.

2. When considering the more abstract "contract theory" deployment of hypothetical consent, Thomson seems to have a slightly more benign, but ultimately rather deflationary attitude: Her view is that the appeal to what would (or would not) be agreed to by somewhat idealized participants in a hypothetical deliberation procedure is "epiphenomenal." The principles that emerge from the hypothetical procedure are not to be regarded as principles of right and of justice because they would have been agreed to; what really matters and what is really "doing the moral work" are the reasons why the participants in the procedure would (or would not) have agreed to them. It is these reasons that warrant our regarding the principles as appropriate and that justify the claim that the participants in the idealized procedure would have agreed to them as well.

To respond to Thomson's challenges and keep discussion within reasonable length, the remainder of this essay will focus on two contexts: (1) surrogate decision making in medical ethics (scenarios 1 and 2 as sketched out in section 1 and subsequently discussed in sections 4–10); and (2) hypothetical contract theory (scenario 6 as described in section 1 and subsequently discussed in section 11). Section 12 provides a summation.

3. The Overall Shape of the Discussion to Follow

What shall we make of these challenges? At least four possible positions are available:

1. Hypothetical consent plays a significant, and in some cases, essential role in certain kinds of morally relevant deliberation.
2. Though not essential, the appeal to hypothetical consent can and often does help us to develop ideas and insights whose practical import would be more difficult for us to appreciate fully otherwise.
3. Hypothetical consent is completely irrelevant.
4. What relevance hypothetical consent might have is entirely parasitic upon other claims that must be defended more directly in any event. Once those claims are plausibly in view, the appeal to hypothetical consent is superfluous.

Contrary to Thomson, I shall suggest that statements such as (1) and (2) accurately represent the role played by hypothetical consent in at least some familiar and important contexts. In certain other contexts, however, statements such as (3) and (4)—which either dismiss or seriously deflate the significance of the appeal to hypothetical consent—have considerable plausibility.

I develop these points:

1. First, in the context of medical ethics—citing cases such as *Brophy* and *Conroy*—I show how the appeal to what a patient would have authorized can and does play a significant role in determining what medical personnel and others ought to do. In contrast, in cases such as *Saikewicz* (and other cases of "never-competent" patients), I explain how the appeal to hypothetical consent is inappropriate.

2. Second, in the context of social contract theory, I suggest that while Thomson's complaint that hypothetical consent is merely "epiphenomenal" is inappropriate when lodged against *some* versions of contract theory, it may well be on target when we consider yet other versions. In particular, I argue that it misses the mark with respect to Rawls's "contractarianism" as he developed it in *A Theory of Justice.*[6]

4. Hypothetical Consent in Medical Ethics: The Thomson Critique

Let's look more closely at the details of Thomson's thought-provoking discussion. Thomson imagines the case of David, a presently unconscious individual whose life can only be saved by amputation of a leg. David is also known to be a clearly committed Christian Scientist. To many people, a very good reason to believe that it is *im*permissible to amputate David's leg—even if it is the only way to save his life—is that David himself, had he been in full possession of his mental faculties, in touch with his own most deeply held beliefs and values, free from undue threats and pressures, and cognizant of the circumstances he is now in, *would have refused to consent* to such a procedure.

In contrast, Thomson sets out to show that David's hypothetical refusal to consent is *not sufficient* to establish that proceeding with the amputation is impermissible. It's not that Thomson believes David's commitment to Christian Science is irrelevant; rather, as we shall see, Thomson offers a *different* interpretation of how his being a Christian Scientist bears, or ought to bear, on our deliberations about the matter—an interpretation in which whether David *would or would not have consented* to the amputation procedure does not really play a significant role.

Thomson also imagines a variant of David's case—in which he is not a Christian Scientist or a Jehovah's Witness or in any other way committed to an outlook that would incline him to refuse permission for the life-saving amputation procedure. Once again, Thomson understands how we may be tempted to "conclude that if it is permissible for you to proceed, then that is because David would consent to your proceeding . . . . But can this be right?" (pp. 187–88). On Thomson's alternative interpretation of how we should decide what to do in such situations, the answer is "no"—it is not right.

To sum up, according to Thomson, the hypothesis, however well founded on evidence it might be, that David would have refused to consent is not sufficient to render the amputation procedure impermissible. And the hypothesis, however well founded, that David would have consented is not necessary for the permissibility of the procedure. On the basis of these two claims, Thomson is prepared to infer that hypothetical consent is not a morally significant notion after all.

There are *two major problems* with Thomson's critique of hypothetical consent:

1. While it may be true that hypothetical consent is neither necessary nor sufficient to establish permissibility, the arguments advanced by Thomson to prove these points simply miss their target.
2. From the claim that hypothetical consent is neither necessary nor sufficient for permissibility, it simply does not follow that hypothetical consent is irrelevant or superfluous, and hence has no morally significant role to play. This is a non sequitur as can be seen by considering the parallel case of *actual* consent.

Taking these two points in turn:

Not sufficient? Thomson begins by observing that "It might be true of a man that he would consent to your slitting his throat" because "he has the mad idea that he killed Cock Robin, and deserves the throat slitting for it." But in such a case "the fact that he would consent does not make it permissible for you to proceed." For Thomson, the lesson to be drawn from this is that "hypothetical consent is not sufficient for permissibility" (p. 188).

Unfortunately, this way of making the point misses the mark. To see why, consider a person who actually, not merely hypothetically, utters the words "I consent to having my throat slit" because he has "the mad idea that he killed Cock Robin." This person's *apparent* "consent" is defective because it is the product of a psychotically deluded mind. His uttering the words "I consent to your slitting my throat" is not tantamount to his giving valid, permission-granting consent. But if *actually* being in a psychotic state and saying "please slit my throat" does not count as valid consent, then, by the same token, the "hypothesis" that someone *would* have uttered such words *were* he to be in such a state *is not the hypothesis* that the person in question *would have given nondefective consent* to having his throat slit. Defective consent, whether actual or hypothetical, is *devoid* of permission-granting force. Defective consent, whether actual or hypothetical, is clearly insufficient for "permissibility."

To sum up, Thomson's argument does not address the question of whether *nondefective* hypothetical consent might be, in at least some cases, sufficient to establish the permissibility of treating the individual in question in a certain way.

Not necessary? Thomson also wants to prove that the amputation procedure might be permissible even without its being the case that David would have consented to it. The point, of course, is that hypothetical consent is not necessary for "permissibility." To support this claim, however, Thomson deploys, once again, an example that is really beside the point. She plausibly (but irrelevantly) suggests that *if* we had been able to awaken David from his unconscious state, he might well have been too groggy to think clearly and so would not have been able to give or withhold consent at all. Alternatively, he might have been so disoriented and disgruntled that he would have explicitly refused any medical procedure.

The problem here is that, once again, Thomson takes as the *hypothetical* condition a condition that would render even actual (apparent) consent (or refusal of consent) defective. Those who believe that actual consent can have an important role to play in medical ethics cases are not asking, "What did, or does, this person have to say while groggy or disoriented?" Rather, they look for what the person has said or does say while clear-headed; cognizant of the diagnosis, the prognosis, and the reasonably expected risks and benefits associated with different treatment options; and aware of his or her own needs, interests, values, and commitments. Words uttered in a groggy state of mind and/or without relevant factual information, a reasonable degree of self-awareness, and so forth, do not count as permission-conferring, nondefective consent.

Clearly, obtaining someone's (actual but) defective consent is hardly a necessary condition of establishing the permissibility of treating him in a certain way. By the same token, however, the truth of the *hypothesis* that (something superficially like) "consent" would have been given but under comparably consent-invalidating circumstances cannot be counted as a necessary condition for establishing the permissibility of a proposed course of treatment. Whether actual or hypothetical, defective consent is hardly necessary for "permissibility."

To sum up, Thomson's argument does not address the question of whether a well-supported inference to *nondefective* hypothetical consent might, in at least some cases, be among the necessary conditions for permissibly proceeding with a certain course of treatment.

A Non Sequitur: "If a Condition is Neither Necessary nor Sufficient for Moral Permissibility, Then it is Morally Irrelevant"

Suppose that (for reasons *other than* those Thomson advances) we do come to the conclusion that the consent hypothesis is neither necessary nor sufficient for the permissibility of a certain way of treating someone who presently lacks decision-making capacity. What relevance does this have? The same can be said of actual consent. *Actual* consent is neither necessary nor sufficient for the permissibility of treating someone in a certain way. But it *does not* follow that actual consent is irrelevant or without any moral relevance or significance.

Actual consent is *not always sufficient for permissibility.* For example, a prenuptial agreement apparently granting a husband the right to batter his wife would lack legal (and moral) force. There are certain rights—we call them "inalienable"—that a person simply has no right to give up or give away. Thus, not even the consent of the victim is a sufficient defense.

Actual consent is *not always necessary for permissibility.* Medically treating (or refraining from treating) someone in a certain way can be morally appropriate (even mandatory) even without that individual's authorization. There appear to be at least *two kinds of situations* in which this might be the case:

1. Emergency situations involving patients who previously had, but presently lack, decision-making capacity. In cases of this sort, it is sometimes very difficult or even impossible to establish that a prior directive actually exists, to access the document, and to interpret its application to the case at hand before it is too late. (Similarly, even if some other individual had been vested with durable power of attorney, it is sometimes difficult or impossible to identify, locate, and communicate with that individual within the window of time available before either death or irreversible injury results.)

2. Situations in which the patient has *never had* decision-making capacity and has *never* developed well-formed beliefs and values. It simply makes no sense to require "actual consent" when the capacities essential to giving or withholding consent have *never actually* been present.

To sum up, *actual* consent is not always necessary for the permissibility of treating someone in a certain way; nor is it always sufficient. But it does *not* follow from all this that *actual* consent is irrelevant. There are many circumstances in which someone's actual consent (or refusal to give consent) carries significant weight in the scales of legal, as well as moral, deliberation.

5. A Comparable Role for "Hypothetical Consent"?

I suggest that (*1*) the *same* reflections that lead to the conclusion that *actual* consent is not always necessary and not always sufficient "for permissibility" *also* explain why hypothetical consent is not always necessary and not always sufficient either. And in a similar vein, (*2*) from the fact that it is neither necessary nor sufficient, it simply does *not* follow that hypothetical consent is irrelevant. Thus, when family, friends, and medical personnel are grappling with the difficult decision of how to treat a person who *previously had, but presently lacks*, decision-making competence and who has left no prior directive, a well-grounded hypothesis about what that individual would (or would not) have authorized can, and usually should, weigh significantly in their deliberations.

Why is hypothetical consent not always sufficient? For the same reason that actual consent is not always sufficient. Some rights are inalienable. Thus, what the individual would have consented to might not have been within his (or anybody's) right to grant.

Why is hypothetical consent not always necessary? For the same two reasons that explain why actual consent is not always necessary: (*1*) there will be individuals who were never capable of forming values and commitments and who always lacked decision-making capacity and (*2*) there will be emergency situations in which there is insufficient time to establish what the individual would have authorized.

Of course, even in some emergency situations, as well as in other, less time-sensitive medical circumstances, it might still be possible to obtain clear and compelling evidence of how the person in question (who is presently incapable of deciding) *would have* decided, if only she had retained (or temporarily regained) decision-making capacity, understood the facts of the case, and so forth. In other words, there are at least some circumstances in which "hypothetical (nondefective) consent" can be reasonably inferred.[7] But what would be the point of such an exercise? What makes it appropriate to try to do so in the first place?

6. Three Real-World Cases

We have seen how hypothetical consent cannot be dismissed as morally irrelevant just because it is neither necessary nor sufficient for permissibility. But this insight does not by itself establish that hypothetical consent is indeed morally relevant, and in what way. Here, then, we might do well to consider:

A provisional thesis: There are cases in which (*1*) inferring, and then (*2*) invoking, hypothetical consent is a reasonable way of (*3*) extending *respect for someone's right to decide what will happen in and to his or her own body,* (*4*) even in circumstances in which that person's capacity for decision making *cannot* be *concurrently* exercised.

To appreciate the *force* of this claim and the *limits* of its application, let's briefly examine three actual cases.

1. A case in which the notion of "hypothetical (refusal to) consent" played a decisive role[8]

Paul Brophy, aged 46, was a fireman and an emergency medical technician in the town of Easton, Massachusetts. On March 22, 1983, a blood vessel in his brain ruptured. He became unconscious and never regained consciousness again. He was diagnosed as being in a "persistent vegetative state." Prior to this tragedy, according to several people who knew him well, including his wife, Brophy had expressed ideas that convinced them he *would not* wish to be maintained in a vegetative state by artificial means (such as a feeding tube).

The Supreme Judicial Court of Massachusetts authorized the removal of the feeding tube on the ground that this is what Brophy would have requested if only he could have regained consciousness and decision-making capacity. Twelve days later Brophy died. In effect, Brophy's right to decide, in accordance with his own values and convictions, what was to be done in and to his own body was extended to a situation in which he could not concurrently exercise decision-making capacity. The court relied on the idea of a "substituted judgment": It would be right to discontinue such medical interventions because, to the best of their ability to determine, that is what Brophy would have authorized.

Now it might be objected that what the court did here was to rely on Brophy's *actual* refusal of consent, albeit issued "in advance," rather than to deploy the notion of his hypothetical refusal of consent. But the fact is that Brophy had only made informal remarks on prior occasions. He had *never* issued a more formal, legally binding directive. Indeed, he "never had discussed specifically whether a G-tube or feeding tube should be withdrawn in the event he was diagnosed as being in a persistent vegetative state following his surgery" (p. 428). And of course, people sometimes do change their attitudes and values; they sometimes fail to anticipate all the relevant features of future predicaments. So it was at least logically possible that Brophy's attitudes had somehow changed enough in the meantime, or would change if only he could *temporarily* regain consciousness and carefully contemplate his actual circumstances, to support the claim that he would not consent to discontinuation of artificial hydration and nutrition. The court ruled, however, that the evidence convincingly pointed in the opposite direction: Given all that was known about his beliefs, attitudes, and values, the court affirmed the hypothesis (the "substituted judgment") that Brophy would have refused those measures.

2. A case in which "hypothetical consent" (and/or refusal) was a relevant but inconclusive consideration[9]

Claire Conroy, aged 84, suffered from heart disease, hypertension, and diabetes mellitus. She was no longer ambulatory, was unable to move from a semi-fetal position, could not speak, and had limited ability to swallow. She had a urinary catheter in place and could not control her bowels. Her left leg was gangrenous to her knee. Her left foot, leg, and hip were covered with bed sores. Her nephew and guardian sought permission to have a nasogastric feeding tube removed. If it were removed, doctors estimated she would die of dehydration in about a week. The nephew had known her for 50 years, and had visited her regularly both before and after her placement in a nursing home. The court determined that he "had good intentions and had no real conflict of interest due to possible inheritance."

The court affirmed the principle that treatment may be "withheld or withdrawn from an incompetent patient when it is *clear* that the *particular* patient would have refused the treatment under the circumstances involved" (emphasis added). The nephew had argued that Conroy would have refused to be maintained in such a condition and that she would have refused the insertion of the nasogastric feeding tube in the first place. He testified that to the best of his recollection, she had never even been to a doctor (until after she became incompetent in 1979); that she had rejected the idea of bringing in a doctor to treat her for pneumonia; and that when his wife brought her to an emergency room, she refused to sign herself in and was of a mind to get herself back home, as soon as she felt strong enough to get away.

So there was at least *some* evidence in support of the claim that Conroy would not have wanted to be subjected to such extensive medical measures, but the court contended that such evidence, though not irrelevant, was not in this particular case sufficient by itself to settle the matter. It remained, at least in the court's opinion, a somewhat open question as to what Conroy would have decided in full awareness of the specific (and unanticipated) circumstances in which she was presently situated. The court then distinguished three different approaches to decision making on behalf of a presently noncompetent person and discussed when each approach would be most appropriate. What it called the "subjective test"—and what we have been calling "hypothetical consent"—*would* be the guiding standard if and when there is sufficient evidence to establish what the particular patient would and would not have authorized. The guardian must try to decide as the patient would have decided, if only she been able to exercise her decision-making capacity with adequate information concerning her present, incompetent state. The "objective test" would come into play "in the absence of trustworthy evidence, or indeed any evidence at all, about what the patient would have decided." On this test, even life-sustaining treatment may be "withheld or withdrawn from a formerly competent person like Claire Conroy if . . . the net burdens of the patient's life with the treatment should clearly and markedly outweigh the benefits the patient derives from life." The court tried to fill in this notion of what is "objectively" good or bad by alluding to such burdens as "recurring, unavoidable, and severe pain" and noting that in some cases proposed medical treatment would have to be regarded as plainly "inhumane." In cases in which there is some evidence of what the patient would have decided, but not enough evidence to settle the matter, the court prescribed a mixed test—what it called "the limited objective test." On this approach, relevant but insufficient evidence about the individual's values and about what the individual would have wanted done is to be weighed on the scales of deliberation along with more "objective" claims about what is typically beneficial or burdensome to a human being, quite apart from more specific attitudes and values (presently unknown) that this particular patient may have held.

3. A case in which the concept of hypothetical consent (and/or refusal) was mistakenly deployed[10]

Joseph Saikewicz was 67 years old, with an IQ of 10 and a mental age of approximately 2 years and 8 months. He was profoundly mentally retarded all his life. He had recently been diagnosed with leukemia. Previously he had "enjoyed generally good health. He was physically strong and well built, nutritionally nourished, and ambulatory. He was not, however, able to communicate verbally—resorting to gestures and grunts to make his wishes known to others and responding only to gestures or physical contacts." A regimen of chemotherapy would afford him a modest chance of living for 1 to 2 years longer but would also cause him to suffer significantly. In reflecting on "the unique considerations arising in this case by virtue of the patient's inability to appreciate his predicament and articulate his desires," the court noted that since Saikewicz "had no capacity to understand his present situation or his prognosis," the treatment in question would immerse him, as the guardian ad litem had argued, "in a state of painful suffering, the reason for which he will never understand. Patients who request treatment know the risks involved and can appreciate the painful side-effects when they arrive. They know the reason for the pain and their hope makes it tolerable." But Saikewicz could not. For this reason, the "evidence that most people choose to accept the rigors of chemotherapy has no direct bearing *on the likely choice that Joseph Saikewicz would have made*" (emphasis added). The court ruled that chemotherapy could be refused on Saikewicz's behalf.

A misguided formulation of what was ultimately at issue: To ground its decision, the court thought it needed to invoke the "substituted judgment standard," calling upon the guardian to choose as Saikewicz would have chosen. But the court's effort to deepen our appreciation for that standard only made its application to Saikewicz's case all the more puzzling: As the court went on to explain, the substituted judgment standard "commends itself simply because of *its straight-forward respect for the integrity and autonomy of the individual*" (emphasis added). The problem here is that since Joseph Saikewicz was *never* capable of autonomous choice, it is difficult to see how respect for *his autonomy* (as opposed to concern for his well-being) could make much sense in this unfortunate case.

Fortunately, the court articulated other key ideas that do make good sense. For example, it affirmed how even a person who is "incompetent" has the right "to be spared the deleterious consequences of life-prolonging treatment." This crucial point is not, however, equivalent to the notion that a never-competent human being is entitled to respect for his or her autonomy. On the contrary, it expresses the thought that even someone who has always been without the capacity to choose nevertheless has the right to have his or her needs and interests carefully considered and effectively represented. Indeed, it was in this very vein that the court spoke of the need "to determine with as much accuracy as possible the wants and needs of *the individual* involved" (emphasis added). In Saikewicz's case this would include paying close attention to the limited benefits and serious adverse side effects of the proposed treatment, the difficulty he would have had cooperating with the treatment, and the absence of any possibility of his drawing solace and courage from hopeful anticipation of a remission.

To sum up, the Saikewicz court considered a case in which the standard of what is in the "best interest of the patient" ought to have been (and in practical reality, actually was) the controlling consideration; in some passages in its opinion, however, the court misleadingly wrote as though it was applying the "substituted judgment" standard.

7. Thomson's More Deflationary Account of Hypothetical Consent

Thomson wants to suggest that appearances not withstanding, the appeal to hypothetical "consent" is not doing any real "moral work." As we have seen, however, from the fact that hypothetical consent is not always necessary and not always sufficient "for permissibility," it does *not* follow that hypothetical consent does no moral work. To support her more deflationary view, there-fore, Thomson needs to offer us an alternative account of what is "really doing the moral work," and this is precisely what she sets out to do.

Thomson understands how people who take hypothetical consent ser-iously are not usually asking, "What would this person have to say if we woke him up and he refused to consent because he could not think clearly, could not grasp the factual realities of his situation, and was not in touch with his own values and commitments?" Rather, the question they think they must try to answer is more like, "What would this person authorize or refuse to authorize if he or she were thinking clearly, were in touch with his or her own values and commitments, and were cognizant of the diagnosis, the prognosis, the various treatment (and nontreatment) options, and their likely benefits, associated risks, and so forth?"

It is Thomson's thesis, however, that once these further stipulations are made explicit, we will be able to see more clearly that what is "really doing the moral work" is not hypothetical consent, but something else instead.

1. What is doing the work is *not* the fact, *if* it is even a fact, that this man "would consent to your proceeding" with the operation, "but rather *what it is about him* in virtue of which he would consent" (if indeed he would) (p. 188) (emphasis added).

2. *What it is about him* turns out to be *what, on balance, is good for him.*

Thus, Thomson writes that "what makes it permissible for you to proceed in David's case, if proceeding is permissible, is this: it is on balance good for David that you proceed" (p. 191). On the other hand, *if* David's being a Christian Scientist means "that your proceeding is bad for him, sufficiently bad to outweigh the good of living," then *that's why* you shouldn't proceed to amputate. By good for him, Thomson hastens to add, she means what is (to the best of our ability to discern) on balance "objectively good for him."

Going to the trouble of figuring out whether the person in question would or would not have consented *if only* he were in a clear-thinking, informed, self-aware state of mind turns out to be just a *roundabout* way of figuring out what is and is not objectively good for this person. The under-lying idea is that what is good for him *will be evident* upon *a clear and accurately informed* examination of the facts about him and his situation— *no matter who* undertakes this examination. There is a value-fact-of-the-matter that will be accessible to *anyone* (the person himself *or anybody else*) appropriately *equipped* with what it takes to know what is good.

So it might be true that under the stipulated conditions the individual himself would have consented, but that is *only* a (trivial) consequence of the fact that anyone who really knew the whole story, who could think clearly and cogently (and who, by hypothesis perhaps, genuinely cared about that individual's well-being), would have prescribed the same course of treatment and urged the doctors to proceed (or refrain from proceeding) accordingly. On this way of thinking, an *individual's* convictions, commitments, volitions, and the like turn out to be just some of the (many) facts that bear (in greater or lesser degree) on what is and is not going to be *good for* that individual.

But there is another, very different way of looking at the matter and of appreciating the significance of (at least some of) a person's volitions and decisions. On this way of thinking, an individual who has decision-making capacity is to be respected, not as a mere locus or "repository" of good and bad states of affairs, psychological or otherwise, but as an "autonomous agent"—with the right to decide what will happen in and to his or her own body. Thomson very briefly mentions, but then dismisses, a way of thinking about the case at hand that *might seem* to reflect this other, more "autonomy-respecting" approach. She writes, "It could be said that what bars operating on a deeply committed Christian Scientist is not that it is bad for him to do so, but the very fact that it contravenes his deeply held moral beliefs. It could be said that operating *is* in a measure bad for him but that what bars operating is not that the bad outweighs the good you would do by operating but rather just (or in addition) the fact that the Christian Scientist deeply believes it wrong to operate" (p. 190).

Curiously, however, Thomson does not even attempt to elaborate on this alternative perspective. In particular, she does not even mention, let alone analyze, the possibility that *what matters here is not what is on balance good for him, but rather what is appropriately respectful of his right to determine what is going to happen in and to his own body* (insofar, of course, as other people's rights would not thereby be violated or jeopardized). Thomson does allow that this other line of thinking raises a question that is "both deep and interesting," but she believes that her own way of "characterizing the case" is "very plausible" and so proposes to "take it." In other words, she proposes that what "bars your proceeding if David is a deeply committed Christian Scientist is that it would be on balance bad for him if you proceeded."

8. An Important Distinction Overlooked

In opting for this account, and virtually ignoring the autonomy-respecting approach, Thomson has insufficiently distinguished cases of two very different kinds, and this has allowed her to blur the distinction between two importantly different principles for deciding how to treat an individual who presently cannot decide for himself: (*1*) cases of the sort illustrated by *Saikewicz,* an individual who *never had* decision-making capacity, and (*2*) cases of the sort illustrated by *Brophy,* an individual with well-formed and well-known convictions, values, attitudes, and so forth.

1. In cases of the first sort, the overriding concern is and ought to be to "protect and promote the best interests of the patient."
2. In cases of the second sort, however, a major concern is and ought to be "to respect his right of self-determination, even though he cannot presently exercise decision-making capacity."

The error here is the inverse, so to speak, of the mistake that the Saikewicz court had made: That court tried to interpret all surrogate decision-making cases as cases covered by an extended version of the "right to self-determination"; in her zeal to deny any fundamental moral significance to "hypothetical consent," Thomson is prepared to subsume all such cases under the "best interests of the patient" principle. Lost in the shuffle is the idea that individuals who meet, or who once did meet, a modest threshold of "decision-making competence" have the right to make certain choices themselves, or to have certain matters decided *on their behalf* in reflection of how they *would have* chosen. Moreover, this right is to be respected even when the choices in question do not accord with what other people (perhaps very thoughtfully and even correctly) believe to be (objectively) *best* for that individual. A person has the right, for example, to live his life as he chooses, even if living it differently would afford him a longer life filled with what he acknowledges would have more good in it on balance. Alternatively, he has the right to decide that he will give priority to advancing the good of others, less fortunate than himself, or to upholding their rights, even though he runs, and knows that he runs, a significant risk of losing his own life much earlier than he would otherwise.

9. Contrast and Comparison; Some Unresolved Issues

In recent years, persons who are concerned to affirm their right to bodily self-determination, even in respect to circumstances in which they may later lack decision-making capacity, have been encouraged to pursue either, or both, of two different strategies: (1) to issue a detailed advance directive; (2) to appoint a health care agent with durable power of attorney (whose primary responsibility will be to arrive at a decision that reasonably approximates what the patient himself would have decided).

Giving (or withholding) "actual consent" through a detailed prior directive might seem to be a wiser course to take than burdening someone else with the task of *hypothesizing* consent. Following instructions contained in an *actual* document would seem to be a more easily and reliably executed task than trying to confirm the hypothesis that consent would have (or would not have) been given. But matters may not be quite so simple. In the urgency of the present situation, it may not be at all clear that any such directive even exists. And if and when it does, it may be difficult to access it soon enough and/or to interpret its implications for the circumstances at hand. In addition, there is the (perhaps deeper) question of how well the individual was able to anticipate the facts of the present situation and understand their significance for the needs and interests he might *later* have developed. Such difficulties are likely to be exacerbated as the temporal distance between the document and the present predicament grows greater. These problems might be classified as "epistemic" (that is, having to do with what can be known or justifiably believed).

Aside from these epistemic issues, however, there are other still more profoundly ethical concerns as well. For one thing, there is a question about the extent to which the self at an earlier stage *can rightfully* exercise authority over the self at a much later stage. When is a prior directive an exercise in trans-temporal "self-unification" and when is it a kind of cross-temporal "tyranny"? Should respect for the trans-temporally "unified" agent override or outweigh compassionate concern for the still conscious but psychologically much less complex human being who is present to us now? Sometimes an individual who has lost decision-making capacity is very clearly comfortable and content with his more limited existence, with the range of experiences and activities of which he is capable, despite the fact that his self in its earlier stages would have rejected such a life as deficient in quality and lacking in dignity. In these cases, what is the right course for a guardian to take? To comply with the directives of the earlier (more "rational" stage of the) self, however detrimental to the needs and interests of the present (stage of the) self? Or, to satisfy the consistently manifested needs and interests of the more psychologically limited, present (stage of the) self?

These are profoundly difficult questions. The notion of "hypothetical consent"—and the appointment of an agent well equipped and well positioned to infer such "consent"—*can be helpful* in overcoming *some*, but certainly not all, of these difficulties. Thus, in contrast with a prior directive, a health care agent should be able to talk to the medical experts on the scene and arrive at a more adequately informed understanding of the patient's current situation. If selected from among friends and relatives who have been in a continuously close relation to the patient, such an agent should also be more vividly aware of the patient's more recently manifested attitudes and values. This in turn should allow for a more accurate inference to what treatment the patient would (or would not) *now authorize—if only he or she could temporarily regain decision-making capacity.* For these reasons, having the decision made in this "hypothetical consent"-attributing way may be less "cross-temporally tyrannical" than issuing a prior directive. It may be more adequately reflective of how individuals can and do evolve over time.

Of course, relying on hypothetical consent attributions can have serious drawbacks as well. Much depends on the transparency of the patient's attitudes, values, and commitments, as well as on the designated agent's character and intelligence. Moreover, this approach cannot by itself resolve the heartrending conflict that sometimes arises between earlier and later stages of the self. It reflects the ideal of respect for a person's autonomous choices, but it cannot tell us how to balance respect for autonomy (as exercised previously) with compassionate concern for the emotional and experiential needs of the noncompetent self in its later stages.[11]

10: Medical Ethics and Hypothetical Future Consent

Recall the case of the mother who wants her child to be immunized against a deadly or debilitating disease and in the face of the child's present resistance comforts herself with the thought that her child will some day retrospectively endorse what she has done and even go on to consent to comparable future measures. (For the sake of simplicity, we can leave aside whether there is anything potentially damaging to the child in undergoing the vaccination.) The question here is whether the mother's appeal to what the child *will* later think, approve, and so forth, is what helps to justify her conduct.

Lurking here in the wings is an entirely different interpretation of such cases—an interpretation of precisely the sort that Thomson was offering us. In other words, it might be said that in order for us to be able to make the right distinctions here, we need to insist that eventual "consent" is not "really doing the work" at all—and that something else instead is what validates the mother's behavior.

I believe that for cases of the sort we are discussing now, Thomson's approach does come *closer* to providing the right account, *but* that we may also have to *modify* that approach in one important way: shifting from an appeal to "what is on balance *good* for someone" to the idea of what is, all things considered, most *respectful* of that individual's *rights*.

It will be helpful to begin by recalling a different sort of case altogether. Victor Frankl was a prisoner in Nazi concentration camps. Despite extreme hardship, he survived and went on to become an important author and respected psychologist. His book, *Man's Search for Meaning*,[12] inspired millions of people. By his own account, his experiences in the concentration camps somehow helped Frankl to become more deeply understanding of the human condition, more insightful about what gives life meaning and purpose, and much more compassionate toward fellow human beings than he would have been otherwise. Frankl could honestly say that he didn't "regret" the horrible experiences and degradations he had sustained during his imprisonment and enslavement—for otherwise he would most likely never be the human being he had actually become.

What, then, does this prove? Not that the Nazis behaved appropriately. From the fact that someone doesn't "regret" how he or she was once treated, it doesn't follow that the behavior in question was therefore right and justifiable. In Frankl's case, he did not regret what happened, but he did not condone what was done either. And even if someone less wise than Frankl had said, "Well, they did the right thing by me, didn't they?" that judgment would have been mistaken.

But what about the case of the mother and child? Could her expectation that the child will later be grateful—and not "regret" what she has done for him—be what is "really" doing the justificatory work? Instead of taking that route, I suggest that what we need here is a *variation* on the analysis Thomson would apply (mistakenly) to *all* cases in which hypothetical consent is attributed. Thus, *as a first approximation*, the mother might be represented as saying:

> This vaccination is so clearly and compellingly for the benefit of my child that if and when he reaches an age when he too *can* think clearly, have and understand the relevant information, and so forth, he will be able to see for himself why I am doing what's *best* for him. As a very young child, of course, he cannot be reasonably expected to see such things for himself.

On this way of thinking, then, there is a fact—the *fact* that the mother is doing what is for the greater good of the child. *Anybody* who can think clearly and knowledgeably about such matters will be able to grasp this fact and hence will be able to approve what the mother is doing. To claim that the adult the child grows up to become "will" see this fact and approve of his mother's previous conduct is just a consequence of this same fact—but a consequence that will not result unless the child also grows up to be clear-thinking, well informed, and so forth.

But why say that the mother's statement given previously is (only) a "first approximation" to what might need to be said? Why not say that it's got the matter just right? Well, for one thing, of course, she does have to accept the *possibility* that the child will not grow up to have what it takes to "know" what is for a person's greater good. But there is another possibility to be reckoned with as well—namely, that the adult the child grows into might subscribe to some view (of which Christian Science is but one example)—in light of which vaccinations and other medical procedures are not conducive to a person's good.

Is the mother then necessarily banking on the further illiberal thought, "If that were to happen, my child would have grown up to become ill-equipped to know what is good"? Not necessarily. The mother could well say something along these lines instead:

> My child might some day grow up to believe that vaccinations are bad. I admit that I believe that such a view is mistaken. But what I am doing now is *not* intended to prevent him from engaging in such reflections and deliberations as an adult in his own right—an adult who might opt for Christian Science rather than medical science. On the contrary, I am acting now so that, to the best of *my* present ability to figure such things out, my child can go on to live long enough to be able to form such convictions and make such decisions *for himself.*

On this more complicated analysis, there is something ("objectively") *right* about what the mother is doing even if the son later embraces a different conception of what is *good.* And in a way that is comparable to Thomson's claim about the good, it might well be thought that anyone sufficiently equipped to think clearly and intelligently about what is right and just will be able to recognize that what the mother is doing is right. The mother's confidence that her child will grow up some day to endorse what she has done is confidence that he will grow up to be able to tell what is *right* from what is wrong. If he grows up to reject what his mother has done *as not having respected his rights, then he will have made a moral mistake.*

Of course, prior to her child's growing up and freely becoming a Christian Scientist, the mother has no way of knowing that the child *will* in fact come to have such an attitude. Thus, the adult that the child grows into might look back and say, "I'm sorry my mother had an incorrect idea about what's good and bad in this world." But he *cannot rightly* say, "My mother treated me wrongly." In a sense, this case is the mirror image of the Frankl case: looking back on his earlier life, Frankl did not regret being in a concentration camp, but he did rightly condemn what the Nazis did as a profound violation of basic human rights. The young adult who has come to reject medical science in favor of faith can retrospectively *regret* what his mother did, but *cannot* reasonably condemn his mother for not respecting his rights.

On this account, as with Thomson's, there *is a moral fact* that is *more fundamental* than hypothetical consent—a fact more fundamental than whether this mother's child will some day grasp that fact and retrospectively "consent" to what the mother has done. But the difference is that it is not primarily a fact about what is, on balance, *objectively for the greater good of her son*. Rather, it is a fact about what *rightly* protects and preserves *his eventual right to decide for himself* what is *good* and what is *not*.

Thomson herself says casually and without much explanation that the Christian Scientist has the right to reject a life-saving measure for himself but not for his own child. The rights-based account suggested here goes some of the way toward explaining this distinction; it is not clear whether the alternative account, which stresses what is on balance good for a patient, can explain and justify this distinction as clearly and compellingly.

11. The "Epiphenomenal" Character of Hypothetical Contract Theory?

There is a tradition in moral and political thought that represents the principles of justice as the terms of a hypothetical "contract"—a contract to which individuals who were deliberating (and bargaining) with one another under certain very special (but somewhat hypothetical) conditions would agree.

Thomson's complaint is that the principles that emerge from such hypothetical "contract"-making models are *not* to be considered principles of right and of justice *on the ground that* individuals hypothetically situated would have agreed to them; rather, what really matters and what is really "doing the moral work" are *the reasons* why the participants in the procedure would (or would not) have embraced those principles. Once these reasons are in view—as they would have to be in order to justify the claim that the

participants in the idealized procedure would have agreed to them as well—
the idea of the hypothetical agreement drops out of the picture.

This, at any rate, is the *general* form of her concern. Let's look at the
specifics:

> I confess to a strong suspicion that hypothetical consent is an
> epiphenomenon throughout current political theory. It is argued
> that such and such are just rules because people would consent to live
> by them if asked. But would they? Perhaps some among them are
> confused or full of envy, or for some other reason would not consent.
> What the theorist typically does in face of these possibilities is to
> impose constraints: we are not to ask whether people (warts and all)
> would actually consent . . . *but whether people would consent if they
> met certain conditions, such as being clear-headed, free of envy and the
> like* [emphasis added]. How do we know they would consent if they
> met those conditions? Well, *living by those rules is to their
> advantage—their real advantage, as opposed to what they might in the
> circumstances (and given their warts) think to be to their advantage*
> [emphasis added]. But then *that* [emphasis in original text] is what
> does the moral work of justifying the thesis that those rules are just.
> The theorists argue from "It is to their real advantage" to "The rules
> are just" via the intermediary "They would consent to the rules"; but
> the intermediary is mere epiphenomenon (pp. 188–89).

There are two problematic elements to this critique:

1. First, consider the more specific claim that what makes rules just is that
   they are to the "real advantage" of the people who, if only they had been
   sufficiently clear-headed, would have chosen them. There are many
   different ways of developing the theme that justice is "what would have
   been agreed to"; what Thomson has to say here makes some sense in
   connection with contract theories of *one* particular sort but does *not*
   apply very well to the quite different approach exemplified by such
   contemporary contract theorists as Rawls and Scanlon.
2. Second, consider Thomson's more general thesis that whatever the
   reasons that the hypothetical contractors would have for agreeing to
   certain principles are the reasons we have for appreciating those
   principles more directly in the first place.

Taking these points in turn: 1. The strand of contractarian thought that
most closely resembles Thomson's remark is essentially egoistic: Justice is

what people would agree to if only they were more rationally and realistically self-interested. The key thought is that despite differences in strength and intelligence, no human being is invulnerable to suffering harm at the hands of another. The advantages in advancing one's ends at the expense of others (for example, through force and fraud) are outweighed by the disadvantages of being subjected to such behavior on the part of others. The prudent decision is for people to renounce the liberty to inflict harm (or perpetrate fraud) on others in return for the comparable renunciation by others. In addition, it will be necessary to cooperate together in setting up a system that ensures compliance with this agreement. The rules thus chosen are *just* precisely because their effective enforcement *is* (in Thomson's words) a "real advantage" for everyone. A theory along these very lines is offered but not fully endorsed by Socrates's interlocutors, Glaucon and Adeimantus, in Book One of *The Republic* by Plato.

Understood in this way, justice makes sense because people *are* roughly equal in threat advantage. It would seem to follow that the less vulnerable that people are to certain other people, the less just they need to be in relation to those people. In circumstances of very low visibility (for example, if one were to have the mythic "ring of Gyges"!) and limited vulnerability, "justice" would seem to lose much of its point. Well aware of this concern, Plato—through the words of Socrates—devoted much of the rest of the *Republic* to developing a rather different notion of justice and to arguing that even when there is the opportunity to commit injustice *without* external sanction, it *is* nevertheless to a person's real (and much deeper) advantage to be just.

A fundamentally different "contract" approach to justice can be found in the writings of such thinkers as Rousseau and Kant, and more recently, Rawls and Scanlon. In theories of this sort, persons are to be respected as having an equality of moral status that is *not* contingent upon roughly equal power or threat-advantage. Instead, what more fundamentally matters is that they have lives to lead and the capacity to regulate their pursuits in accordance with mutually acceptable "terms of association." The central question becomes, Are there "terms of association" to which persons so conceived could and would agree? Justice is not represented as the result of an agreement between individuals who prudently recognize one another's equal threat-advantage, but rather, as a reflection of a certain ideal: equal respect for persons as leaders of lives and as citizens of society.

Of course, the ideal of equal respect for persons is inspiring but problematically vague. Thus, in his earlier masterwork, *A Theory of Justice*,[13] Rawls hit upon an interesting heuristic device: a *hypothetical* bargaining situation (dubbed the "original position") in which persons who are symmetrically situated and equally represented as choosers and pursuers of ends are to work out the most fundamental terms of their political association with one another. The most striking feature of this hypothetical decision-making model is that the parties to it must deliberate under a constraint that Rawls called "the veil of ignorance." What this means is that they must ignore (or still more graphically, not even be permitted to "know") their own particular identities—their natural features, their social positions, and their respective values or "conceptions of the good." (A subsequent refinement—not relevant to our present discussion—that Rawls added to this model was to think of each party to this "original position" as a representative of some particular individual in society.)

The parties to this imaginary situation do know that they (or the individuals they represent) do have two capacities: the capacity to form and pursue a conception of the good and the capacity—a "sense of justice"—to lead their lives in accordance with mutually acceptable terms of association. And they have access to all "general knowledge" about the human condition that might be available through such fields of study as psychology, sociology, economics, and the like.

Subject to these constraints, the imaginary parties to this hypothetical "bargaining" situation must try to do the "best" they can for "themselves." Though they are also described as "nonenvious," they are not specifically motivated by altruistic concerns either. Instead, they are said to be "mutually interested." For Rawls, this means that they take "no interest in one another's interests."

On the surface, Rawls's hypothetical contract model might appear to be just another version of an essentially "egoistic" approach to justice. But since none of the parties can identify (either self or "client" represented) with any *particular* individual in the real world, they will, in effect, have to deliberate with equal concern for any of the individuals in whose shoes they might find themselves (or find their "clients") once the imaginary "veil of ignorance" is "lifted." Thus, as Rawls was at pains to point out, "The feeling that this conception of justice is egoistic is an illusion fostered by looking at but one of the elements of the original position" (*TJ*, p. 129).

Why, then, did Rawls construct the hypothetical deliberation procedure in a way that could give rise to such an illusion? The answer has to do with his sense that if we had tried to develop a theory of justice more directly from the ideal of "respect for persons" or from the assumption that the parties to the original position are moved by "benevolence plus knowledge" of the world, such notions would not have provided us with an adequate basis for sufficiently clear and precise reasoning. People of good will can often agree on such ideas as "respect for persons" or the need to "care" about one another as they care about themselves but still manage to disagree about which more practical behaviors and policies are required by such attitudes. Rawls's theory does not dismiss such notions, but it does claim that "they call for interpretation" (p. 513). In Rawls's view, "the aims of benevolence and the requirements of respect" are "undefined" until we can formulate appropriate principles of justice that give them specificity and content. Rawls's hope was to construct an idealized deliberative model that "combines the requisite clarity with the relevant ethical constraints" (p. 512). The "clarity" is provided, at least to some degree, by representing each of the parties to the original position as interested only in one "self" but then effectively inducing, through the constraint of the veil of ignorance, an equally profound interest in the fate of *any* self. It is as though, starting with a very vague idea of equal respect for each and everyone, we pressed decision theory and game theory into service to help us develop in a more rigorous way the practical implications of that idea. That at least was the hope. As Rawls himself puts this point, "I have avoided attributing to the parties any ethical motivation. They decide solely on the basis of what is calculated to further their interests so far as they can ascertain them. *In this way we can exploit the idea of rational prudential choice.* We can, however, define ethical variations of the initial situation by supposing the parties to be influenced by moral considerations. *It is a mistake to object that the notion of the original agreement would no longer be ethically neutral. For this notion already includes moral features*" (p. 512, emphasis added).

2. Concerning the question of why real people in the real world should take any interest in the principles that would have been "chosen" under highly artificial circumstances, the answer is not as simple as the one Thomson suggests. The hypothetical contract makers choose on the basis of "self"-interest. But a truly *egoistic* individual could not rationally desire to be constrained to deliberate in the way the "original position" requires its "participants" to do, let alone to be committed to living in accordance with the principles that would thus be chosen. "Self"-interested choosers under the constraints of the original position have to be concerned with the fundamental plight of each and every "self" in society. This is not egoism, enlightened or otherwise.

So persons who in real life *are willing to simulate* the deliberations of the hypothetical parties to Rawls's hypothetical situation and to put stock in the principles thus chosen show that *they* are prepared to adjust *their* ends and constrain *their* conduct out of *respect* for one another's equal status as leaders of lives and as citizens in political society. Contrary to Thomson's representation of the matter, the reasons the *parties* to the "original position" have for agreeing to certain principles are *not* exactly the same reasons we ourselves have for considering those principles to be *fair* terms of political association and for striving to have the design of the basic political structure of our society accord with those principles. Our reasons have to do with our sense that the constraints under which the parties to the original position deliberate, successfully model or reflect important moral concerns over and above prudence.[14]

None of this is to deny that we *might* be able to develop the same theory of justice by starting with the (somewhat vague) idea of equal respect for persons. But since different philosophers have long argued about just what such respect entails, the device of an "original position" may help us to focus on just what (further) assumptions about the basic moral status of human beings each such view of "equal respect" is implicitly making.[15] It is for this reason perhaps that Rawls himself suggests that we might want to explore various possible "ethical variations" of the "initial situation."[16]

12. Summation

We began with the observation that there are several different contexts in which, though consent *has not actually been given,* it nevertheless seems to be both reasonable to infer and *relevant* to insist that if certain conditions (1) had obtained, (2) were to obtain, and/or (3) will yet obtain, then someone's consent (1) *would have been,* (2) *would be,* and/or (3) *will yet be* given.

We have now explored two major contexts in which the hypothesis of consent *is* relevant and *does* play a significant role in our moral reflections: (1) in medical contexts involving surrogate decision makers, the point of trying to establish what would or would not have been authorized by an individual who previously had decision-making capacity is to extend to that individual a measure of autonomous control over what shall happen in and to that person's own body despite the lack of decision-making capacity under the circumstances that actually obtain; and (2) in moral and political philosophy, the purpose of such a hypothesis—for at least *one version* of "contract theory"—is to "model" certain basic but otherwise vague and abstract *moral assumptions* (for example, about the equal status of persons as leaders of lives and as citizens in political society) and hence to assist, whether as a fruitful expository device or as an essential tool, in a fuller, more precise articulation of what is implied by those assumptions.

We have also considered two other kinds of cases—cases exemplified by Saikewicz and cases illustrated by the mother-and-child scenario—in which what is "really" doing the "moral work" *is* something *other than* consent, whether hypothetical or actual. In the first kind of case, the fact that the individual *has never had* (and *never will have*) decision-making capacity makes it difficult to talk about respect for that individual's *right to decide* such matters. Thus, the surrogate's responsibility is to try to determine what is in that individual's "best interests" rather than what *that* individual *would have* authorized. In the second kind of case, the guardian's hypothesis that the ward *will* later "consent" to (or endorse) what the guardian has previously done is not necessarily misplaced or inappropriate; the hypothesis may or may not be true. But if it is true and *if* its truth has moral relevance, it is only because of the way in which it "piggy-backs" on a deeper, hypothetical-consent-*independent* moral fact. (Rather than somehow constituting or creating it in the first place, the individual's later "consent" or endorsement reflects appreciation of that fact.) In contrast with Thomson's way of interpreting such cases, however, what is "doing the moral work" in the mother-and-child case is not primarily a fact about what is, on balance, *for the greater good* of her son. Rather, it is a fact about what rightly preserves and protects *his eventual right to decide for himself* what *is good* and what is *not*. [17]

Notes

1. *Riggs v. Palmer*, 115 N.Y. 506 (1889).
2. Cf. D. Wendler and C. Grady, "What Should Research Participants Understand to Understand They Are Participants in Research?" *Bioethics* 28 (2008): 203–08.
3. Cf. J. Rawls, *A Theory of Justice.* Cambridge: Harvard University Press, 1971, revised 1999 and T.M. Scanlon, *What We Owe To Each Other.* Cambridge: Belknap Press of Harvard University Press, 1998).
4. Judith J. Thomson, *The Realm of Rights* (Cambridge, MA: Harvard University Press, 1990). Subsequent parenthetical page references in the main text are to *this* work.
5. Many people have had doubts about whether "hypothetical consent" really ought to play any role at all in our moral deliberations. Thomson's discussion provides us with what is perhaps the most philosophically sophisticated critique thus far presented.
6. It may, however, gain some purchase in respect to the approach Rawls took much later on in his second book, *Political Liberalism* (New York: Columbia University Press, 1993), and related writings. See Note 16.

7. Sometimes, perhaps especially in emergency situations, the hypothesis of consent is based on facts about human beings more generally rather than on attitudes and values specific, or indeed idiosyncratic, to the person in question. Thus, for example, unless we do have evidence of person-specific attitudes to the contrary, it is reasonable to hypothesize (or "presume") that the person on whose behalf we must decide would direct us to spare him from paraplegia. It might be useful, then, to reserve the expression "presumed consent" for hypotheses of consent grounded in such general assumptions about human nature rather than in more individual-specific knowledge.

8. *Patricia E. Brophy v. New England Sinai Hospital, Inc.*; No. N-4152, Supreme Judicial Court of Massachusetts, 398 Mass. 417; 497 N.E.2d 626 (1986).

9. *In the Matter of Claire C. Conroy*, Supreme Court of New Jersey, 98 N.J. 321, 486A. 2d 1209 (January 17, 1985).

10. *Superintendent of Belchertown State School et al. vs. Joseph Saikewicz*, 373 Mass. 728.

11. For competing views on these difficult matters, see Ronald Dworkin, *Life's Dominion* (New York: Alfred A. Knopf, 1993), ch. 8 ("Life Past Reason"), and Rebecca Dresser, "Dworkin on Dementia: Elegant Theory, Questionable Policy," *Hastings Center Report* (November–December 1995): 32–38.

12. Victor E. Frankl, *Man's Search for Meaning* (1946) (Washington Square Press, 1984).

13. John Rawls, *A Theory of Justice,* rev. ed. (Cambridge, MA: Harvard University Press, 1999); hereafter "*TJ*"; subsequent parenthetical page references in the text are to this edition.

14. The hypothesis that consent *would have* been given under certain conditions (that did not in fact obtain) is sometimes advanced—not in order to support general principles of right and of justice, but to establish that particular individuals have an *obligation* to obey particular governments. Given space limitations, I will not explore this variant of hypothetical contract theory here. For criticism of the idea that a person can be under an obligation to comply with an institutional arrangement simply because under certain hypothetical circumstances he or she would have agreed to do so, see Ronald Dworkin, "The Original Position," *University of Chicago Law Review* 40 (Spring 1973): 500–33, and reprinted in Norman Daniels, ed., *Reading Rawls* (Palo Alto, CA: Stanford University Press, 1989), 16–53, esp. 18–19. As we shall see (in Note 14), Dworkin *does* go on to endorse *Rawls's* use of a hypothetical contract model, not as a way of establishing obligations, but as a way of lending support to *general principles* of right and of justice (including, one might add, principles that specify when and why people can be said to have incurred various obligations and when, leaving obligation aside, they could be said to have a "natural duty of justice" to cooperate in support

of existing institutional arrangements). For more extensive discussion of why "hypothetical consent" cannot establish *political obligation*, see Cynthia Stark, "Hypothetical Consent and Justification," *Journal of Philosophy* xcvii, 6 (June 2000): 313–34. Like Dworkin, Stark believes that hypothetical consent under certain idealized conditions "has the power to justify" general principles. But she holds that this justificatory role presupposes a "meta-ethical principle" that "denies the existence of an independent order of value . . . to which we could appeal to determine what is just" ("Hypothetical Consent and Political Legitimacy," *The Paideia Archive* [Twentieth World Congress of Philosophy, August 1998], 6, available at: www.bu.edu/wcp/Papers/Poli/PoliStar.htm). Rawls's considered position is that the use of the contract model does not presuppose the truth of any such controversial meta-ethical assumption. Indeed, an "overlapping consensus" in support of Rawlsian justice could well include those who believe that the original position deliberation procedure is significant precisely because it reflects certain very basic (and "independent") moral "truths" (for example, that there is, as Dworkin asserts, a "natural right" to equal respect and consideration in the design of the basic political structure) and *not* because it somehow "constructs" such ideas.

15. Thus, Ronald Dworkin has observed how exponents of otherwise competing political theories nevertheless often share the belief that people have "a right to equal concern and respect in the design and administration of the political institutions that govern them" but disagree about what that right entails. Dworkin contends that the "original position may now be seen as a device" that affords these theorists the opportunity, "rare for them," to "submit" their competing political views to "some form of philosophical examination" ("The Original Position," loc. cit., 50–53).

16. By the time he published his second book, *Political Liberalism* (1993), Rawls had modified his account of what motivates the parties to the original position thought experiment in a way that might allow for Thomson's "epiphenomenalism" complaint to gain more purchase. The parties are depicted as concerned above all else with ensuring the fully adequate development and informed exercise of "two moral powers": (1) the capacity to form and pursue *a conception of the good* and (2) the capacity to have and to exercise *a sense of justice*. From this perspective, it is hardly surprising that the hypothetical contract makers would opt for principles that assigned high priority to freedom of the person; freedom of conscience; freedom of expression; the right to participate, directly or indirectly, in the processes by which public policies are made; and so forth. Thus, it might now seem plausible to suggest that the contract apparatus has become a cumbersome distraction rather than a useful tool—that what is "really doing the work" in Rawls's theory of justice is not the hypothesis that certain principles would be

agreed to in the original position but the thesis that to respect one another as *leaders of lives and as citizens* in political society, people must cooperate in support of the development and exercise of one another's "two moral powers."

17. *If,* however, there is no reasonable prospect of the child's developing into a person with decision-making capacity, then this becomes a case like *Saikewicz*. The surrogate's responsibility is to protect and promote the child's well-being.

7

Consent to Harm

Vera Bergelson[1]

Introduction

The case of Oliver Jovanovic, dubbed by tabloids the "cybersex torture" case,[2] began in November 1996, when Jamie Ruzcek, a 20-year-old Barnard student, reported to the police that she had been sexually assaulted by Oliver Jovanovic, a 30-year-old doctoral candidate at Columbia University. The alleged assault happened during the first "live" date between Jovanovic and Ruzcek, which took place after weeks of their online conversations and e-mail correspondence. According to Ruzcek, "Jovanovic had hogtied her for nearly twenty hours, violently raped and sodomized her, struck her repeatedly with a club, severely burned her with candle wax, and repeatedly gagged her with a variety of materials."[3]

Jovanovic was prosecuted, convicted of kidnapping, sexual abuse, and assault, and sentenced to a term of 15 years to life. He was released from prison 20 months later when the appellate court ruled that the trial judge had improperly denied admission of portions of Ruzcek's e-mails to Jovanovic in which she discussed her sadomasochistic interests and experience. The court explained: "Because the jury could have inferred from the redacted e-mail messages that the complainant had shown an interest in participating in sadomasochism with Jovanovic, this evidence is clearly central to the question of whether she consented to the charged kidnapping and sexual abuse."[4] Since nonconsent is an element of each offense—kidnapping and sexual abuse—the appellate court predictably reversed Jovanovic's convictions on both charges. But the court did not stop there; it also reversed Jovanovic's conviction of assault in the second and third degree.

Under New York law, a person is guilty of second-degree assault when, "[w]ith intent to cause physical injury to another person, he causes such injury to such person . . . by means of a deadly weapon or a dangerous instrument."[5] A person is guilty of third-degree assault when, "[w]ith intent to cause physical injury to another person, he causes such injury to such person."[6] Neither statutory provision lists the lack of consent as an element to be proven by the prosecution, or allows the defense of consent. So the appellate court did something quite remarkable: It reversed the assault conviction and, at the same time (albeit in a footnote only), reiterated the traditional rule that "[t]here is no available defense of consent on a charge of assault."[7] The court elaborated:

> Indeed, while a meaningful distinction can be made between an ordinary violent beating and violence in which both parties voluntarily participate for their own sexual gratification, nevertheless, just as a person cannot consent to his or her own murder, as a matter of public policy, a person cannot avoid criminal responsibility for an assault that causes injury or carries a risk of serious harm, even if the victim asked for or consented to the act.[8]

In his opinion, concurring in part and dissenting in part, Judge Mazzarelli pointed out the obvious discrepancy between the majority's holding (consent is not a defense to assault) and decision (reversal of the assault conviction).[9] He also opined that the evidence produced at the trial was sufficient to support the defendant's conviction of assault,[10] and the majority did not dispute that conclusion.[11]

Technically, Judge Mazzarelli was right, and the majority was wrong. The decision defied both formal logic and established legal rule.[12] But, from the perspective of fairness and internal consistency of criminal sanctions, the *Jovanovic* appellate decision was entirely warranted. Indeed, if Jovanovic actually caused Ruzcek a lot of pain and anguish, why should her consent shield him from criminal liability for sexual violence and kidnapping, but not for assault?[13] Clearly, this is not because rape or kidnapping is a less serious offense than assault. In fact, a person in danger of being raped or kidnapped may use any physical force, including deadly force, to protect himself against that danger, whereas a person in danger of a simple assault does not have the same right. And yet, consent of the victim "turns a rape into love-making, a kidnapping into a Sunday drive, a battery into a football tackle, a theft into a gift, and a trespass into a dinner party,"[14] but, except in a couple of narrowly defined circumstances, it is powerless to change the moral and legal character of assault.

The Origins and Current Boundaries of the Rule of Consent

Historically, the special rule of consent to physical harm originated in Anglo-American jurisprudence in the seventeenth century. Prior to that, an individual was free to acquiesce practically to anything, and consent was viewed as a complete ban on prosecution. As the famous maxim goes, *volenti non fit injuria*: "a person is not wronged by that to which he consents."[15] Changes came as a result of monopolization of the system of punishment by the state. While in the early ages of criminal justice the victim was the central figure in the prosecution and settlement of any nonpublic offense,[16] in the normative and centralized judicial structure the victim became almost entirely excluded from the criminal process.[17] "In contrast to the understanding of crime as a violation of the victim's interest, the emergence of the state developed another interpretation: the disturbance of the society."[18] An increasing number of historically "private" offenses were reconceptualized as "public."[19] The state (or king) became the ultimate victim and the sole prosecutor of a criminal act.[20] Consequently, an individual lost the power to consent to what the state regarded as harm to itself.

In one of the earliest English cases that rejected consent of the victim as a defense to serious bodily harm, the court opined that the defendant was guilty because, by maiming the willing victim, he deprived the king of the aid and assistance of one of his subjects.[21] Three centuries later, an American court used a very similar argument, explaining that the "commonwealth needs the services of its citizens quite as much as the kings of England needed the services of theirs."[22]

Today, American law continues to maintain that one's life and body do not quite belong to him. Courts habitually disregard the voluntary nature of private harmful actions, citing various public policies. Among those are concerns that private violence may disturb peace; that the injured person may become public charge; and that harmful conduct has no social utility, is immoral, and expresses the parties' disrespect to law and social order. Accordingly, the individual's power to authorize an act that may affect his physical well-being remains strictly limited. For example, the Model Penal

Code (MPC) views consent of the victim as a defense "if such consent negatives an element of the offense or precludes the infliction of the harm or evil sought to be prevented by the law defining the offense."[23] This general rule, however, does not apply to offenses involving bodily harm. In those cases, consent of the victim exonerates the perpetrator only in three sets of circumstances: (1) when the injury is not serious, (2) when the injury or its risks are "reasonably foreseeable hazards" of participation in a "lawful athletic contest or competitive sport or other concerted activity not forbidden by law," and (3) when the bodily harm was inflicted for the purpose of a "recognized form of treatment" intended to improve the patient's physical or mental health.[24]

This specific rule, which reflects the law in the absolute majority of states,[25] has been criticized for its narrow scope and arbitrary boundaries. As one judge remarked, it is "very strange that a fight in private between two youths where one may, at most, get a bloody nose should be unlawful, whereas a boxing match where one heavyweight fighter seeks to knock out his opponent and possibly do him very serious damage should be lawful."[26] Examples of the law's arbitrariness are abundant. Consider just a few.

Familial Breast Cancer Syndrome, Body Integrity Identity Disorder, and Gender Identity Disorder

A woman who carries a breast cancer gene may choose to have a preventive mastectomy. This surgery, although quite lawful, is considered controversial in medical literature: There is little proof that, for purposes of cancer prevention, it is superior to less extreme and disfiguring alternatives.[27] For women with familial breast cancer syndrome, a condition indicating a high risk for developing breast cancer, the primary advantage of the surgery is that it helps to relieve chronic stress and anxiety over the substantial likelihood of developing the disease.[28]

Yet, analogous considerations of emotional pain fail to legitimize an elective surgery on a patient with body integrity identity disorder (BIID), a rare ailment whose victims seek to become amputees.[29] The limited statistics seem to indicate that, if BIID patients succeed in their pursuit, their quality of life improves dramatically.[30] A surgeon who agrees to perform such an amputation, however, opens himself up to criminal liability because his patients' consent is legally invalid.[31]

The BIID patients often compare themselves to those suffering from gender identity disorder (GID), describing the common experience as "being trapped in the wrong body."[32] The law, however, treats the two groups very differently: The GID patients can consent to a sex change operation, which often involves removal of healthy sex organs, whereas the BIID sufferers cannot consent to amputation of an arm or a leg.

Sadomasochistic Beating, Religious Flagellation, and Ritual Mutilation

Under the current rule, consensual infliction of pain during a sadomasochistic encounter is illegal and constitutes assault. Courts have held that it may not be classified as a "sport, social or other activity" permitted under the state penal code.[33] Religious flagellation, on the other hand, enjoys considerably more deferential treatment by authorities. In a nineteenth-century Scottish case, the court opined that "[i]n some cases, a beating may be consented to as in the case of a father confessor ordering flagellation; but this is not violence or assault, because there is consent."[34] More recently, some courts have said that the law "may prohibit religiously impelled physical attacks,"[35] but research has revealed no actual legal cases. Some states even include the element of nonconsent in the definition of ritual mutilation. The Illinois Criminal Code, for instance, provides that

> A person commits the offense of ritual mutilation, when he or she mutilates, dismembers or tortures another person as part of a ceremony, rite, initiation, observance, performance or practice, *and the victim did not consent or under such circumstances that the defendant knew or should have known that the victim was unable to render effective consent.*[36]

The italicized language suggests that if the religious mutilation, dismemberment, or torture is done *with* the consent of the victim, such activity should be lawful.

Consensual Transmission of HIV

Even though sadomasochistic sex constitutes a crime, consensual intentional transmission of HIV is not punishable in a significant number of states. The phenomenon, known as "bug chasing," involves "bug chasers" (HIV-negative men who actively seek out infection by having unprotected sex with infected partners) and "gift givers" (HIV-positive men willing to infect "bug chasers"). According to a source, this practice is the cause of 25% of all new infections among American gay men.[37] These statistics have been questioned, but even if they are not entirely accurate, there is a general consensus that "bug chasing" and "gift giving" present a serious problem for the gay community.[38] Nevertheless, out of 24 states that have statutes criminalizing the act of knowingly exposing another human being to HIV, 8 states explicitly recognize consent of the victim as an affirmative defense,[39] and another 10 reach the same outcome by making failure to disclose one's HIV status an element of the crime.[40]

What Constitutes "Serious" Harm

Since any harmful act that does not fit into the "athletic" or "medical" exception is, by definition, criminal, unless the inflicted injury is not serious, assessment of the seriousness of the victim's injury determines the outcome of many cases involving consensual harm. A typical penal statute classifies bodily injury as serious if it "creates a substantial risk of death or . . . causes serious, permanent disfigurement, or protracted loss or impairment of the function of any bodily member or organ."[41] Pursuant to this definition, any short-term, non-life-threatening injury should not be deemed "serious." Yet, as the MPC acknowledges, the evaluation of the seriousness of harm is often affected by judges' "moral judgments about the iniquity of the conduct involved."[42] Courts tend to inflate the risk and harmfulness of an activity they want to denounce. For example, almost any injury inflicted during a sadomasochistic encounter has been consistently classified as serious.

In *State v. Collier*, the defendant was convicted of assault resulting in a serious injury, under a typical statute described earlier.[43] The victim's injuries consisted of "a swollen lip, large welts on her ankles, wrists, hips, buttocks, and severe bruises on her thighs."[44] Although none of these injuries could possibly be qualified as life threatening or permanent, the appellate court affirmed the conviction.[45]

Some state penal codes include physical pain in the definition of "bodily harm."[46] In *State v. Guinn*, the defendant was convicted of inflicting "serious physical injury" in the course of a sexual encounter.[47] There was no evidence that the victim "ever required any medical attention or suffered any wounds of any sort."[48] Yet the appellate court sustained the assault conviction, reasoning that the sadomasochistic paraphernalia used by the defendant must have caused serious physical pain (candle wax was "hot and it stung" and nipple clamps were "tight and cutting"), and "physical pain" satisfied the definition of "physical injury."[49] Naturally, under a statute of this type, practically any sadomasochistic activity may be characterized as criminal.

The current rule of consent to harm is problematic on many levels: Not only is it arbitrary and strict, but it is also autocratic and absolute. People are allowed to consent to harm only if their activities are on the list of things approved by the state. The law envisions no balancing or accommodation of conflicting interests of an individual and society. The disregard for an individual, inherent in this rule, goes against the basic principles of autonomy and personal responsibility defining American criminal law. Moreover, the authoritarian presumption that it is not the individual, but rather the state that is the victim of every crime is plainly wrong because, if that were so, then consent would not be a defense to any harm.[50] Yet we know that individuals are free to consent to all kinds of harm—emotional, financial, or reputational—as long as those harms are not physical.

This critique prompts two questions: One, why do we perceive consent to bodily harm so differently than consent to any other activity; specifically, why does consent preclude such offenses as theft, rape, or kidnapping but not murder or battery? And two, if we were to revise the current law of consent, where should we draw the line between permissible and impermissible bodily harm?

Why Consent to Physical Harm Is Treated Differently Than Consent to Any Other Limitation of Rights

To have a right means to have a certain moral status. Consent is a way to change this status unilaterally by transferring to another person a claim, privilege, power, or immunity.[51] For example, by promising a neighbor to sell him my car, I give him a claim against me with regard to that promise. By consenting to a root canal procedure, I give my dentist a privilege to perform it. By inviting a friend to dinner, I give him a power to visit me. In all those instances, I waive a right I used to enjoy and give other people rights they did not have before. And yet there is an important difference in *how* consent changes the relevant relationship between the parties in some of these scenarios.

Recall the MPC consent provisions. Under the MPC, voluntary consent of a legally competent individual may trigger two different rules, either the general rule or the specific rule for consent to bodily harm. We already reviewed the latter; now let's take a closer look at the former. The MPC general rule of consent provides that consent of the victim is a defense if it either *negatives* an element of the charged offense or *precludes* the harm or evil sought to be prevented by the law defining that offense.[52] What is peculiar in this rule is that both grounds for the defense have little to do with the theory of defenses.

Any defense presumes that a criminal act has been committed; however, it was committed under the circumstances that may either justify or excuse the perpetrator. An act is criminal only if it encompasses all elements of the offense. If an element is missing, no defense is needed simply because the perpetrator is not guilty even of a *prima facie* criminal wrongdoing.[53] For example, each of the offenses of rape, kidnapping, and theft includes in its definition the element of nonconsent.[54] If that element is negated by the victim's acquiescence, the defendant is completely exonerated by the so-called failure of proof. In these circumstances, consent of the victim does not serve as a defense; instead, it defeats the very possibility of an offense.

The second, alternative ground for the MPC defense of consent is also puzzling: On the one hand, it almost verbatim repeats a segment of Section 3.02, which summarizes general requirements for a defense of justification; on the other hand, it differs from Section 3.02 in a meaningful way. Section 3.02 maintains that conduct is justifiable if "the harm or evil sought to be avoided by such conduct is greater than that *sought to be prevented by the law defining the offense* charged."[55] The italicized words coincide with the language of Section 2.11 (Consent). However, if the general justification provision requires only that the inflicted harm or evil be *lesser* than the harm or evil that was avoided, the consent provision talks about complete *preclusion* of any harm or evil sought to be prevented by the law defining the offense. The consent provision, thus, exculpates the defendant only when social harm is entirely avoided. But if there is no social harm, why should the defendant even need a defense? Isn't this provision merely a broader version of the first part of the section (that is, negation of an element of the offense charged)?

The materials of the American Law Institute (ALI) proceedings confirm this hypothesis. According to the MPC Reporter Herbert Wechsler, the alternative ground for relief in Section 2.11(1) was intended to cover a situation when the definition of an offense, which logically should have incorporated the nonconsent language, by legislative oversight or for some other reason omitted it:

> There are also cases where in the definition of a crime the words
> "without consent" have not been put in, but where it is perfectly clear
> that in the legislative conception of the offense the idea it is intended,
> and that's the purpose for the rest of part (1), that if consent

precludes the infliction of the harm or evil sought to be prevented by the legislature, then even though it doesn't negative the formal element, it still ought to be a defense.[56]

In other words, the defense of consent set forth in Section 2.11(1) of the MPC is *not* a defense at all. Instead it is another way to state the rule that a person is not guilty of an offense unless each element of the offense is proven beyond a reasonable doubt.[57] In that sense, Section 2.11(1) is redundant, and the drafters of the MPC have largely acknowledged that by calling it "merely tautological"[58] and contrasting it with the specific rule of consent to bodily harm stated in Section 2.11(2):

> Now, the second part is more than tautological. There is a real need to indicate when and how far consent should be a defense to the bodily injury crimes, because again you wouldn't draft a murder statute in terms of killing somebody without his consent. Obviously, the idea is that it's a crime whether he consents or not, and how far consent to bodily injury should go involves some deep questions of policy.[59]

The conceptual imprecision of Section 2.11 would not be that interesting had it not reflected an important intuition of the MPC drafters apparent in their attempt to differentiate between two entirely different roles of consent in criminal law. Compare cases of rape, kidnapping, or theft on the one hand, and cases of killing or maiming on the other. In the first group of cases, the *act itself* does not violate a prohibitory norm. Having sex, transporting someone to a different location, or taking other people's property is not bad *in itself*. It becomes bad *only* due to the absence of consent. In other words, no matter how we draft the statute, in cases of theft, rape, or kidnapping, the absence of consent is *inculpatory*—nonconsent is a part of the definition of the offense.[60]

In contrast, causing pain, injury, or death is not morally neutral; it is regrettable.[61] Bringing about a regrettable state of events is bad and should be avoided.[62] Therefore, the law should promote a conduct rule that prohibits the very *act* of killing or hurting, providing, of course, for the necessary exceptions, such as self-defense. However, the fact that a person may be legally justified in killing an aggressor does not make the killing as morally neutral as borrowing a book—it is still regrettable. It is still regrettable that a dental patient has to suffer pain, even though the dentist is justified in causing it,[63] whereas there is nothing regrettable in consensual sex or consensual change of ownership. To lose or reduce its inherent wrongfulness, the act of killing or hurting requires justification. The role of consent here is *exculpatory*; it may only serve as a defense.

In his influential work, *Rethinking Criminal Law*, George Fletcher has insightfully observed that, to distinguish a definition from a defense, we need to identify a prohibitory norm, which "must contain a sufficient number of elements to state a coherent moral imperative."[64] In the case of killing or inflicting pain, this imperative is quite straightforward: Do not kill, do not inflict pain. But what conduct rule do we want to convey to the community in cases of rape, theft, or criminal mischief? Should it say: Do not have sex? Do not take other people's possessions? Do not break other people's property? Certainly not. Even the last rule, the most controversial of the three, would be unmerited and impracticable. There is nothing wrong with breaking things. People may need to break things, including those belonging to others, in the process of construction, repair, cleaning, cooking, or just having fun. We do not want to prohibit useful or morally neutral activities. What we want to prohibit is engaging in these activities *under the circumstances* that make such activities wrongful. Accordingly, the conduct rule applicable to killing or hurting does not require the nonconsent language, whereas the conduct rule prohibiting rape, theft, or criminal mischief simply makes no sense without the nonconsent element.

In practical terms, this distinction means that consent precludes even a *prima facie* case of rape, theft, or criminal mischief, regardless of whether the consensual act brings about more good than harm, and regardless of whether the defendant is aware of the victim's consent. Significantly more is required to establish a successful defense, and a failure to satisfy the requirements is significantly more costly. For example, under the current law, as Paul Robinson correctly pointed out, the defendant's lack of knowledge of a legally relevant fact has different consequences in cases of "impossible" attempts on the one hand and cases of "unknowingly justified" actors on the other.[65] In cases of the first kind, the most serious offense of which the defendant may be convicted is attempt (e.g. a perpetrator who proceeds with intercourse while—mistakenly—believing his partner to be a minor is guilty of attempted statutory rape), whereas in cases of the second kind, the defendant is guilty of a completed offense (e.g. a perpetrator who shoots his enemy to death is guilty of murder even if, unbeknownst to the perpetrator, the enemy was about to attack him with a deadly weapon). Since in most jurisdictions a completed offense is punished more severely than an attempt,[66] the perpetrator who was unaware of a "lucky" fact that negated an element of an offense is treated better than the perpetrator who was unaware of a "lucky" justifying fact.

Why is that so? Mainly because we view a defense of justification as a limited license to commit an otherwise prohibited act in order to achieve a socially and morally desirable outcome.[67] For instance, if a group of mountaineers, caught by a snowstorm, took refuge in a deserted cabin and consumed the owner's provisions, they would be justified under the defense of necessity.[68] This limited license is teleological in nature; it presumes an objective need to seek rescue, an objectively preferable outcome, and the good faith of the actors. If, say, the mountaineers committed the break-in because, in their minds, it was a lesser evil than remaining hungry for the next few hours, they would not be entitled to the defense.[69] Nor would they be justified if the reason for breaking in was a desire to have an impromptu party in the cabin. The mountaineers would not be justified even if, unknowingly, they in fact saved their lives by hiding from the upcoming snowstorm.[70]

Thus, in order to be justified, the mountaineers must establish three elements:

1. the basis for the defense (actual necessity);
2. an objectively preferable outcome (a positive balance of harms and evils); and
3. the subjective awareness of the justifying circumstances and belief in the necessity to overstep a prohibitory norm in order to achieve the preferable outcome.[71]

Similarly, to be justified for hurting someone in self-defense or defense of another, the defendant must establish:

1. the basis for the defense (immediate necessity to fend off an unlawful attack);[72]
2. an objectively preferable outcome (it is preferable to harm an aggressor rather than allow the aggressor to harm an innocent victim); and
3. the subjective awareness of the attack and belief in the necessity to use force in order to achieve the preferable outcome.

If the perpetrator used force in the absence of an attack (no basis for self-defense or defense of another) or injured several innocent bystanders in order to immobilize the aggressor (not an objectively preferable outcome), he would not be justified.[73] Nor would he be justified if he merely used the attack as a ploy to harm the aggressor (bad faith).

The last point may be illustrated by the following example: Suppose person A hates his enemy B and wants him dead. Knowing that B frequents a certain bar, A spends night after night outside the bar waiting for an occasion. While he is waiting, he witnesses numerous fights, sexual assaults, even murders; however, he never interferes, until finally one day he sees B attacking another patron *C* with deadly force. Knowing the law of defense of another,[74] *A* intervenes and kills *B*. At his trial, *A* honestly tells his story of patience and determination. Should he be rewarded for these qualities and completely exonerated, even though we know that he would not have defended *C* but for his desire to kill *B*?

Although technically *A* is entitled to an acquittal, I think most of us would view such an outcome as a mockery of justice. Justification defenses are not intended to provide people with convenient opportunities to commit crimes. Any justifiable conduct requires good faith; and, in the context of a limited license to overstep a prohibitory norm, the requirement of good faith should be satisfied only when the subjective purpose of the perpetrator is directed toward the goals for which that license is granted.

Furthermore, under the MPC, the "choice of evils" is not available as a defense against a reckless (or negligent) crime if the defendant was reckless (or negligent) in bringing about the situation that made the injurious choice necessary.[75] Similarly, the MPC and the law of most states deny the perpetrator the justifications of self-defense and defense of another in prosecution for a reckless (or negligent) crime, if the belief that would otherwise justify his actions was held recklessly (or negligently).[76] Under this logic, should not a defendant who *intentionally* placed himself in a situation in which he would be able to use the defense of another as a cover-up for *intentional* homicide be denied the defense of justification? The language of the MPC certainly suggests this conclusion: In determining the perpetrator's eligibility for self-defense and related defenses, the MPC addresses only the actor who "*believes that the use of force upon or toward the person of another is necessary for any of the purposes for which such belief would establish a justification.*"[77]

Applying the same principles to the defense of consent, we, therefore, should only grant complete justification to the perpetrator who can establish all requirements of the justificatory defense, namely:

1. the basis for the defense (valid consent of the victim);
2. an objectively preferable outcome (a positive balance of harms and evils); and
3. the subjective awareness of the victim's consent and belief in the necessity to hurt the victim in order to achieve the preferable outcome.

In what follows I consider these requirements and their application in more detail.

The Defense of Consent

Valid Consent of the Victim

The first requirement of the successful defense is the presence of the victim's legally valid consent, factual or imputed.[78] Conceptually, factual consent may be understood in one of two ways: either as the consenter's subjective state of mind, that is, his willingness to agree with what another person proposes (factual attitudinal consent), or the consenter's expression of acquiescence by words or conduct (factual expressive consent).[79] Which meaning of consent lies in the foundation of legal consent?

It appears that the answer to this question depends, once again, on the role of consent with respect to a particular offense: If nonconsent plays the inculpatory role, then either attitudinal or expressive consent should suffice as a predicate for a legally valid consent and preclude the offense. For example, the charge of rape would be unwarranted if a legally competent person voluntarily expressed his willingness to engage in a sexual act, regardless of how closely that willingness reflected his true feelings. That charge would be equally unwarranted if a legally competent person wholeheartedly welcomed the sexual intimacy, yet never outwardly expressed his feelings.[80] In contrast, when consent plays the exculpatory role, only expressive consent may provide the basis for legally valid consent. This stricter requirement is necessitated by the last element of the defense: The perpetrator must be aware of the victim's consent, and it is impossible to be "aware" of someone's state of mind unless that person has somehow expressed his preferences.

Naturally, not any factual expression of consent is recognized by law. To be valid, consent must be rational and voluntary, that is, freely given and informed.[81] Consent obtained by duress or fraud regarding the nature of the perpetrator's act is void *ab initio*,[82] and so is consent given by a person who cannot understand the nature of that to which he consents. Certain groups of people (e.g. children, mentally ill, intoxicated), in most instances, are deemed incapable of granting valid consent.[83] In addition, there is a strong argument that courts should require higher levels of rationality and voluntariness of the victim's decision as the amount of inflicted or risked harm increases.[84] For example, a simple "sure, why not?" may be sufficient to constitute consent for piercing one's ears but not for cutting them off. Particularly dangerous or irreparable decisions (e.g. consensual homicide) may even be presumed involuntary until proven otherwise.[85]

Factual consent of the victim provides one way to satisfy the requirement of legally valid consent. Another way to reach the same objective is by establishing imputed consent. Species of imputed consent include constructive consent (the victim's acquiescence to one act presupposes acquiescence to some other act too); informed consent (the victim voluntarily assumes the risk of a certain harm); and hypothetical consent (the victim is incompetent and determination is made for the victim, based on what the victim would have consented to had he been competent or based on the victim's best interests).[86] The first two types of imputed consent involve a person who validly agrees to a certain injurious act (e.g. plastic surgery). In addition to the explicitly authorized actions, this person is deemed to have constructively agreed to all other actions of the medical personnel that are necessary or incidental to the surgery (constructive consent). This person is also deemed to have voluntarily assumed the risk of certain disclosed complications and side effects (informed consent).

The third type of imputed consent is different. It comes into play when an individual is not capable of giving legally valid permission due to temporary or permanent incompetence, and others have to determine what the individual would have wanted. For example, in the case of Terri Schiavo, who had spent the last 15 years of her life institutionalized with a diagnosis of persistent vegetative state, Terri's husband petitioned the court to authorize removal of her life-sustaining feeding tube. He argued that, under the circumstances, Terri would not have wished to continue life-prolonging measures and the court agreed with his arguments.[87] When a decision is made for an individual who has never been competent, the test for imputed consent is somewhat different; in that case, the decision is made in the "best interests" of the incompetent individual.[88]

One could argue that, when the perpetrator, acting in the best interests of *any* victim—competent or incompetent—produces a measurably positive outcome, the victim's consent is immaterial. And indeed, sometimes the law justifies a benevolent action even though it overrides another person's autonomy. For example, it is permissible to use force against a person in order to stop his suicidal attempt. At least in part, this rule reflects societal perception of suicide as inherently irrational. Whether this perception is accurate and the rule is morally sustainable is a question open for debate. It is clear, however, that the application of the rule is quite limited. It is impermissible to force-feed a competent, free individual who wishes to starve himself to death. It is impermissible to perform a surgery on an unwilling patient, even if that surgery is beneficial for the patient's health. And, it is certainly impermissible to perform involuntary euthanasia on any conscious human being in any circumstances.

Consider *Gilbert v. State*, in which the court convicted a 75-year-old man of first-degree murder for shooting his wife to death.[89] Roswell and Emily

Gilbert had been married for 51 years. For the last few years of her life, Emily suffered from osteoporosis and Alzheimer's disease, and her condition rapidly deteriorated. Testifying at his trial, Roswell Gilbert said: "there she was in pain and all this confusion and I guess if I got cold as icewater that's what had happened. I thought to myself, I've got to do it... I've got to end her suffering...."[90]

As dramatic and sad as this case is, the appellate court was right to affirm the defendant's conviction. Roswell Gilbert was motivated by compassion and the desire to protect his wife from suffering and, in fact, he did everything in his power to make her death as painless as possible.[91] But even if her condition were so desperate that Roswell objectively benefited Emily by cutting short her agony, he should not be entitled to justification. Unauthorized homicide of an autonomous human being is, and should be, murder. No one has the right to decide for another person that his life is not worth living, or, citing the words of the *Gilbert* opinion, " '[g]ood faith' is not a legal defense to first degree murder."[92]

A Positive Balance of Harms and Evils

The requirement to achieve a positive balance of harms and evils raises a complicated question of law and policy. Traditionally, criminal harm is understood as *wrongful* interference with the victim's essential welfare interests.[93] The interference is deemed wrongful if it violates the victim's rights. From this perspective, consensual physical harm presents a problem: Since consent constitutes a waiver of rights, the perpetrator who kills or injures a willing victim does not violate the victim's rights.[94] But can we say that cases of voluntary euthanasia, consensual cannibalistic killing, and sadomasochistic beating are equally free from criminal wrongdoing?

In an attempt to resolve this problem, a number of scholars have recently suggested that the concept of criminal harm should not be limited to violation of one's autonomy.[95] In their view, such acts as, say, consensual gladiatorial matches are impermissible because they violate the participants' dignity, and dignity is so essential to our humanity that, in cases of a conflict between autonomy and dignity, the former ought to yield.[96] For that reason, consent may not serve as a defense to the violation of dignity.

I share the view that certain degrading behavior may be wrongful even when it does not violate the victim's rights. Society may be concerned about human dignity in various circumstances, including those in which a prohibitory norm does not originate in a rights violation. Consider experiments conducted in the 1980s that involved the use of fresh cadavers as "crash dummies."[97] When those experiments became known, they caused public outrage. But why? We usually do not feel offended by autopsies or post-mortem organ donation. Perhaps, as Joel Feinberg suggested, the answer has something to do with the perceived symbolism of the different uses:

> In the air bag experiments cadavers were violently smashed to bits, whereas dissections are done in laboratories by white-robed medical technicians in spotless antiseptic rooms, radiating the newly acquired symbolic respectability of professional medicine.[98]

Or perhaps the difference is not merely symbolic, and violently smashing cadavers to bits is, in fact, disrespectful—disrespectful of our only recently shared humanity? An act of autopsy or removal of an organ for transplantation is not qualitatively different from a regular surgery. Extracting a kidney, inter vivo or postmortem, does not reduce one's moral status to that of a thing. Smashing a body in an industrial experiment or using human remains to manufacture soap does have this effect. In other words, even when an act of indignity is committed on an unconscious or dead body or when the victim does not perceive an assault on his dignity as such, a wrongful act has been done.

What is at stake here is people's moral dignity, or dignity of personhood, as opposed to social dignity, or dignity of rank. Social dignity is nonessential; in a society that permits social mobility, it can be gained and lost. Moral dignity, by contrast, is an essential characteristic of all human beings.[99] It is so important for our collective humanity that we extend it to all those who satisfy "the minimum requirements of personhood,"[100] and even beyond that, to those who closely miss them.

And yet, as important as moral dignity is, its violation should not be criminalized lightly. Whenever the state prohibits consensual behavior, for the sake of dignity or any other reason, it suppresses individual liberty and autonomy—partly paternalistically, but mostly for the benefit of society at large.[101] Therefore, the threat to society should be serious enough to warrant use of criminal sanctions. For instance, the careless attitude to human dignity exhibited by "Fear Factor," a popular television reality show, has raised concerns of a number of its viewers. One journalist commented: "Do we really need to see people buried under 400 rats, each biting the exposed body parts of the desperate contestants? No. And it doesn't get any more palatable when someone yells out, 'Keep your butt cheeks clenched!'"[102]

It is understandable that those pictures may disturb some members of the public, but the nature and magnitude of the personal and societal harm brought about by the show did not rise to the level that would justify a criminal ban—that harm was simply "not the law's business,"[103] at least, not the criminal law's business. Anthony Duff has accurately observed that not punishing someone's conduct does not mean approving of it; instead, that can mean the lack of standing to judge or condemn such conduct.[104] We do not have to approve of radical cosmetic surgery, religious flagellation, or sadomasochistic brutality; however, society may be better served by not prosecuting those consensual activities.

In other words, not every violation of human dignity deserves criminal punishment, but only such that affects society at large. As I argued in more detail elsewhere, to avoid overcriminalization yet capture the most egregious cases, the criminal doctrine should be revised to explicitly include dignity violation in the concept of wrongdoing.[105] Criminal harm then would retain its current meaning as a wrongful setback to an important welfare interest, but "wrongful" would mean either (1) such as violates the victim's autonomy or (2) such as violates the victim's dignity.[106] The two kinds of criminal harm comprise the same evil—objectification of another human being. That evil may be brought about by an injury to a vital human interest, combined with either a rights violation (e.g. theft) or disregard of the victim's dignity (e.g. consensual deadly torture). The absolute majority of criminal offenses, being *nonconsensual*, include both kinds of harm.

As for *consensual* physical harm, it should be punishable only when an important welfare interest normally protected by criminal law is set back in a way that denies the victim his equal moral worth. A recent German case, in which Armin Meiwes was prosecuted for killing his willing victim, Bernd Juergen Brandes, and cannibalizing on his flesh, may serve as an example.[107] By killing Brandes, Meiwes did not violate Brandes's right to life. However, he not only defeated the most essential interest of Brandes (his interest in continued living) but also used Brandes as an object, a means of obtaining the desired cannibalistic experience, and thus disregarded his dignity. In contrast, consensual mercy killing destroys the patient's interest in continued living but, when warranted by the patient's condition and motivated by compassion, respects and preserves his dignity. Such killing, therefore, should not be subject to criminal sanctions. Unfortunately, the current law does not recognize this difference. In *Michigan v. Kevorkian*, for example, the state prosecuted Dr. Kevorkian for administering a lethal injection to a former racecar driver who, due to advanced Lou Gehrig's disease, was no longer able to move, eat, or breathe on his own.[108] Even the patient's family had accepted his choice to escape the suffering and indignity of the slow demise. But not the trial court or the appellate court: Dr. Kevorkian was convicted of second-degree murder, and his conviction was affirmed.[109]

To summarize, in order to satisfy the second requirement of the defense of consent, the perpetrator must establish that, to the extent he set back the victim's welfare interests and, at the same time, disregarded the victim's dignity (i.e. caused criminal harm), the harmful act nevertheless produced an objectively positive outcome. The more serious—disabling and irreversible—the harm to the victim, the more serious must be the benefits brought about by the injurious action. A sadomasochistic beating, which leaves no permanent damage, should be justified by the mere fact that its participants desired it. Even those who believe that such a beating offends the victim's dignity would probably agree that it does not significantly affect the victim's long-term interests. On the other hand, only extraordinary circumstances might be able to justify consensual deadly torture.

The Subjective Awareness of the Victim's Consent and Belief in the Necessity to Hurt the Victim in Order to Achieve an Objectively Preferable Outcome

Finally, for complete justification, the perpetrator would have to establish that, not only did he act with the victim's consent (factual expressive or imputed) and achieve a positive balance of harms and evils, but he also intended that outcome while causing harm. This subjective requirement, common to other justification defenses, is particularly appropriate in the case of the defense of consent. Just like in cases of necessity or self-defense, consent of the victim does not impose on the perpetrator an *obligation* to act; it merely provides the perpetrator with an *option*. However, a natural disaster or a life-threatening attack creates a compelling reason for exercising that option. We cannot say the same about one's consent. For example, I may request (and simultaneously consent to) a surgery. If my doctor does not believe I need one or is reluctant to perform it himself, he is under no duty to do so.

When a child breaks a rule, we demand: "Why did you do that?" This is a question about a moral reason for action and effectively about the availability of a defense. What we want to know is whether the child had a good reason for violating the rule of conduct. We are unlikely to accept "because such-and-such told me to" as a valid reason or defense. The classic parental reply to that would be: "And what if he told you to jump off the Brooklyn Bridge?" By this reply, we in fact say: "You are a free moral agent. Why, being a free moral agent, did you choose to break the rule (cause harm)?"

In other words, one's consent creates a very weak content-independent reason for action, and thus cannot eliminate the wrongfulness of overstepping a prohibitory norm.[110] The perpetrator would not be justified if he simply followed the victim's self-destructive wish without the ultimate goal to achieve a benevolent result. In fact, he would not be even excused by a mere expression of acquiescence by the victim. Of course, an emotional plea, a request combined with a threat, or an order by authority can have significant coercive power and can make a person of reasonable firmness agree to an action that he would not have performed otherwise.[111] These reasons for action can provide grounds for the defense of duress; however, they are extraneous to the theory of consent.

Partial Defense of Consent

The proposed conceptualization of the defense of consent has two normative consequences. One is that consent alone does not suffice to justify the victim's death or injury; the other is that consent should always be at least a partial defense, because it defeats at least one aspect of harm, namely, violation of rights. A partial justification does not make a wrongful act right; it only makes it *less wrongful* compared to an identical but nonconsensual act.[112] Take a lifeboat scenario, in which all will die unless a few sacrifice their lives by jumping overboard. Assume that the necessary number of people have volunteered, but for whatever reason (perhaps they are too weak to be able to move), they cannot complete the suicidal act on their own. Would it be wrong to push them off? I believe that even if it were wrong, it would certainly be less wrong than drowning those who have not volunteered.[113] It would be less wrong because the person who threw the victims over did not violate their rights. Accordingly, he brought about less harm than in an identical but nonconsensual act and, thus, should deserve a lesser punishment.

The notion that a less harmful act deserves a lesser punishment, although not unanimously accepted, has strong support both in our law and our morality.[114] We decide whether people deserve praise or penalty based, in part, on the end result of their actions. A sprinter who almost won the race does not deserve the same medal as the sprinter who, in fact, came in first. Similarly, a driver who almost hit a pedestrian does not deserve the same punishment as a driver who did, in fact, hit and kill someone. Many criminal law doctrines implicitly or explicitly draw on the moral significance of harm. For example, the defense of necessity justifies the actor who has violated a prohibitory norm in order to avoid a greater harm.

The moral significance of harm makes the attribution of harm essential to the idea of fair punishment. In a nonconsensual act, the perpetrator bears full responsibility for the harm. When the act is consensual, however, the victim shares the responsibility and the perpetrator's criminal liability should reflect that. Naturally, the extent of partial justification attributed to the victim's consent should depend on the facts of each case and, at a minimum, be affected by the importance of the victim's interests (both harmed and intended to be harmed); the extent of the actual and intended damage to the victim's interests and dignity; and the actual and intended balance of harms/evils and benefits. In many instances, partial justification will reduce the perpetrator's punishment to the minimal level. For example, a person who euthanized a willing, terminally ill patient out of sheer hatred for him and his family does not deserve full justification, but this does not mean he ought to go to jail. He did not violate the victim's rights or dignity, and while destroying the victim's interest in continued living, he advanced his interest in avoiding pain and suffering. Accordingly, community service or its equivalent may be a more appropriate sentence. Conversely, someone like Armin Meiwes is guilty of a serious wrongdoing, and his partial justification should not translate into the same mitigation of punishment as in the preceding example.

Conclusion

Intentionally injuring or killing another person is presumptively wrong. To overcome this presumption, the perpetrator must establish a defense of justification. Consent of the victim may serve as one of the grounds for such a defense. For complete justification, the perpetrator's reasons for a consensual injurious act must be subjectively benevolent and the act must produce an overall positive balance of harms and evils, including harm to the victim's welfare interests and dignity. If these requirements are not met, the defense should be only partial.

The proposed rule makes sense both theoretically and practically. From the theoretical perspective, it places consent squarely within the family of justification defenses. All of them, from self-defense to necessity, seek to overcome the deontological constraint against intentional infliction of harm. These defenses may be granted to a person who chose a certain course of action *despite* its negative effects (as opposed to *for the sake* of its negative effects) and succeeded in producing a better outcome. From the practical perspective, this rule leaves room for balancing the harms and benefits caused by the perpetrator. This is an important difference from the current law, which is absolute in what it allows and disallows. Overall, adopting a rule based on a uniform principle common to other justification defenses would lead to more fair, consistent, and morally sustainable verdicts.

Notes

1. Professor of Law, Robert E. Knowlton Scholar, Rutgers School of Law-Newark; J.D., University of Pennsylvania; Ph.D., Institute of Slavic and Balkan Studies at the Academy of Sciences of the Soviet Union. This article is based, in part, on Vera Bergelson, "The Right to Be Hurt: Testing the Boundaries of Consent," *George Washington Law Review* 75 (2007): 165–236. It has also been reprinted in a symposium issue of *Pace Law Review* (2008). I am grateful to the participants of the Victims and Criminal Justice System symposium at Pace Law School for their thoughtful comments, and to the deputy director of Rutgers Law Library Paul Axel-Lute and my research assistant Linda Posluszny for their massive help in researching this project.
2. *Jovanovic v. City of New York*, No. 04 Civ. 8437, slip. op. at 1 (S.D.N.Y. Aug. 17, 2006).
3. Ibid., 4.
4. *People v. Jovanovic*, 263 A.D.2d 182, 197 (N.Y. App. Div. 1999).
5. *N.Y. Penal Law* § 120.05(2) (McKinney Supp. 2008).
6. *N.Y. Penal Law* § 120.00(1) (McKinney 2004).
7. *People v. Jovanovic*, 263 A.D.2d 182, 198 n.5 (N.Y. App. Div. 1999).
8. Ibid. (citations omitted).
9. Ibid., 207 (Mazzarelli, J., concurring in part and dissenting in part).
10. Ibid. Judge Mazzarelli wrote:

    [T]he complaining witness's testimony was sufficient to support both of these convictions, and, in the circumstances, hot candle wax was appropriately considered a dangerous instrument. Moreover, the complainant's testimony was corroborated by a neighbor who heard sounds as if someone were "undergoing root canal" from defendant's apartment at the time in question, by the complaining witness's prompt outcries to five individuals, some of these individuals' observations of the complaining witness's injuries, the lab results as to her clothing, and the e-mails sent between the complaining witness and defendant subsequent to the incident.

    Ibid. (citations omitted).
11. See, e.g., ibid., 198 n.5 (accepting the jury finding that the victim was physically injured during her encounter with the defendant).

12. See, e.g., *State v. Van*, 688 N.W.2d 600 (Neb. 2004) (extending the principle that consent is not a defense to an assault to bodily injury inflicted during a sadomasochistic beating); *State v. Collier*, 372 N.W.2d 303 (Iowa Ct. App. 1985) (noting that "to allow an otherwise criminal act to go unpunished because of a victim's consent would not only threaten the security of society but would also undermine the moral principles underlying the criminal law").

13. In fact, there are serious doubts about the truthfulness of Ruzcek's allegations. Quoting the court in the recent civil case,

> The physical evidence did not match Ruzcek's assertions. A comprehensive gynecological examination of Ruzcek on November 27, 1996 found no bleeding, teeth marks, bruises, scratches, swelling, redness, or burn marks, all of which would be expected if Ruzcek's account were true. . . . No traces of Jovanovic's DNA were found on the victim, her clothing, or any of the undergarments she wore on the night of the alleged assault. No blood was found on any of the victim's clothes, no ligature marks upon her body, and no abrasions about her mouth. Hair and fiber tests showed no signs of a violent struggle or sexual assault. Ruzcek's allegations were questionable in other ways as well. She had given contradictory accounts of the alleged assault . . ."changing critical facts every time she recounted the event."

> *Jovanovic v. City of New York*, No. 04 Civ. 8437, slip. op. at 4–5 (citations omitted).

14. Heidi M. Hurd, "Blaming the Victim: A Response to the Proposal that Criminal Law Recognize a General Defense of Contributory Responsibility," *Buffalo Criminal Law Review* 8 (2005): 504.

15. See Terence Ingman, "A History of the Defence of Volenti Non Fit Injuria," *Juridicial Review* 26 (1981): 8–9.

16. See Harry Elmer Barnes and Negley K. Teeters, *New Horizons in Criminology*, 2nd ed. (New York: Prentice Hall, 1951), 342 (explaining that public offenses were those that exposed a "group to spiritual or human enemies, particularly the former"). "Crimes against persons were not controlled by the tribe or the family but by the clan under the principle of blood feud." Ibid.

17. See Clarence Ray Jeffery, "The Development of Crime in Early English Society," *Journal of Criminal Law, Criminology, and Police Science* 47 (1957): 662. ("By 1226 an agreement between the criminal and the relatives of a slain man would not avail to save the murderer from an indictment and a sentence of death. The state no longer allowed a private settlement of a criminal case.").

18. Stephen Schafer, *Victimology: The Victim and His Criminal* (Reston, VA: Reston, 1977), 22.

19. By the eighteenth century, all crimes and misdemeanors were regarded as public wrongs. See William Blackstone, *Commentaries on the Laws of England* (Philadelphia: J.B. Lippincott, 1904), 4:*5 (explaining that "public wrongs, or crimes and misdemeanors, are a breach and violation of the public rights and duties due to the whole community").

20. See ibid., *5–6.

21. Ibid., *205.

22. *State v. Bass*, 120 S.E.2d 580, 586 (N.C. 1961).

23. *Model Penal Code*, § 2.11(1) (1980).

24. Ibid., § 2.11(2).

25. Thirteen states explicitly recognize a general defense of consent in their statutes. See, e.g., *Ala. Code* § 13A-2-7 (2005). Other states have incorporated the concept of consent in the Special Part of their penal codes, making nonconsent an element of an offense or providing for the defense of consent with respect to specific crimes. See, e.g., 720 *Ill. Comp. Stat.* 5/12-17 (2002) ("It shall be a defense to any [sexual offense] where force or threat of force is an element of the offense that the victim consented."). Where the statute does not explicitly mention consent, case law usually defines in what circumstances consent may function as a defense. See, e.g., *People v. Gordon*, 11 P. 762, 762 (Cal. 1886) (stating that victim's consent negates the charge of assault).

26. *R v. Brown*, [1994] 1 A.C. 212, 278 (H.L.) (Lord Slynn's opinion).

27. Lane D. Ziegler and Stephen S. Kroll, "Primary Breast Cancer After Prophylactic Mastectomy," *American Journal of Clinical Oncology* 14 (1991): 453 (discussing controversial nature of prophylactic mastectomy and comparing it with less radical alternatives).

28. See Mal Bebbington Hatcher et al., "The Psychosocial Impact of Bilateral Prophylactic Mastectomy: Prospective Study Using Questionnaires and Semistructured Interviews," *British Medical Journal* 322 (2001): 76–81.

29. "When It Feels Right to Cut Off Your Leg," *Geelong Advertiser* (Australia), July 4, 2005, 15.

30. Ibid.

31. See generally Tim Bayne and Neil Levy, "Amputees by Choice: Body Integrity Identity Disorder and the Ethics of Amputation," *Journal of Applied Philosophy* 22 (2005): 75.

32. Carl Elliot, "A New Way to Be Mad," *Atlantic Monthly*, December 2000, 73–74.

33. See *State v. Collier*, 372 N.W.2d 303, 307 (Iowa Ct. App. 1985).

34. "Consent in the Criminal Law," *Law Commission Consultation Paper*, No. 139, London: H.S.M.O., 1995, 10.1–10.4 (internal citation omitted).

35. *United States v. Meyers*, 906 F. Supp. 1494, 1496 (D. Wy. 1995). See *Ogletree v. State*, 440 S.E.2d 732, 733 (Ga. Ct. App. 1994) (opining that, even had the

victim consented, the severe beating ordered by a pastor would still constitute battery).

36. 720 *Ill. Comp. Stat. Ann.* 5/12-32(a) (West 2005) (emphasis added).

37. Gregory A. Freeman, "Bug Chasers: The Men Who Long to Be HIV+," *Rolling Stone*, February 6, 2003.

38. Amanda Weiss, "Criminalizing Consensual Transmission of HIV," *University of Chicago Legal Forum* (2006): 389–90.

39. Those states are Florida, Idaho, Illinois, Iowa, Nevada, North Dakota, South Dakota, and Tennessee. Leslie E. Wolf and Richard Vezina, "Crime and Punishment: Is There a Role for Criminal Law in HIV Prevention Policy?" *Whittier Law Review* 25 (2004): 854.

40. Those states are Arkansas, California, Georgia, Louisiana, Michigan, Missouri, New Jersey, Ohio, Oklahoma, and South Carolina. Ibid.

41. *Model Penal Code,* § 210.0(3) (1980). Following the Model Penal Code (MPC), many states have adopted an identical or similar definition. See, e.g., *N.J. Stat. Ann.* § 2C:11-1(b) (West 2005); *Tex. Penal Code* § 1.07(46) (Vernon 2005).

42. *Model Penal Code,* § 2.11 cmt. 2 n.8 (1980). The Commentary points out that the MPC provision does not explicitly foreclose resort to such judgments, though the envisioned emphasis is on the amount of injury itself. Ibid.

43. 372 N.W.2d 303 (Iowa Ct. App. 1985).

44. Ibid., 304. See *R v. Donovan,* (1934) 2 Eng. Rep. 498, 503 (K.B.) ("seven or eight red marks" on the body of a participant of a sadomasochistic encounter found to be sufficient for an assault conviction); *R v. Emmett,* [1999] EWCA (Crim) 1710 (Eng.) (bloodshot eyes and a burn, which had completely healed by the time of the trial, sufficed for an assault conviction of a participant of consensual sado-masochistic sex).

45. *Collier,* 372 N.W.2d at 309 (Schlegel, J., dissenting) (pointing out that the inflicted bodily harm did not constitute a serious injury within the meaning of the state statute). The relevant statute qualified a physical injury as serious if it "create[d] a substantial risk of death," "cause[d] serious permanent disfigure-ment," or "cause[d] protracted loss or impairment of the function of any bodily member or organ." *Iowa Code* § 702.18 (2008).

46. See, e.g., *Model Penal Code,* § 210.0(2) (1980); *Wash. Rev. Code* § 9A.04.110(4)(a) (2004) ("'Bodily injury,' 'physical injury,' or 'bodily harm' means physical pain or injury, illness, or an impairment of physical condition."). In *State v. Guinn,* the relevant statute did not define "serious physical injury." No. 23886-1-II, 2001 Wash. App. LEXIS 502, at *33 (Wash. Ct. App. March 30, 2001). But "substantial bodily harm" was defined as "bodily injury which involves a temporary but substantial disfigurement, or which causes a temporary but substantial loss or impairment of the function of any bodily part or organ, or

which causes a fracture of any bodily part." Ibid. (citing *Wash. Rev. Code* §
9A.04.110(4)(b) (2004)). And "great bodily harm" was defined as "bodily injury
which creates a probability of death, or which causes significant serious permanent disfigurement, or which causes a significant permanent loss or impairment
of the function of any bodily part or organ." Ibid. (citing *Wash. Rev. Code* §
9A.04.110(4)(c) (2004)).

47. Ibid., *1.
48. Ibid., *34.
49. Ibid.
50. See Markus Dirk Dubber, "Toward a Constitutional Law of Crime and
Punishment," *Hastings Law Journal* 55 (2004): 570 (pointing out that, "if the
state were indeed the victim of every crime, then consent should be a defense to
none").
51. See generally Wesley Newcomb Hohfeld, *Fundamental Legal Conceptions* (New
Haven, CT: Yale University Press, 1923). See also Judith Jarvis Thomson, *The
Realm of Rights* (Cambridge, MA: Harvard University Press, 1990), 360–61.
52. *Model Penal Code*, § 2.11(1) (1980).
53. "Justification and excuses do not seek to refute any required element of the
prosecution's case; rather they suggest further considerations that negate culpability even when all elements of the offense are clearly present." Sanford H.
Kadish, Stephen J. Shulhofer, and Carole S. Steiker, *Criminal Law and Its
Processes: Cases and Materials*, 8th ed. (New York: Aspen Publishers,
2007), 737.
54. See, e.g., *Model Penal Code*, §§ 212.1, 213.1, 223.2 (1980).
55. *Model Penal Code*, § 3.02(1)(a) (1980) (emphasis added).
56. American Law Institute, *39th Annual Meeting*, 1962, 90–91. A typical case
envisioned by the drafters of the MPC would involve damage of property with
the owner's consent. Ibid., 91 ("Obviously the whole idea of the crime is misusing
somebody else's property.").
57. *Model Penal Code*, § 1.12(1) (1980) ("No person may be convicted of an offense
unless each element of such offense is proved beyond a reasonable doubt. In the
absence of such proof, the innocence of the defendant is assumed.").
58. The American Law Institute, 39th Annual Meeting, *Proceedings* (May 1962), 90.
59. Ibid., 91.
60. See George P. Fletcher, *Rethinking Criminal Law* (Boston: Little, Brown, 1978),
705; Bergelson, "Right to Be Hurt," 202–06.
61. See, e.g., *R v. Brown*, [1994] 1 A.C. 212, 250 (H.L.) (Lord Lowry's
opinion) (opining that "for one person to inflict any injury on another
without good reason is an evil in itself (malum in se) and contrary to public
policy").

62. See, e.g., Joel Feinberg, *The Moral Limits of the Criminal Law: Harmless Wrongdoing* (New York: Oxford University Press, 1988), 18 (defining evil in the most generic sense as "any occurrence or state of affairs that is rather seriously to be regretted").

63. Peter Westen has correctly pointed out that consent to injury does not eliminate its harmfulness. Peter Westen, *The Logic of Consent* (Burlington, VT: Ashgate, 2004), 115 (observing that it would be "patently false to say that a person who consents to conduct, e.g., a medical patient who consents to surgical amputation of an eye or limb or a breast, suffers no burdens or setbacks to her interests of any kind from it").

64. Fletcher, *Rethinking Criminal Law*, 568.

65. See Paul H. Robinson, "Competing Theories of Justification: Deeds v. Reasons," in *Harm and Culpability*, ed. A.P. Simester & A.T.H. Smith (Oxford: Clarendon Press, 1996), 45.

66. The MPC and a substantial minority of states that follow the MPC impose the same punishment for an attempt as for the crime attempted (except for the crimes punishable by death or life imprisonment). See, e.g., *Model Penal Code* § 5.05(1) (1980); *Conn. Gen. Stat. Ann.* §53a-51 (West 2008); 18 *Pa. Stat. Ann.* § 905 (West 2007). In these states, the defendants guilty of an "impossible" attempt and the "unknowingly justified" defendants would be, in most instances, treated identically.

67. Fletcher, *Rethinking Criminal Law*, 565 (arguing that justification is an exception to a prohibitory norm and, as such, should be available only to those who merit special treatment).

68. See, e.g., *Model Penal Code,* § 3.02 cmt. 2 (1980), 9.

69. See ibid., § 3.02 cmt. 2, 12 (pointing out that "one who takes a life in order to avoid financial ruin does not act from a justifying necessity").

70. But see Paul H. Robinson, "A Theory of Justification: Societal Harm as a Prerequisite for Criminal Liability," *UCLA Law Review* 23 (1975): 288–91 (arguing that claims of justification should prevail regardless of the actor's state of mind).

71. See *Model Penal Code,* § 3.02 cmt. 2 (1980) ("It is not enough that the actor believes that his behavior possibly may be conducive to ameliorating certain evils; he must believe it is 'necessary' to avoid the evils.").

72. The MPC is different: Its self-defense provision is entirely subjective. As long as the actor *believes* his use of force to be necessary to fend off an unlawful attack, he is justified. See ibid., § 3.04. The actor may still be responsible for reckless (or negligent) homicide or injury if his beliefs were held recklessly (or negligently).

73. Although under these circumstances the perpetrator may not be justified, he may be excused.

74. See, e.g., *Model Penal Code*, § 3.05.

75. Ibid., § 3.02(2). In a number of states, the rule is even stricter: The defense of necessity is completely foreclosed for an actor who was at fault in bringing about the situation requiring the choice of harms or evils. See ibid., § 3.02 cmt. 5 n.27.

76. *Model Penal Code*, § 3.09 (1980). See, e.g., *Ark. Code Ann.* § 5-2-614 (2008); *Ky. Rev. Stat. Ann.* §503.120 (LexisNexis 2008); *Neb. Rev. Stat. Ann.* § 28-1414 (2007).

77. *Model Penal Code*, § 3.09(2) (1980) (emphasis added).

78. See Westen, *The Logic of Consent*, 4–10.

79. Ibid., 4–5.

80. Although the actor would not be guilty of rape in either case, in the second, unlike in the first one, he would be guilty of an attempted rape.

81. See, e.g., Joel Feinberg, *The Moral Limits of Criminal Law: Harm to Self* (New York: Oxford University Press, 1986), 316.

82. See, e.g., *Model Penal Code*, § 2.11(3) (1980). See also *Model Penal Code*, § 2.11(3) cmt. 3 (1980), 398–99.

83. See Feinberg, *Harm to Self*, 316 ("If he is so impaired or undeveloped cognitively that he doesn't really know what he is doing, or so impaired or undeveloped volitionally that he cannot help what he is doing, then no matter what expression of assent he may appear to give, it will lack the effect of genuine consent.").

84. See ibid., 117–21.

85. Ibid., 124–27. Feinberg wrote:

In the cases of "presumably nonvoluntary behavior," what we "presume" is either that the actor is ignorant or mistaken about what he is doing, or acting under some sort of compulsion, or suffering from some sort of incapacity, *and* that if that were not the case, he would choose not to do what he seems bent on doing now.

Ibid., 124.

86. See Westen, *The Logic of Consent*, 269–72.

87. William R. Levesque, "Schiavo's Wishes Recalled in Records," *St. Petersburg Times Online*, November 8, 2003.

88. See Westen, *The Logic of Consent*, 290–91.

89. *Gilbert v. State*, 487 So. 2d 1185, 1186–87 (Fla. Dist. Ct. App. 1986).

90. Ibid.

91. Ibid. (defendant explained that he used a gun because it causes instantaneous death).

92. Ibid.

93. Joel Feinberg, *The Moral Limits of Criminal Law: Harm to Others* (New York: Oxford University Press, 1984), 62. Those include "interests in the continuance for a foreseeable interval of one's life, and the interests in one's own physical health and vigor, the integrity and normal functioning of one's body, the absence of absorbing pain and suffering or grotesque disfigurement, minimal intellectual acuity, emotional stability." Ibid., 37.

94. Obviously, this problem does not exist for those who see at least some rights of people as inalienable. Inalienability of the right to life, however, is a hard position to maintain, particularly for those who tolerate death penalty. As Joel Feinberg correctly warned,

    Those who believe in the inalienability of the right to life . . . might well think twice before enforcing its forfeitability. . . . Whenever the right in question can be thought of as burdensome baggage, it cannot be made inalienable *and* forfeitable without encouraging wrongdoing—the pursuit of relief through "error, fault, offense, or crime."

    Joel Feinberg, "Voluntary Euthanasia and the Inalienable Right to Life," *Philosophy and Public Affairs* 7 (1978): 112.

95. See, e.g., Meir Dan-Cohen, "Basic Values and the Victim's State of Mind," *California Law Review* 88 (2000): 770; Dubber, "Toward a Constitutional Law of Crime," 568; R.A. Duff, "Harms and Wrongs," *Buffalo Criminal Law Review* 5 (2001): 39–44; R. George Wright, "Consenting Adults: The Problem of Enhancing Human Dignity Non-Coercively," *Boston University Law Review* 75 (1995): 1399.

96. Wright, "Consenting Adults," 1399. See also Dan-Cohen, "Basic Values," 777–78; Dubber, "Toward a Constitutional Law of Crime," 568 (arguing that personal autonomy includes dignity, and that the concept of criminal harm should be based on protection of a person rather than a state).

97. Joel Feinberg, "The Mistreatment of Dead Bodies," *Hastings Center Report* 15 (1985): 31–32.

98. Ibid.

99. See Dubber, "Toward a Constitutional Law of Crime," 535. Dan-Cohen makes a similar point when he observes that the term "dignity" should be understood as "moral worth" and not "social status." See Meir Dan-Cohen, *Harmful Thoughts: Essays on Law, Self, and Morality* (Princeton, NJ: Princeton University Press, 2002), 169 n.23.

100. Dubber, "Toward a Constitutional Law of Crime," 535.

101. Feinberg, *Harm to Self*, 172.

> When B requests that A do something for (or to) him that is directly harmful or
> dangerous to B's interests, or when the idea originates with A and he solicits and
> receives B's permission to do that thing, then (in either case) B can be said to
> have consented to A's action. If nevertheless the criminal law prohibits A from
> acting in such cases, it invades B's liberty (by preventing him from getting what
> he wanted from A) or his autonomy (by depriving his voluntary consent of its
> effect).

102. Tim Goodman, "Reality TV Hits a Tailspin with NBC's 'Fear Factor.'" *San Francisco Chronicle,* June 11, 2001, section E-1, Final edition.

103. *The Wolfenden Report: Report of the Committee on Homosexual Offenses and Prostitution* (New York: Stein and Day, 1963), 133.

104. Duff, "Harms and Wrongs," 37.

105. Bergelson, "Right to Be Hurt," 219–21.

106. Interestingly, the Universal Declaration of Human Rights makes this distinction quite clear when it states in Article 1: "All human beings are born free and equal in dignity and rights." *Universal Declaration of Human Rights*, G.A. Res. 217A, at 71, U.N. GAOR, 3d Sess., 1st plen. mtg., U.N. Doc. A/810, Art. 1 (December 12, 1948).

107. See Michael Cook, "Moral Mayhem of Murder on the Menu," *Herald Sun* (Melbourne), January 15, 2004, 17, http://www.australasianbioethics.org/ Media/2004-01-16-MC-cannibal.html.

108. *People v. Kevorkian*, 639 N.W.2d 291, 298 (Mich. Ct. App. 2001).

109. Ibid., 296.

110. See, e.g., Joseph Raz, *The Morality of Freedom* (New York: Oxford University Press, 1988), 437. Based on Raz's definition, a "reason is content-independent if there is no direct connection between the reason and the action for which it is a reason. Ibid., 35.

111. See, e.g., *Model Penal Code,* § 2.09(1) (1980).

112. Douglas N. Husak, "Partial Defenses," *Canadian Journal of Law and Jurisprudence* 11 (1998): 170.

113. See Michael Moore, *Placing Blame* (New York: Oxford University Press, 1997), 708 (making a similar argument).

114. Compare Michael Moore, "Victims and Retribution: A Reply to Professor Fletcher," *Buffalo Criminal Law Review* 3 (1999): 70 (arguing that "[i]t's not culpability alone that counts in determining desert.... Rather, the amount of harm caused determines the seriousness of the wrong done, and the amount of wrong done does affect desert") with H.L.A. Hart, *Punishment and Responsibility* (Oxford: Clarendon Press, 1968), 131 ("Why should the

accidental fact that an intended harmful outcome has not occurred be a ground for punishing less a criminal who may be equally dangerous and equally wicked?"). The debate over the moral and legal significance of the resulting harm has a long history and still continues. For an insightful analysis of the advocated positions on both sides of the debate, see, e.g., Moore, *Placing Blame,* 191–247.

PART TWO

Domains of Consent

8

Consent to Sexual Relations

Alan Wertheimer

Introduction

It is commonly thought that we should regard it as morally and legally permissible to engage in sexual relations if and only if the parties consent.[1] With appropriate qualifications, I think this view is correct. But, as with many other principles, it raises more questions than it resolves. Among those questions are the following.

First, in what does consent fundamentally consist? Is consent (solely or primarily) a state of mind or is it an action? Can one consent to sexual relations by adopting the relevant mental state? If an act of consent is necessary, is it sufficient? Can one consent to sexual relations without the relevant mental states?

Second, when does someone's "token" of consent to sexual relations render it permissible for the other party to proceed? It is sometimes said that the cardinal rule in sexual relations is that "no means no." Although I don't dispute that rule, it does not solve the problem as to what to say when a person says yes. When should a token of consent be regarded as transformative for moral or legal purposes? To use terminology developed in Chapter 4, it is often said that morally transformative (MT) consent must be competent, voluntary, and informed. How should we understand those criteria? Can minors give MT consent to sexual relations? The mentally retarded? Can one give MT consent while intoxicated? What about coercion? It is uncontroversial that one's consent is not MT if it is offered in response to the use or threat of physical force. But what about other threats? Is one coerced by the threat to be abandoned in a remote area? By the threat to end a dating relationship? By the threat to be fired (or not promoted)? Can one be coerced by an attractive offer? And what about deception? Does fraud or misrepresentation negate moral transformation? If not, why not? If so, when?

In this chapter, I sketch answers to some of these questions or, when I have no answers, try to illustrate what issues must be resolved in order to develop proper answers. The most important task is to develop a general account of what I call the criteria of moral transformative consent (CMT), a set of criteria that itself can take two forms: the criteria of morally transformative consent for the law (CMT_L) and the criteria of morally transformative consent for morality (CMT_M). Both versions of CMT are moral criteria, but the criteria that indicate when consent should—as a moral matter—be regarded as legally permissible are not identical to the criteria that indicate when a person's consent renders another's action morally permissible.

Although I will not always explore the differences between these two versions of CMT in this chapter, there may, for example, be good reason to treat consent induced by certain forms of deception as legally transformative while also insisting that it does not render sexual relations morally permissible.

Some believe that we can develop CMT through an analysis of the concept of consent. We ask, in effect, "When is it proper to say that someone consents to do X?" Given an answer to that question and given the premise, we can then say when sexual relations are morally and legally permissible. This picture greatly exaggerates what a certain kind of conceptual analysis can do. The criteria for what constitutes MT consent will always involve moral argument and empirical evidence that is sensitive to the reasons for adopting a more or less rigorous view of CMT_L and CMT_M. And the reasons go both ways. It is often said that we require consent out of respect for a person's autonomy. That is true. But there is a deep tension between what we might call the positive and negative dimension of autonomy. We respect an agent's negative autonomy when we say that it is legally or morally impermissible for others to have sexual relations with her without her competent, informed, and voluntary consent. We respect an agent's positive autonomy when we make it possible for her to render it permissible for others to engage in sexual relations with her if she consents. Unfortunately, we cannot simultaneously maximize both dimensions of autonomy. To the extent that we seek to protect an agent's negative autonomy, we should set high standards for what qualifies as MT consent. On the other hand, setting high standards for what qualifies as MT consent may encroach on the agent's ability to realize her own goals and desires. The distinctiveness of the two dimensions of autonomy is well illustrated by a moral or legal regime that rigorously protects everyone's right to refuse sexual contact, but places extensive restrictions on one's right to engage in sexual contact, such as restrictions on nonmarital sex or homosexual relations. Under this regime, there is extensive negative autonomy, but less positive autonomy than we might want.

As I use the terminology in this chapter, to say that B's consent is morally transformative is to say that, *ceteris paribus*, B's consent renders it permissible for A to proceed. It is not to say that B's consent is sufficient to an "all things considered" moral assessment of A's actions. Even when consent establishes permissibility, it hardly establishes that sexual relations are morally worthy. Exchanging money for sexual relations may be morally problematic even if the prostitute consents. Indeed, it might remain impermissible for reasons that have little to do with its consensuality. Still, the prostitute's consent is morally transformative because it removes one important reason for regarding A's behavior as wrong.

Although this chapter focuses on consent to sexual relations, I believe that the general structure of the argument is generalizable to any context in which issues of consent arise. As I argued in Chapter 4, it is possible that CMT remain relatively constant at an extremely abstract level across contexts, but they will demonstrate considerable variability when applied in different contexts. There is, for example, no reason to assume that the informational requirements of MT consent to a medical procedure (where we use the phrase "informed consent") are identical to the informational requirements of MT consent to sexual relations. And we would hardly want to require that such consent be given in writing.

A few preliminary points. First, in what follows, I will bracket questions about the "ontology" of consent, whether consent is, at its core, a mental state or an action. I will assume that B tokens consent in an appropriate way. I also set aside cases in which B does not token consent at all, as in cases of pure force and unconsciousness, where A penetrates B without any willed acquiescence or cooperation on B's part, as in these cases.

Pure Force. A and his accomplices tie B's arms and legs to a bed. A penetrates B while B screams, "No, please stop."

Anesthesia. A, a dentist, penetrates B while she is unconscious from anesthesia.

I will be interested in cases where B explicitly tokens consent but where it may be argued that B's consent is not MT on grounds of coercion, deception, incompetence, or intoxication.

Second, I will assume for analytical purposes that A is male and that B is female. Although the CMT are, in principle, gender neutral, the standard cases in which we worry about consent are heterosexual relations in which the alleged perpetrator is male and the alleged victim is female.

Third, the question throughout is whether B gives MT consent to sexual relations and not whether B is "raped." We may think that consent induced by certain forms of deception is not morally transformative and should not be treated as legally transformative, but we may want to reserve the term "rape" for cases in which the perpetrator uses or threatens physical force or renders the victim unconscious.

Coercion

Let us now consider coercion. When does A coerce B in a way that renders B's consent nontransformative? I have argued elsewhere that A coerces B into sexual relations when (1) A proposes to make B worse off relative to the appropriate baseline if she does not acquiesce to the act *and* (2) it is reasonable for B to succumb to A's proposal rather than suffer the consequences.[2] The point of criterion (1) is to establish whether A's proposal is coercive. The point of criterion (2) is to establish when a coercive proposal actually coerces. If A's proposal is not coercive, then CMT will generally regard B's token of consent as MT even if (as in 2) it is reasonable for B to succumb to A's proposal rather than suffer the consequences.

> *Debt.* A, who owes B $500, says, "Have sexual relations with me and I will repay my debt. Otherwise, ciao."

> *Abandonment.* A and B drive to a secluded spot in A's car. B resists A's advances. A says, "Have sexual relations with me or I will leave you here."

> *Tickle.* A knows that B is ticklish. A says he will tickle B if she does not have sex with him.

Even if A's proposal is coercive in these cases, it does not follow that we will regard B as having been coerced if we do not think that the threat is sufficiently grave to render B's consent ineffective. If A threatens to break B's arm unless B kills C, A's proposal is coercive, but we would not say that A has been coerced into killing C and is therefore not responsible for C's death. Similarly, if A proposes to harm B in some way unless B consents, it does not necessarily follow that she is not responsible for the normal consequences of her consent. Few would claim that A commits a criminal *sexual* offense in *Tickle*, and some might say the same in *Abandonment* or *Debt* if B acquiesces. Although I note this issue here, I set such issues aside and focus exclusively on the question as to whether A's proposal is coercive and not whether B is ultimately coerced.

I said that A coerces B only if A proposes to make B worse off. But worse off than what? For present purposes, I consider two possibilities: (*1*) A may propose to make B worse off than B's status quo or preproposal baseline if she refuses; (*2*) A may propose to make B worse off relative to where B has a *right* to be vis à vis A, what I call B's *moralized* baseline.

I believe that (*2*) is the right approach for our purposes. The single most important element in determining when coercive proposals nullify the transformative power of consent is whether A proposes to make B worse off than her *moralized* baseline, whether A's "declared unilateral plan"—what A proposes to do if B does not accept A's proposal—would violate B's rights or, where "rights" discourse is inapposite, whether A proposes not to do for B what A has an obligation to do for B. Consider *Weapon*.

> *Weapon*. A, a stranger, says, "Do not resist me or I will kill you with this gun."

In many cases, such as *Weapon*, the two baselines converge, for A's declared unilateral plan would make B worse off than her preproposal status quo and would also violate B's rights. To see why the moralized baseline provides the better criterion for evaluating the validity of consent, we must consider cases where the various baselines do not converge.

To explore this issue, consider two cases in which B's status quo differs from her moralized baseline. In some cases, A may have an obligation to render B *better* off than her status quo, in which case A's declared unilateral plan—to do nothing—may actually be coercive.

> *The Opportunistic Lifeguard*. A is a professional lifeguard at B's country club. He sees that B, who he knows to be very wealthy, is in trouble. He proposes to help B only if B agrees to pay him $10,000. B accepts, and, after being saved, refuses to pay on grounds that she consented under duress.

If A has an obligation to attempt to rescue B, then A's proposal is coercive because A proposes to make B worse off than her moralized baseline if B rejects A's proposal, even though he proposes to make her *better* off than her status quo. B's consent would not be MT. By contrast, it is sometimes permissible for A to propose to render B worse off than her preproposal status quo baseline.

> *Plea Bargaining.* A, a prosecutor, says, "Plead guilty to a lesser offense and take a 1-year sentence or I will prosecute you on a more serious charge, for which you will receive 5 years if you are convicted." B accepts and then claims she was coerced into the agreement.

On my approach, A's proposal is *not* coercive because he has not proposed to make B worse off than she has a right to be, assuming that the prosecutor is acting reasonably in proposing to put B on trial for the more serious charge. Relative to her status quo, A is threatening to make B worse off if she does not plead guilty, but relative to B's moralized baseline, A is offering to make B better off than she has a right to be if she accepts A's proposal.

To say that we should evaluate the coerciveness of A's proposal by reference to B's moralized baseline does nothing to define that baseline. It is *neutral* with respect to the specification of A's obligations or B's rights. That is an issue for moral theory.

Although it is clear that A's declared unilateral plan would violate B's rights in *Opportunistic Lifeguard*, where rescuing people is a responsibility of A's job, it is not clear that A's declared unilateral plan would violate B's rights in the *Opportunistic Samaritan*.

> *The Opportunistic Samaritan.* A, a stranger, is walking by B's country club and hears B shout for help. A proposes to rescue B only if B agrees to pay A $10,000. B accepts and then refuses to pay on grounds of duress.

If A's declared unilateral plan (not to rescue B for free) would violate B's rights or fail to fulfill his obligations to B, then A's proposal is coercive. If not, then A's proposal is not coercive, although it might be exploitative.

It is sometimes argued that offers can be coercive. As a general proposition, this is false. Offers expand a person's options even if, as in the case of an unattractive offer, a person prefers the status quo. But recalling a phrase from *The Godfather*, it is often said that A coerces B when A makes an offer that is "too good to refuse," perhaps forgetting that Don Corleone "offered" the target a choice between signing a contract and having his brains on the contract, a proposal whose declared unilateral plan would appear to violate the target's right not to have his brains on the contract (to say the least)! So this hardly shows that genuine offers can be coercive.

Pseudo-offers aside, B may find A's offer too good to refuse for two different reasons, and it is important to distinguish between them. First, A's proposal may create a set of alternatives in which one option is so clearly superior that it would be irrational for B to choose otherwise. Call this an *attractive offer*. There is nothing necessarily problematic about such offers despite the "overpowering factors" favoring B's decision, as when A offers B a new job that would render her so much better off than her eminently acceptable status quo that she says with a smile on her face, "Your offer is too good to refuse." Other cases are more difficult. B may find A's offer too good to refuse because the short-term benefits contained in A's proposal may be so tempting or irresistible that they distort B's judgment and motivate B to accept an offer that she is likely to regret. Call this a *seductive offer*. Consider two cases.

> *Indecent Proposal.* A, who is very rich, says to B, "I'll give you $1,000,000 if you spend the night with me."[3]

> *Lecherous Millionaire.* B's child needs expensive medical treatment. A proposes to pay for the treatment if B will meet him for sex twice a week for 1 year.[4]

Given the distinction I have drawn, it is not clear whether *Indecent Proposal* or *Lecherous Millionaire* constitutes an attractive offer or a seductive offer. That depends on a complicated calculation of its long-term consequences. But suppose that one or both are seductive offers. I believe that CMT may well hold that A's "seductive offer" can compromise the transformative power of consent in a way analogous to defects in competence or information because, by definition, B's judgment is distorted. Even when that is so, however, seductive offers are not helpfully described as coercive, because A does not threaten to violate B's rights in *Indecent Proposal* or *Lecherous Millionaire* if B declines the offer.

Still, it might be said that I am missing something important. Although A does not propose to violate B's rights in these cases if B rejects his proposal, it may be claimed that A's offer is coercive because B has *no reasonable alternative* to accepting A's proposal. I readily admit that there is a *sense* in which one is "forced" to do that which there is no reasonable alternative to doing, but this is not the sort of "force" or coercion that undermines moral transformation. The problem is that many people have been misled by the paradigmatic (gunman) examples of coercion. It is true that B has no reasonable alternative in *Weapon*, and so we might think that B is coerced *because* she has no reasonable alternative. That is false. To see why, consider a case in which B faces a choice between having surgery for cancer and probable death; she may reasonably feel that she has no reasonable alternative to surgery. But this is precisely the point. We do *not* say that B's consent to surgery is invalid just because she has no other reasonable choice. We would hardly charge her oncologist with battery because he operated without her "voluntary" or "uncoerced" consent.

The previous lines of analysis might be subject to another objection. Suppose that B has a *right* to care for her child in *Lecherous Millionaire*. Does it not follow that A's proposal to leave B below her moralized—rights defined—baseline is coercive? It does not. Rights are specific to relationships. Whereas B may have a right that the society or government provide her child with medical care, she has no right that *A* provide her child with medical care. A does not propose to violate B's rights if she rejects his offer if we assume that A is not morally or legally required to help out B's child without demanding anything in return. I do not deny that there is something unseemly about the agreement in *Lecherous Millionaire*, but I do not think that such unseemliness amounts to coercion or compromises the transformative power of B's consent.

Let us now consider some cases of putative sexual coercion. Some cases are, as they say, no-brainers. It is beyond question that B's consent is not MT in *Weapon* or in a case such as this.

> *Texas.* A, a complete stranger, enters B's apartment and waits for B to come home. When B arrives, A threatens to stab B unless B succumbs to sexual relations. B pleads with A to wear a condom, falsely telling A that she has AIDS.[5]

On the moralized baseline view, it seems that A also makes a coercive proposal in other cases we have seen such as *Abandonment, Lower Grade*, and *Debt*. By contrast, it seems that A does not make a coercive proposal in the following cases.

> *Dating.* A and B have been dating for some time, but have not had sexual relations. A says, "I'm not willing to continue dating you if we don't have sex, so either we have sex or stop dating."

> *Escape.* B is in prison for life. A, a prison guard, offers to help her escape if she has sexual relations with him.

> *Landlord.* A owns the apartment that B rents. B is several months behind on her rent, and with few prospects of being able to pay.

A tells B, "Have sex with me once a week until you pay up, or I'm going to have you evicted."

Higher Grade. A, a professor, says, "Have sexual relations with me and I will give you a grade two grades higher than you deserve. Otherwise, you'll get just what you deserve."

In the first set (*Abandonment, Lower Grade, Debt*), A's declared unilateral plan violates B's moral or legal right not to be abandoned or to receive the grade she deserves or to have her loan repaid. By contrast, A's declared unilateral plan does not violate B's rights in the second set of cases, because B has no right that A continue their dating relationship on her preferred terms or receive a higher grade than she deserves or not to be evicted or to be allowed to escape.

My analysis of *Higher Grade* and *Escape* should not be misunderstood. It is clearly *wrong* for A to make his proposal in these cases, even though A does not propose to violate B's rights if B rejects the proposal, and even though such bribes might be welcomed by B. A professor violates his responsibility to his institution and to other students by offering to trade grades for sex, and may deeply insult B by suggesting that she does or might think about her sexuality in ways she may abhor.[6] A prison guard violates his obligation to society if he helps a prisoner escape and commits an additional wrong if he trades that favor for sexual services. But insults and bribes do not coerce. Assuming that the proposals in *Higher Grade* and *Escape* are honest and credible (and are understood that way by B), we should not treat B's consent as not transformative on grounds of coercion.[7]

In my view, *Hiring* is a more difficult case.

Hiring. A is the sole owner and proprietor of a restaurant, at which the tips are very good. B applies for a job as a waitress. A says that he will hire her only if she has sex with him.

Hiring exemplifies what is often called quid pro quo sexual harassment. Although A's proposal strikes me as coercive, it poses a problem for my analysis, for A's declared unilateral plan does not appear to violate B's rights. I assume that A is under no obligation to hire B even if she is the most qualified. A could hire his less-well-qualified daughter if he preferred. A might say, "I'm not proposing to harm B. Having sex with me is just a condition of employment, as is wearing the designated uniform. If she doesn't like the terms, that's fine with me. I'll find others that do." If this is right, then the prohibition of quid pro quo sexual harassment must be justified on grounds other than straightforward coercion.

If *Hiring, Lecherous Millionaire,* and *Indecent Proposal* all involve non-coercive quid pro quo offers, can we distinguish among them such that B's consent is not MT in *Hiring,* but is MT in *Lecherous Millionaire* and *Indecent Proposal?* I believe so, and I believe that this is to be explained, at least in part, in terms of the social consequences of recognizing consent as MT in the various contexts. Consider CMT from an *ex ante* perspective. It seems likely that the class of potential employees will be *better off* if we disallow such arrangements and refuse to treat B's consent as MT. If, as in *Hiring,* sole proprietors are not permitted to make such offers, they will still need to hire and promote employees and will probably hire them without the sexual quid pro quo. By contrast, it is not clear that the class of potential offerees will be better off if proposers are barred from making their offers in *Lecherous Millionaire* and *Indecent Proposal,* for if A cannot demand a quid pro quo, it is unlikely that A will make any offer at all.

Deception

Although deception typically nullifies the transformative power of consent in commercial contexts, *caveat amator* has been the traditional principle for sexual relations. Several states criminalize deception with respect to a sexually transmitted disease or impersonation of a husband. But such exceptions aside, the law has been quite permissive with respect to sexual deception, and prevailing moral norms somewhat but perhaps not all that much less so. It is not clear why this is so. If we think that deception undermines one's capacity to act autonomously, then we ought to take sexual deception more seriously.

There is some controversy as to the relative wrongness of various forms of deception. We can distinguish between a statement (lie) that is technically false and intended to deceive, a statement that is literally true but is intended to deceive, and a failure to disclose relevant information. I am inclined to think that the moral importance of differences between these forms of deception is often exaggerated. Nonetheless, I will set this issue aside, save to note that in some contexts—such as medicine and the sale of a home—we require the physician or the seller not only not to deceive but also to positively disclose relevant information. It is an open and interesting question as to whether and when we should adopt a similar view about sexual relations.

Consider the following cases.

Gynecologist. A tells B that he will be inserting an instrument into her vagina. Instead, he inserts his penis.

Twins. A, whose identical twin is married to B, slips into B's bed while she is half asleep. B believes that A is her husband.

Talent Scout. A meets B, an aspiring actress. A falsely tells B that he is a talent scout for a Hollywood producer. A makes no quid pro quo demands, but A believes (correctly) that B accepts his advances only because she believes his story.

Sister. A has been having sexual relations with B's sister, unbeknownst to B. Although B would have rejected A's advances if she knew about this relationship, he says nothing.

HIV. A makes advances. B asks A if he has been tested for HIV. A, who has tested positive for HIV, tells B that he had a negative test 1 month ago.

Love. A and B are dating. A makes advances. B says, "I don't want to go further unless you really care about me." A says that he does, but later tells mutual friends that he was lying.

Marriage. A and B have been dating for some time, but have not had intercourse. B tells A that she is "saving herself" for her husband. A likes B but is a committed bachelor. A tells B that he intends to marry her.

Vasectomy. A makes advances. B tells A that she has a problem with the pill, so she'll accept only if A wears a condom. A falsely tells B that he had a vasectomy.

Single. A and B meet in a night class, and have several dates. B makes it clear that she refuses to have sex with married men. A falsely tells B that he is not married.

Cure. A, a hospital employee, tells B her blood tests indicate that she has a serious disease, and that it can be cured by expensive and painful surgery or by intercourse with an anonymous donor (who turns out to be A) who has been injected with a serum. A and B meet in a hotel and have intercourse.[8]

Pro Choice. A is a strong "right to life" advocate. B is strongly pro choice and chooses not to be intimate with those who do not support a woman's right to choose. In response to B's inquiry, A lies about his view.

B consents in response to A's deception in all of these cases. In which cases should we regard B's consent as MT? The law has long distinguished between *fraud in the factum* and *fraud in the inducement*. A commits fraud in the factum when B is deceived as to what is done, as exemplified by *Gynecologist*. A commits *fraud in the inducement* when B consents to what she believes to be intercourse, but does so for mistaken reasons, such as (1) the purpose of intercourse (*Cure*), (2) A's nominal identity (*Twins*), (3) A's characteristics (*Single, Talent Scout, Vasectomy, Pro Choice, HIV*), or (4) A's mental states (*Marriage, Love*).

Fraud in the factum is generally regarded as the more serious form of fraud, although I think that "fraud" misdescribes a case such as *Gynecologist*. It's not that B is defrauded into consenting to sexual relations. She does not consent to sexual relations, period. By contrast, the law has been reluctant to regard *fraud in the inducement* as negating the transformative power of consent. When an identical twin impersonated his brother, the woman's consent was considered sufficient "because she knew she was agreeing to an act of intercourse."[9] Richard Posner conjectures that if a woman is not "averse to having sex with a particular man, the wrong, if any, is in the lies . . . rather than in an invasion of her bodily integrity."[10] On this view, *Vasectomy* or even *Cure* are not properly regarded as sexual offenses because B is not averse to having sex with A. Posner also argues that there is less need to protect targets from sexual deception than commercial deception, because prospective sexual partners can choose to prolong courtships and investigate the personal qualities of a suitor, whereas waiting and investigating are less viable and too costly in the more hurried and impersonal relationships of the marketplace.

I am less sure. Consider *Odometer*.

Odometer. A sets back the odometer on a car before selling it to B.

We do not say that there is no criminal fraud in *Odometer* because B is not averse to buying the nominal car from A and (merely?) misrepresents the *characteristics* of the car. Posner might reply that A's fraud in *Odometer* is serious because B has suffered an identifiable economic loss, whereas B got the sexual experience that she sought, say, in *Single* or *Pro Choice* or *Sister*. But that does not show that sexual deception is not seriously wrong nor that it fails to cause harm. Rather, it requires us to determine whether A's action could be wrong or harmful even if the deception does not detract from the synchronic experience, say, because it is a violation of B's autonomy or right to control the terms on which she has sexual relations or will likely lead to subsequent regret.

It is hard to say why and when deception is sufficiently wrong so as to render B's consent nontransformative. Cordial interaction among human beings often seem to require that we make statements that are less than fully honest or that we fail to disclose information in which the other party might be interested. Indeed, we regard some forms of deception as part and parcel of the sexual initiation and negotiation. "Exaggerated praise, playful suggestions, efforts to impress, and promises intended to reassure and trigger emotions (but not to be strictly believed) are all part of the ritual of escalating erotic fascination that makes up a 'seduction' in the colloquial sense."[11] In addition, some forms of deception or exaggeration may be integral to the sexual interaction itself. Do women behave wrongly when they fake an orgasm or overstate their pleasure?

So the problem is this. If some sexual deceptions are to be regarded as morally and legally permissible whereas others are not, how can we distinguish between those two categories? The permissive approach to sexual deception embodied in the law may derive in part from "line-drawing" difficulties. We can probably draw a bright line around disease (*HIV*), pregnancy (*Vasectomy*), and identity (*Twins*). At the same time, although I would regard *Pro Choice, Single, Marriage,* and *Sister* as morally serious deceptions that may compromise CMT_M, they are not easily distinguished from deceptions that are less serious "puffing" or "storytelling."[12] The permissive approach may also derive from evidentiary difficulties. It is often difficult to establish what A said and whether A was intending to deceive when he made his statement. And if we cannot distinguish the serious from the trivial with sufficient clarity or establish who said what, then we must either allow for at least some deceptions that are impermissible or prohibit some that are permissible.

Given all this, there is some tendency to treat the mating game as akin to negotiations in which we simply expect that people are not always truthful. Nonetheless, we must be careful not to draw the wrong moral conclusion from line-drawing and evidentiary difficulties, such as they are. Although there may be good reasons to think that deception does not typically compromise CMT_L, where we may assign the burden to B to protect herself, I believe that many cases of deception may well compromise CMT_M. Even if the law should not regard A's behavior as criminal in the cases just mentioned, we may think that A is not morally entitled to proceed and that doing so is an important violation of B's sexual autonomy.

Competence

As a general rule, B's token of consent is morally transformative only if she is suitably competent, that is, only if she has the requisite emotional and cognitive capacities. There are several ways in which CMT might raise questions about B's competence to consent. Here I consider age and retardation. In the following section, I consider intoxication. Not surprisingly, I will argue that CMT do *not* specify a univocal set of psychological requirements. If a retarded adult with a mental age of 13 can give MT consent to sexual relations, it does not follow that a normal 14-year-old can also give MT consent. As I have argued, CMT are the output of moral argument that will be sensitive to the implications of adopting those criteria in various situations.

Most states forbid sexual relations on the basis of age, even when the younger party gives an unambiguous, undeceived, and uncoerced token of consent. Some states also criminalize sexual relations when there is a significant age differential between an adolescent and the partner. If we map the prevalence of teenage intercourse onto existing statutes, there are at least 7.5 million incidents of statutory rape per year.[13] But positive law aside, when and why should we regard the consent of a young person as invalid?

Consider the following cases

Chat Room. A, 33, and B, 14, have met in an Internet chat room. They agree to meet in a motel and have intercourse.

Sweethearts. A, 15, and B, 15, are high school sweethearts. They frequently have sexual relations.

Spur Posse. A is a 17-year-old member of the "Spur Posse," a group in which boys compete to have intercourse with as many girls as possible. B is a 14-year-old high school freshman who does not know about the group. She is flattered by A's attention and deceptions.

Child. B is a 9-year-old girl. A is an 18-year-old friend of B's older brother. A says, "Did you know that it feels good if I put my penis into your vagina? Do you want to try it?" B says, "OK."

Sitter. B is a 14-year-old who babysits for A's child. B has an enormous adolescent crush on A (34). When A is driving B home one evening, B says, "I'm a virgin, but they say older men are better. Would you teach me about sex?"

In which cases are sexual relations morally permissible? In which cases should we regard sexual relations as legally permissible? These are different questions. I am inclined to think that (barring more details) A's behavior is morally impermissible in all but *Sweethearts* and that *Spur Posse* may compete for low position on the moral ladder. I also think that while A's behavior should be legally impermissible in *Child, Sitter,* and *Chat Room,* it is arguable that the law should go the other way in *Spur Posse* even if it is morally worse.

Our legal and moral practices invoke age criteria because age is a useful *proxy* for psychological capacities that are relevant to the validity of consent and it is not feasible to assess those capacities on a case-by-case basis. The sorts of psychological capacities required for competent consent are always a function of the subject of the consent. We allow youngsters to make many decisions, even given their relatively low cognitive and emotional capacities, so long as we do not think wrongful decisions are likely to be seriously harmful. Is it harmful for young girls to engage in what would otherwise be described as consensual sex? It has been suggested that sex by minors is no big deal, that "coitus occurring after puberty, willingly undertaken by the girl, and representing the fulfillment of a normal physiological need, probably cannot in itself harm her."[14] By contrast, it has been argued that sexual interactions are "by definition, serious undertakings" that are fraught with grave risks of injury and harm to vulnerable girls.

It is an empirical question as to whether sex by young minors carries a high risk of harm and whether, as seems likely, that harm is sensitive to the age disparity between the parties. Here there is some reason to err on the side of protecting negative autonomy. If minors are prohibited from having sexual relations when very young or with older males, we would not be imposing a long-term deprivation. True, they can never recover the lost experiences of sexual encounters that did not occur, but minors will get older and will then be able to have sexual relations more or less as they desire.

Michelle Oberman is concerned that a legal or moral regime that regards an adolescent's consent to sex as invalid might have untoward effects on abortion rights.[15] She is right to be concerned. It is not easy to say why a 14-year-old should be regarded as sufficiently mature to make her own decision about an abortion, but not sufficiently mature to choose to have sexual relations, get a tattoo, or have cosmetic surgery. Although I am not concerned here to defend this combination of policies, my approach to CMT shows why this is at least a coherent position. Although a person's cognitive and emotional capacities are relevant to CMT, there is no one-to-one correspondence between one's capacities and the moral decision as to whether to regard one's consent as MT. And there are several differences between abortion and sexual relations that might justify distinguishing the cases. First, there are practical considerations. Because abortions are relatively infrequent, it is possible to conduct "judicial bypass hearings" that evaluate the minor's ability to choose on an individual basis. It is hard to see such a policy working with respect to sexual relations. Second, there is an important distinction between the "positive autonomy" costs in abortion and sexual relations. To fail to respect a teenager's positive autonomy to engage in sexual relations requires her to abstain. To fail to respect her positive autonomy to secure an abortion is, in effect, to require her to carry a fetus to term. Given this distinction, it is arguable that we have more reason to err on the side of positive autonomy with respect to abortion than with respect to sex.

The main point is that we cannot come to firm conclusions as to whether a minor's consent is MT on the basis of philosophical considerations alone. We need to know more about the decision processes of minors and the extent to which they are capable of making reasonable decisions about their long-term interests. We need to know more about the way minors are affected by sexual relations or would be affected under alternative social arrangements.

Let us now consider retardation. Teresa was 16 years old, enrolled in the eighth grade. She was diagnosed as retarded when she was 3, and had an IQ of 59. She met Adkins, who was 27, in a local mall, where they exchanged telephone numbers. Teresa's mother subsequently overheard a telephone conversation between Adkins and Teresa, took the phone, told Adkins about Teresa's retardation, and also told him to leave her alone. The next day, Teresa phoned Adkins and asked him to meet her at a store. They met, went to Adkins's home, had intercourse twice, ate dinner, watched television, and fell asleep. They were discovered when Teresa's mother notified police that her daughter was missing.[16] Adkins was convicted under a Virginia statute that makes it illegal to have sexual relations with one who has a mental impairment that prevents the impaired person from "understanding the nature or consequences of the sexual act . . . and about which the accused should have known."[17] Bracketing the issue of age, should we regard Teresa's consent as MT?

Consider these cases.

> *Retardation.* A is a somewhat "nerdy" 17-year-old virgin who would like to have his first time with someone nonthreatening. He is friendly with B, a 19-year-old neighbor, who is moderately retarded. A says, "Do you want to see what it's like?" B responds, "OK, if you want to, but don't tell my mother."

> *Friends.* A and B, both 24, are both moderately retarded and like each other. A proposes that they have intercourse.

Should we regard B's consent as MT in these cases? If retarded females typically end up feeling very hurt in such cases because they do not understand how sex will affect them, then there would be reason not to regard their consent as MT. But suppose that they do not. Suppose that most retarded females (at a certain level of retardation) understand the physiology of sexual relationships, that they typically enjoy the sexual encounters that they *experience* as consensual, and that they do not typically regret their sexual encounters. We might have reason to protect them from disease and unwanted pregnancy (for their sake), and we might also worry about the costs to society imposed by disease, pregnancy, and offspring. But under the assumption that allowing retarded females to engage in sexual relations is not (*ex hypothesi*) bad for them, we should expect CMT to regard their consent as MT.

To put the previous point in now familiar terms, we have reason to be concerned to facilitate the (albeit limited) positive autonomy of the retarded as well as to protect them from predators. Although the moderately retarded may have cognitive competence that is no greater than those of nonretarded minors, there is more reason to be concerned about protecting the positive autonomy of the retarded. If we say that minors are unable to give transformative consent, we do not preclude sexual experience over the course of their lives. Minors get older. By contrast, to say that a retarded female cannot give transformative consent is to deny her permanently the opportunity to legitimately experience intimacy and sexual pleasure.

Would CMT draw a distinction between *Retardation* and *Friends*? In *Retardation*, it is arguable that a nonretarded male is "taking advantage" of or exploiting the retarded woman, but there is no coercion. In *Friends*, there is no hint of exploitation, advantage taking, or inequality. Despite these differences, I am not sure that we would want to draw a sharp distinction between the cases with respect to MT. We do not want to say that retarded persons are only permitted to have sexual relations with other retarded persons or, unlike nonretarded persons, that the retarded are only permitted to have sexual relations in the context of an enduring relationship.

Intoxication

The question is this: Is it permissible for a male to have sexual relations with a woman who consents after becoming voluntarily intoxicated? For present purposes I shall assume that B gives an unambiguous (verbal or behavioral) token of consent. I set aside those cases where B consumes or (knowingly or unknowingly) ingests a substance that renders her unconscious or semiconscious. I also set aside cases such as *Partying*, where B gives sober consent at Time 1, which is followed by intoxicated consent at Time 2.

Partying. A and B have dated, but have not had sex. A says, "Is tonight the night?" B says, "Yeah, but let's have a few drinks first." Later on, B gets quite high and responds positively to A's advances.

Now some think that if a woman consents while she is (severely) intoxicated, her consent is *necessarily* invalid because intoxication undermines the capacity requirements of MT consent. End of story.[18] Call this the *intoxication claim*. By contrast, some think that if a woman is responsible for her intoxicated behavior, it follows that she is responsible for what she does while intoxicated and, therefore, that her intoxicated consent must be treated as MT. Call this the *responsibility entails MT claim*. I will argue that we are not required to accept either claim.

To fix ideas, consider the case—I shall refer to it as *Brown*—of Adam Lack and Sara.[19] Sara (a pseudonym), a Brown University freshman, consumes approximately 10 shots of vodka in her dorm room one Saturday night. She walks a few blocks to a Brown crew party, then to a fraternity house to see someone she had been dating. Adam finds Sara in a friend's room lying next to some vomit. Adam asks Sara if she wants a drink of water. Sara says yes. Adam gets her some water. They talk. Adam asks Sara if she wants to go to his room. She says yes. Sara follows Adam to his room without assistance, kisses him, and begins to undress him. Sara asks Adam if he has a condom. He says yes. They have sex. They talk, smoke cigarettes, and go to sleep. In the morning, Adam asks Sara for her phone number, which she provides. "It took a while for it to actually set in," Sara says. "When I got home, I wasn't that upset. The more I thought about it, the more upset I got." Three weeks later, and after Sara sees a "women's peer counselor" in her dormitory, Sara brings charges against Adam Lack. According to the Brown University Code of Student Conduct, one commits an offense when one has sexual relations with another who has a "mental or physical incapacity or impairment of which the offending student was aware or should have been aware."

The present question is not whether Adam Lack violated the Brown University Code of Student Conduct. It is arguable that if, as Adam claimed, Sara asked if he had a condom, then she could not have been *that* intoxicated. That issue aside, the present question is whether we should accept the animating principle of this provision: Should it be regarded as morally, institutionally, or legally impermissible to have sexual relations with a woman who consents to sexual relations while intoxicated?

Consider the following cases.

Inhibitions. A and B have dated. B has said that she's not ready for sex. From her own experience and from other sources, B knows that alcohol consumption distorts her judgment. B consumes several drinks at a party. When A proposes that they have sex, she feels much less inhibited than usual and half-heartedly says, "There has to be a first time."

Fraternity Party. B is a college freshman. She has never had much to drink. She attends her first fraternity party and is offered some punch. She asks, "Does this have alcohol?" A responds, "Absolutely." She has several glasses and becomes quite high for the first time in her life. When A proposes that they go to his room, she agrees.

Spiked. B attends a fraternity party for the first time. There is a keg of beer and a bowl of punch that has been "spiked" with vodka but is labeled nonalcoholic. B has several glasses of punch, and becomes quite high. When A proposes that they go to his room, she agrees.

Dutch Courage. A and B have dated. B is a virgin, and feels frightened about sex. Believing that she will never agree to sex if sober, she consumes four drinks in an hour. After some kissing and petting, A says, "Are you sure it's OK?" B holds up her glass, smiles, and says, "It is *now.*"

I will not pursue in detail the question as to why intoxication might compromise the transformative power of consent. We may, for example, think that B is not acting as fully autonomous when intoxication weakens her ability to govern her actions by the reasons that she accepts. And I will assume for the sake of argument that B's judgment is sufficiently distorted by her consumption of an intoxicant that her consent would not be MT if the intoxicant had been surreptitiously administered to B by A, as in *Spiked.*

As we have seen, cases of intoxicated consent come in various degrees of voluntariness or self-inducement. In some cases, B consumes the substance with the specific intention that it alters her psychology (*Dutch Courage*). In other cases, B intentionally consumes a substance with the knowledge that it may affect her desire or judgment but does not intend this effect (*Inhibitions*) or, perhaps, anticipate its effect (*Fraternity Party, Brown*). As a matter of positive law, the voluntariness of B's intoxication has generally been regarded as constituting a defense for the defendant.[20] But the question for us is normative: *Should* B's consent be treated as MT if B is voluntarily intoxicated?

Let us assume that B is responsible for becoming intoxicated and can also be held responsible (at least in a general way) for what she does while intoxicated even if she then lacks the mental capacities that are normally assumed as required for ascriptions of responsibility. If we are justified in treating B as morally responsible for her decision to become intoxicated or for her (voluntary) intoxicated behavior, then we can reject the intoxication claim. It is perfectly *coherent* to claim that if B is responsible for her intoxicated behavior, then CMT *can* treat B's intoxicated consent as MT. Should we then accept the responsibility entails MT claim? If we *can* say that B is responsible for her intoxicated consent, does it follow that we *must* treat her consent as MT?

Heidi Hurd believes so. She argues that if we hold people responsible for their criminal behavior, then we should treat B's consent as MT. "On pain of condescension, we should be loathe to suggest that the conditions of responsibility vary among actors, so that the drunken man who has sex with a woman he knows is not consenting is responsible for rape, while the drunken woman who invites sex is not sufficiently responsible to make such sex consensual."[21] I disagree. First, it is entirely possible that the mental capacities that are required for responsibility for criminal wrongdoing are different from and less robust than the mental capacities that are required for responsibility for consent. Second, and more generally, the normative upshots of ascriptions of responsibility are fundamentally open-ended. It is a mistake to think that to be held morally responsible for one's choices is to be required to internalize *all* the consequences of that behavior. If I choose to ski or eat ice cream, I assume an extra risk of a broken leg or heart disease. It does not follow that I should bear all the medical costs of such conditions. Similarly, it is perfectly coherent to argue that B is responsible for her intoxicated behavior, but not for all of its possible upshots and, in particular, not for rendering it permissible for A to take advantage of her intoxicated consent.

Given this, I believe that we can reject both the intoxication claim and the responsibility entails validity claim. I believe that it is an open question as to whether we should regard intoxicated consent as MT and that it will not be settled by "moral logic." To see how we might answer that (open) question, it will be helpful to step back from sexual relations and consider other contexts of consent. Consider consent to a medical procedure.

Cancer. B has an appointment to see A, her physician, where she expects to receive the reports of a biopsy. Because she is very anxious,

she has several drinks before her appointment. A tells B that she does
have cancer and recommends surgery. A presents a consent form.
B signs.

It seems entirely reasonable that B's intoxicated consent in *Cancer* should
not be treated as MT if B's intoxication is or should be evident to the
physician. A cannot say, "She was drunk when she came in to sign the consent
form. She's responsible for her intoxication, not me. End of story." We need
not and do not say that B's responsibility for her intoxication entails that her
intoxicated consent to a medical procedure *must* be treated as MT. Rather,
we ask whether the balance of moral reasons favors treating a patient's
intoxicated consent to major surgery as MT, and (I think) we are inclined
to say it does not.

Consider intoxicated consent in a commercial context.

SUV. A and B go out drinking. When A sees that B is very
intoxicated, A proposes to buy B's car at 50% of its market value.
B accepts.

Although the traditional rule about intoxicated consent to a contract goes
some distance toward treating intoxicated consent as giving rise to a binding
agreement, current doctrine holds that a contract made by an intoxicated
person is voidable "if the other party has reason to know that the intoxicated
person is *unable to act in a reasonable manner* in relation to the transaction."[22]
On this view, the contract in *SUV* might be unenforceable. The contract law
approach is revealing. In deciding whether to treat B's intoxicated consent as
binding, contract law shifts the focus from B's responsibility for her intoxicated behavior to the question of whether the ends served by a regime of free
contracting would be promoted or undermined if intoxicated agents were
held to their bargains. There may be reasons of fairness and utility that favor
treating B's contract as unenforceable if she is severely intoxicated and A
knows or should know this, but not if A cannot reasonably be expected to
know this. If B's intoxication were "sufficient to *diminish* the intelligence, and
the party dealing with the intoxicated person knowingly made use of the
situation in order to induce the bargain," it may be better to assign the burden
of B's intoxicated consent to A and regard such contracts as unenforceable.

We have considered two models—medical consent and contracts—in
which intoxicated consent is not necessarily treated as MT, but they may not
constitute useful models for consent to sexual relations. So consider two
activities that are arguably closer to sex: getting tattooed and gambling.
Many states prohibit tattooing of an intoxicated person.[23] These statutes do

not distinguish between voluntary and involuntary intoxication. If the client is intoxicated, the tattoo cannot be performed. These statutes reflect the view that even if B is responsible for becoming intoxicated, it does not follow that we must treat B's consent as MT.

Would a similar approach make sense with respect to sexual consent? It might be argued that getting tattooed is a more serious matter than having sex. One can have drunken sex and be sober in the morning and arguably no worse off for it. If one gets a tattoo while drunk, one may be sober in the morning but the tattoo will be relatively permanent. On the other hand, sex involves the risk of pregnancy and disease, whereas (sterile) tattoos do not. And so it is not clear that the potential harmful effects of tattoos are more serious. I am not concerned to justify the prohibition of intoxicated consent to tattoos or to argue that CMT would treat the two sorts of consent in a similar fashion. But if one thinks that the states are justified in taking a harder line on intoxicated consent to tattoos than intoxicated consent to sex, one must be prepared to justify that distinction.

Consider gambling. It might be argued that an intoxicated gambler should be able to recover her losses on the grounds that a wager between a gambler and a gambling establishment constitutes an implied contract that is voidable on grounds of intoxication.[24] Not surprisingly, the standard legal view is that the gambler absorbs the risk of her intoxicated judgment, that her intoxicated consent is MT. Is this the right view?

We might consider what rule about intoxicated gambling would be chosen by gamblers *ex ante*. Suppose that potential gamblers were given a choice between a rule that treats gambling losses incurred while intoxicated as recoverable and a rule that treats them as nonrecoverable and that the consequences of adopting both rules were well understood. What would they choose? I suspect that most would choose the nonrecoverable rule, for unless their losses were nonrecoverable, casinos would be reluctant to allow them to both drink and gamble, particularly given that it might be very difficult to monitor a gambler's sobriety before each gambling transaction (imagine a hall of people at slot machines).

Suppose this is right. Is sex like gambling? Sex is not like gambling in some respects that tell in favor of a stricter approach to intoxicated sex than intoxicated gambling. First, people who enter a casino intend to gamble before they become intoxicated, but women who find themselves in sexual situations do not necessarily intend to have sexual relations before they become intoxicated. Second, while it may be unreasonable to expect casino personnel to monitor each gambler's alcohol level before each gambling transaction, it is arguably not unreasonable to expect potential sexual partners to monitor each other's level of intoxication. Third, it is arguable—although by no means certain—that the emotional and physical harms consequent to intoxicated consent to sexual relations are greater than the various harms consequent to intoxicated gambling.

On the other hand, sex is like gambling in some respects that tell in favor of a similar or more permissive rule about intoxicated consent to sexual relations. People do like to gamble, *ex ante*, even when they regret having gambled *ex post*, and much the same is true for sex. Indeed, whereas most gamblers lose on a given day (intoxicated or sober) and almost all gamblers lose over the long run, many intoxicated sexual relationships are pleasurable and do not typically involve significant physical or psychological harm. Rather, drinking to the point of at least moderate intoxication may be crucial to what some regard as a desirable sexual and social experience. Without wanting to minimize either the risks incurred or the distress experienced by women in cases such as *Brown*, we should not focus exclusively on the cases that go badly. We must recognize that many women as well as men intentionally become intoxicated precisely to reduce their inhibitions. Given that a decision to regard intoxicated consent as invalid would limit the positive autonomy of women to engage in sexual relations while intoxicated, if that is what they wish to do, we cannot say that something like the Brown University policy enhances women's autonomy.

Would CMT endorse something like the Brown University policy? We need to know whether women are likely to enjoy sexual relations while intoxicated and, more important, how they tend to feel about it in retrospect, particularly given that sexual relations can lead to pregnancy and disease that would otherwise have been avoided. Here, too, we can ask what rule about intoxicated consent would be chosen by women *ex ante*. If women would prefer a "gambling" regime that allows them to become intoxicated and engage in sexual relations so long as they actually token consent, then that would tell in favor of such a regime. If women would prefer a "tattoo" regime in which their intoxicated consent is never treated as MT, then that would tell in favor of a less permissive regime. We can't decide on the best account of CMT without answering these sorts of questions.

Conclusion

I am painfully aware that I have not resolved the question as to when consent to sexual relations should be regarded as MT, but I hope to have successfully shown that the question as to when we should regard it as morally or legally impermissible to engage in sexual relations will not be settled by metaphysical or conceptual investigations into the meaning of consent or abstract appeals to moral theory. It will be settled by moral reasoning that is responsive to the variety of situations that people encounter and that is informed by empirical investigation.

Notes

1. This chapter is largely based on my book, *Consent to Sexual Relations* (Cambridge: Cambridge University Press, 2003).
2. See my *Coercion* (Princeton, NJ: Princeton University Press, 1987).
3. As portrayed in movie of this name.
4. I borrow this example from Joel Feinberg, *Harm to Self* (New York: Oxford University Press, 1989), 128–29.
5. This is based on a Texas case in which, at first, the grand jury refused to indict the defendant on the grounds that the victim consented when she proposed that the perpetrator use a condom. See the discussion in Peter Westen, *The Logic of Consent* (Burlington, VT: Ashgate Publishing Co., 2004), 9.
6. By contrast, while B may subsequently regret acquiescing in *Dating*, B cannot complain that A has introduced a sexual component into a relationship from which it should be absent.
7. I assume, for example, that A is not making a covert threat to give B a lower grade than she deserves if she rejects his proposal.
8. This is based on an actual case, confirming that the law does not need bizarre hypotheticals. Real cases will suffice. See *Boro v. Superior Court*, 163 Call. App. 1224; 210 Cal. Rptr 122 (1985).
9. Steven Schulhofer, *Unwanted Sex* (Cambridge, MA: Harvard University Press, 1998), 152.
10. Richard Posner, *Sex and Reason* (Cambridge, MA: Harvard University Press, 1992), 392.
11. Jane Larson, "Woman Understand So Little, They Call my Good Nature 'Deceit': A Feminist Rehinking of Seduction," 93 *Columbia Law Review*, 374 (1993): 425.
12. Schulhofer, *Unwanted Sex*, 92.
13. Michelle Oberman, "Regulating Consensual Sex with Minors: Defining a Role for Statutory Rape," 48 *Buffalo Law Review* 703 (2000): 703.
14. 'Forcible and Statutory Rape: An Exploration of the Operation and Objectives of the Consent Standard," 62 *Yale Law Journal* 55 (1952): 77.
15. Ibid., 75.

16. *Adkins v. Virginia* 20 Va. app 332, 457 S.E. 2d 382 (1995).
17. Va. Code §18.2–67.10(3). The conviction was overturned on appeal.
18. According to Joan MacGregor, the fact that a woman "was drunk or high on drugs should naturally lead to the conclusion that she was not consenting, as she was incapable of voluntary consent." "Force, Consent, and the Reasonable Woman," in Jules Coleman and Allen Buchanan, eds., *In Harm's Way* (Cambridge: Cambridge University Press, 1994), 244–45. Laurence Thomas says "it is axiomatic that consent is rendered void if obtained from a person while [s]he was in . . . an utterly inebriated state." "Sexual Desire, Moral Choice, and Human Ends," *Journal of Social Philosophy* 33 (2002): 178–92, 183.
19. This account is based on an article in the *Orange County Register*, January 3, 1997, and is based largely on Adam Lack's account of the facts. The article originally appeared (date unknown) in the *Providence Journal-Bulletin*. For the purposes of this article, I shall assume that this account is correct. Even if it is not correct, we would still have to decide what to say about a case in which something like these facts occurs.
20. For example, the relevant Vermont statute states that one commits a sexual assault if one engages in a sexual act with another person and has "impaired substantially the ability of the other person to appraise or control conduct by administering or employing drugs or intoxicants without the knowledge or against the will of the other person. . . ." Title 13, V.S.A. Section 3252. *Corpus Juris Secundum* maintains that there is no offense ". . . where the female voluntarily drank the substance alleged to have excited **or** stupefied her." *supra*, n. 15, at 483.
21. Heidi Hurd, "The Moral Magic of Consent," 2 *Legal Theory* 121 (1996): 141.
22. Ibid.
23. The Alabama statute says that "A person shall not tattoo, brand, or perform body piercing on another individual if the other individual is under the influence of intoxicating liquor or a controlled substance." Ala. Code 1975 Sec 22-17A-2.

9

Sex, Law, and Consent

Robin West

Liberal legal theory primarily, and liberal feminist legal theory derivatively, have jointly shaped much of our contemporary understanding of the various relations between sex and law. At the heart of that familiar liberal legalist paradigm is the distinction between consensual and nonconsensual sex. That distinction serves two central purposes. First, the absence or presence of consent demarcates, broadly and imperfectly, sex that should be regarded as criminal from that which should not. Nonconsensual sex, generally, ought to be regarded as rape, or, if not rape, as a lesser but still quite serious sexual assault.[1] To whatever degree, and it is still considerable, the law fails to criminalize nonconsensual sex; to that degree, according to liberal legal theorists and reformers, the law should be criticized and changed. So, for example, not only forcible, violent sex between strangers, but also (liberals argue) nonconsensual but nonviolent sex between dates or cohabitants; non-consensual marital sex; sex coerced through particularly egregious fraud; sex imposed upon unconscious, intoxicated, or mentally incapacitated victims; and sex coerced through implied threats of future violence, or of a nonviolent violation of rights—all of this sex should be understood as some degree of criminal sexual assault, regardless of whether or not the sex is accompanied by force, regardless of whether or not the woman resisted, and—at least for some liberal reformers—regardless of whether or not she verbally expressed her nonconsent. Liberal feminists from Harriet Taylor and John S. Mill[2] from the nineteenth century to Susan Estridge, Michelle Anderson, and Stephen

Shulhofer of the twentieth and twenty-first[3] have generally pressed for broader definitions of rape and sexual assault and broader enforcement of existing laws so as to bring the law on the streets and in the bedrooms in line with this basic moral claim: Nonconsensual sex is wrong in all circumstances, and so wrong as to be properly regarded as a serious crime.

The second purpose, implicit rather than explicit, served by the distinction between consensual and nonconsensual sex, within liberal legalism is rhetorical rather than legal, and might best be called that of "legitimation." Liberal legal scholars typically, if not invariably, urge not only that consensual sex should not be criminal, but also that legal regulation of any sort, including the imposition of civil sanctions, and perhaps nonlegal community disapprobation or political critique likewise, is uncalled for. We should loosen, or liberalize, and perhaps entirely prohibit, unduly moralistic regulatory control of all consensual sex, whatever the source of the regulation, and whatever the target. Thus, over the last 30 years, liberal scholars and reformers have argued that the production and consumption of pornography should be insulated against regulation, so long as all sexual acts required for its production (and consumption) were consensual,[4] that obscenity regulations premised on offense to community morality should be likewise eliminated entirely or severely cut back,[5] that prostitution should be decriminalized and if regulated at all only toward the end of protecting the health of participants,[6] that consensual sex between partners of the same gender should be constitutionally protected against state regulation,[7] that the availability of the right to marry should not depend in any way on the sexuality, the gender, or the sexual practices of would-be participants,[8] that contraception and abortion should be freely and fully available and the right to obtain them should be constitutionally protected against regulation,[9] and that sexual harassment laws should be read narrowly so as to protect consensual sex and sexual speech in workplaces and in schools.[10] Consensual sex, perhaps quintessentially for contemporary liberal legalists, wherever it happens, and whatever its form, and whatever the motivation—whether it be in cars, in bordellos, or on screen sets; whether it be between persons of the same sex, opposite sex, or no discernible sex; whether it be anal, oral, vaginal, missionary, marital, nonmarital, vanilla, nonvanilla, sadomasochistic, or something other; whether it be for pleasure, for reproduction, for money, for status, for friendship, or for the approval of one's peers—should be deregulated. It ought to be left alone: by law, by the community, by various would-be moral censors, and by politically motivated interrogators.

Arguments for deregulation of consensual sex vary, depending on different strands of liberalism, but all, in some way, rest on the legitimating function of consent to sex. Within libertarian legal theory, the point is familiarly put in terms of victimless crimes and undue state paternalism: If two or more parties consent to sex, then the sex is victimless, and therefore any state regulation—whether criminal or civil—would be paternalistic and unwarranted.[11] For more traditional Millian liberals, the reason has more to do with individual autonomy, or identity, than with the dangers of state regulation: The sexual activity to which we consent is akin to expression, and is central to one's conception of the good life; to interfere with it is to interfere with an important dimension of individual autonomy.[12] From the sometimes aligned normative law-and-economics camp, the claim is more sweeping: Assuming no third-party effects, and assuming competent parties, *any* consensual sexual transaction—sex for money, sex for pleasure, sex for a favor, sex for protection, sex for shelter, and so on—as is true of any nonsexual consensual transaction, is presumptively of positive value to both parties; if it weren't, why would they consent to it?[13] And, if it is presumptively of positive value to both parties and no one else is hurt, then it is value, wealth, or efficiency maximizing. Liberal feminists add a feminist twist to all three arguments: Denial of the worth of consensual sex has often been accompanied by and sometimes been motivated by a vitriolic denial of the equal worth of women's sexuality and capacity for sexual pleasure.[14]

Thus, consent to sex renders the sex that follows victimless, central to autonomy and identity, of positive economic value, and emblematic of the equal worth of she who gives it. The arguments converge, though, on a common conclusion: Consensual sex, because it is consensual, ought to be not only noncriminal but also shielded from legal regulation and moral or political critique. To regulate consensual sex acts or render them the object of civil sanctions or even community disapproval is at best undue state or community intervention—overly paternalistic, voyeuristic, nanny-state-ish, inefficient, moralistic, or just unnecessary—and at worst disruptive of the creation of value, autonomy sapping, identity robbing, equality compromising, and virtually by definition coercive. Consent legitimates the sex that follows, the effect of which is to insulate it from not just criminalization, but more broadly, from legal regulation likewise.

The liberal (and liberal feminist) reliance on consent as demarcating the distinction between sex and rape has attracted a good bit of critique, not only from defenders of more traditional and more restrictive definitions of rape (that require, in addition to or instead of lack of consent, the use of force by the perpetrator and resistance from the victim, and still impose numerous restraints on the criminality of marital sex), but also from radical strands of feminism, and more recently, from queer theory. The broadly legitimating role consent plays within liberal understandings of sex and law has not attracted nearly as much critical attention, either from feminists, queer theorists, or liberals themselves. In the bulk of this piece I would like to suggest some reasons why it might be worth our while to reverse this trend. Consent works relatively well, I will argue, as the demarcation of noncriminal from criminal sex; or at least, radical feminist and queer theoretic arguments against it are unconvincing. By contrast, the political and moral legitimation of wide swaths of sexual behavior that is affected by the liberal deregulatory projects, more or less given a pass by liberalism's left-wing and feminist critics, has quite real and relatively unreckoned costs.

One such cost, and the only one I will elaborate in this chapter, is that here as in other spheres of life legitimation effectively renders invisible—and in some versions of liberalism, even incoherent—what may be significant harms caused by the conduct so legitimated. More specifically, I will argue that consensual sex, when it is unwanted and unwelcome, often carries harms to the personhood, autonomy, integrity, and identity of the person who consents to it—and that these harms are unreckoned by law and more or less unnoticed by the rest of us. The possibility that the liberal valorization of consensual sex that is so central to liberal deregulatory projects legitimates these harms ought to concern us far more than it has, at least to date. That doesn't mean we should seek to broaden the definitions of either sex crimes or the contours of private law so as to punish or compensate for a wider range of conduct. I do not think we should or could. We do, though, need a better understanding of the relation between our understanding of what is criminal or tortious behavior and why—and what that does, or doesn't, imply about the value, worth, and pleasures of our noncriminal sexual behaviors.

The chapter is organized as follows. As noted, the first part of this four-part chapter argues briefly that both the (relatively new) queer theoretic and the (getting on now) radical feminist arguments against the liberal reliance on consent as the demarcation between rape and sex are misguided. They both fail to grapple with the distinctive harms that come from a sexual perpetrator overriding the will of a weaker partner, although they do so for opposite reasons and with drastically different consequences. The remainder of the chapter concerns the legitimating role of consent in liberal conceptions of law and sex. In the second part, I will describe, or at least delineate, one specific type of harm—the harm caused by unwanted and unwelcome but nevertheless fully consensual sex—that the legitimation of consensual sex has the consequence of denying or at best obfuscating, and argue why those harms are important, even if they are not and should not be the target of criminal sanction. In the third part I will try briefly to account for our relative failures to better understand them. Specifically, I will explore some of the reasons they have generally escaped the notice not only of liberal legalists concerned with rape and rape law reform but also of liberalism's critics, primarily radical feminists and queer theorists. Finally, in the conclusion I will suggest that those are not good reasons, and that we—meaning legal theorists, and not only moral or political philosophers—should focus more than we do on consensual sexual harms and their relation to law, in the intimate sphere, no less than we do in our political and economic lives.

Consent and Rape

As is fairly well known, beginning in the 1980s, radical feminists in law and outside of law, but most forcefully Catherine MacKinnon, have argued in various ways that the sharp line drawn by liberals between consensual and nonconsensual sex falsifies the degree of coercion imposed upon women by men in our ordinary sexual lives.[15] That which is perceived as consensual sex, according to this now familiar radical feminist critique, is more often than widely believed the result of coercive forces, ranging from believable threats of future violence, to social or economic pressures, to a ubiquitous sexualized and pornographic culture that only somewhat paradoxically forces women and girls to consensually give it up, and all the better if they do so desirously. Echoing Marx's parallel accounting of the role of consensuality in labor relations,[16] MacKinnon and other radical feminists argued that in the sexual sphere no less than in the economic, "consent" is not a meaningful marker between autonomy and coercion. Thus, radical feminism tended to conflate consensual and nonconsensual sex, finding all of it the product of coercion.

Radical feminist critiques of consent and of rape law have garnered an enormous response, both from liberals and from liberal feminists, the former arguing that the radical position, if codified in law, would overcriminalize nonviolent and sometimes only reckless or negligent behavior, and the latter that the radical position (whether or not reflected in law) denies women's "agentic" power, feeds pernicious stereotypes of women incapable of saying no to unwanted sex, and implicitly, and wrongly, assumes women's strong aversion to sex generally.[17] I am not going to pursue those arguments here (I have elsewhere).[18] I want to focus instead on what I think is a problematic feature of the radical feminist critique of the liberal paradigm that for various reasons has not been much addressed, either by liberals or liberal feminist theorists, to wit, that the radical feminist critique of rape law denies the distinctiveness of the *experience* of nonconsensual sex, and hence, the distinctiveness of its harms. Even if we assume, that is, that there is a good deal of coercion in the background conditions that produce consent to sex (just as there is a good deal of coercion operating in the background conditions that produce consent to alienating labor, or consent to bad governance), it doesn't follow that consensual and nonconsensual sex are in all ways the same, or that the "coercion" is or feels qualitatively similar, or that the harms they occasion are not different. Thus, there is a quite real felt difference between those coercive forces that elicit consent—no matter how bad the bargain struck—and the coercive force employed by an actor who overrides or ignores the lack of consent. It is *not* necessarily a difference in the degree of harmfulness; as I will argue below, the former might in the long run be more damaging and to more people than the latter. It is, though, a difference in qualitative experience, and there are real costs involved in conflating them.

Being burgled in one's home, or robbed on the street, feels different than being exploited by an unscrupulous employer in an unequal and capitalist economy. Robberies occasion a fear that one will be killed—that one's existence, and not just one's dignity, will be obliterated. It is traumatic and frightening in a way that exploitation is not. It is a departure from the normal course of life, which, however exploitative the conditions of one's life might be, does not include a constant fear that one will be killed in the next few seconds. It is upsetting for just that reason, in a way that exploitation is not; exploitation, after all, may well *be* the norm against which the trauma of a robbery stands in relief. That does not make the robbery, all things considered, *worse* than economic exploitation: Exploitation in an underpaid and alienating job through the course of adulthood might well be far more damaging than having been the victim of a one-time robbery, in the long run. Certainly, exploitation is more insidious, more invisible, and more easily masked—it's harder to name and blame both the harm and the perpetrator. Constant workplace exploitation may also be, in the long run, more important politically than occasional robberies: The very phenomenon of private sphere economic exploitation unchecked and largely unregulated by an unconcerned state suggests the existence of an unjust community, an unjust social structure, and an unjust legal regime, while the robbery or burglary suggests aberrant behavior, against which both the interests of that unjust legal regime and its exploited citizens are jointly aligned. A trauma, once identified, can be recovered from, and both the state and the citizen have a stake in seeing that they don't happen, that they are both deterred and compensated. An unjust social order—maybe not.

The same is true of sex. Heterosexuality may well be compulsory in all the ways argued by Adrienne Rich in her classic mid-seventies essay[19]: Girls are given no or little choice but to enter the world of heterosexuality, the culture willy-nilly propels all of us toward early heterosexual intercourse (social conservative resistance notwithstanding), and men and boys feel an entitlement while women and girls feel an imperative to participate—and all of this is reinforced explicitly by a constant stream of cyber and real-space pornography, and then underscored, rather than meaningfully challenged, by mainstream religion traditions, that may quibble over the timing and circumstances of the compulsion, but hardly over the central command: While pornography pushes girls and women to submit to sex across the board, religious tradition dictates that women should become wives, who then must and should submit to their husbands' sexual demands, virtually world over and for most of recorded history. That's a lot of coercion. If there's any truth at all to this account, then it's sensible enough to say that what that coercion produces is an awful lot of consent to an awful lot of dreadful sex; I'll argue as much explicitly in the next section.

Forcible rape, however, is "coercive" in an entirely different way. The physical invasion of the self and body, the interruption and denial of sovereignty over one's physical boundaries that the invasion entails, the fear of death foremost in the mind of the victim, the sure knowledge that one's will is irrelevant, the immediate and total reduction of one's self to an inanimate being for use by another, and the sustenance of multiple injuries, both vaginal and nonvaginal, internal and external—all of this, simultaneously experienced, typify and constitute the experience. The experience of the compulsion of which Adrienne Rich spoke might share in some of these features, but the contrasts swamp the shared point of contact. The compulsion in "compulsory heterosexuality" creates constricted identities, and expectations, and certainly social roles, all of which in turn might *elicit* consent to sex. The latter—the coercion used by a rapist at knifepoint, at gunpoint, or with overpowering threats of force—overrides the *lack* of it. The sex that results from compulsory heterosexuality, whatever else it is, is consensual, as we normally use the term and certainly as the law understands it. The sex that results from the coercive wielding of knives, fists, and guns is rape. Again, this doesn't mean the latter is "worse" than the former: Compulsory heterosexuality *might* do more widespread and longer-lasting damage both in the individual case and in the aggregate than rape, in the same way that economic exploitation *might* do more widespread and longer-lasting damage, and to more people, than theft. Compulsory heterosexuality that elicits consent to unwanted sex over a lifetime undermines an individual's self-sovereignty even as an ideal, while the traumatic experience of rape might ultimately underscore, for the victim, the importance of both autonomy and self-sovereignty as essential for a well-led life. In the aggregate, compulsory heterosexuality is certainly more pervasive, harder to name and blame, more insidious, and so on. Further, as with economic exploitation, the state has little interest in deterring, addressing, or even noticing "compulsory heterosexuality": Whether or not it does so depends on other state interests entirely—in eugenics, population control, family policy, or the various sorts of bio-projects of which Foucault spoke and wrote. It is not central to the *raison d'etre* of the state to deter compulsory heterosexual intercourse—to deter the conditions that prompt consent to sex. The state has a direct interest, however, in the criminalization of violent rape.

They are, simply, different. Why conflate them? There is not much to be gained by doing so, and I think there is quite a bit to be lost. Let me note two such costs. The first is to the success and even coherence of liberal rape law reform movements. The claim that current definitions of rape undercriminalize, and that a good bit of nonconsensual sex ought to be but currently isn't criminal, and that there is more ordinary rape in the world than most realize or care to admit, is the basis of an important and largely liberal reform agenda. That agenda is not furthered, it is undercut, when it is confused with the claim that rape is ubiquitous. If rape is ubiquitous, the claim that there exists a class of undercriminalized nonconsensual sex that ought to be criminalized becomes trivially true, but inconsequential, if it is viewed as part and parcel of a political view that can't possibly be the basis of a serious reform of the criminal code. If all sex is literally rape, there is no norm against which to define the wrong the code is designed to target.

It is clear now, and it was certainly clear to many of us at the time, that it was never the intention of theorists, particularly Catherine MacKinnon, to expand the criminal code so as to include and prosecute as "rape" all sex, or all heterosexual sex—and MacKinnon is right to insist that she never said as much.[20] Nevertheless, it is also clear that the claim was *heard* in this way. One reason it was so heard is that the claim was made, and often, that the experience of women who are rape victims, conventionally described, and of women having consensual sex within a patriarchal regime is more similar than dissimilar, and that they are so by virtue of the coerciveness of both.[21] It is that claim, I believe, that misdescribes the experience of both. If understood as a call to criminalize far more sex than is envisioned by even the most far-reaching of the reforms of liberal feminist rape activists, it undercuts rather than bolsters liberal rape reform projects.

The second cost of the conflation of compulsory heterosexuality and coercive sex is less immediately felt, but may be more consequential. The rhetorical conflation of the compulsion that sometimes produces consent to heterosexual sex, and hence produces some consensual sex, with the coercion that produces rape overstates the role of rape in the perpetuation of patriarchic hierarchies. Rape, understood either conventionally (as forced sex, with utmost resistance by the victim, imposed on someone other than one's wife) or as liberals would redefine it (as nonconsensual sex), is an aberrational act that violates sovereign interests in social and public stability as well as women's interest in physical security. The state prosecutes it when it can. By contrast, the sex that results from consent that is given within social structures that embed gendered inequality—consensual sex, where the consent is elicited in part through societal compulsion—is, at least arguably, ubiquitous. If we define the latter as "rape," then rape is indeed central to patriarchal control of women by men, and the struggle against "rape" so understood is likewise central to ending it. But there is a danger in putting the point this way. If we reference, either intentionally or not, the conventional, criminal-code definition of "rape" to describe the phenomenon of "compulsory heterosexuality" because coercion is central to both, then we invite the mistaken conclusion that promoting greater enforcement and prosecution of rape crimes, as understood by the state, will end patriarchy.

But this conclusion is just not warranted, and not simply because the sex described by the inclusive definition of "rape" previously is not what the state will prosecute, no matter what the definition of rape. It isn't warranted, more fundamentally, because the compulsory conditions that elicit consent to unwanted sex might be more central to those obnoxious regimes than the knives and fists employed by rapists to override their victims' will. Even if it is true, as MacKinnon begins her most important book, that "sexuality is to feminism what work is to Marxism: that which is most one's own and most taken away,"[22] then the conflation of rape and consensual sex seems all the more particularly ill-advised: Wiping out all theft, through a more aggressive use of the criminal law, will not return their alienated work to laborers, and likewise, ending rape, through a more aggressive use of the criminal law, will not fundamentally return sex to women. Economic exploitation of laborers is not the result of a state's underenforcement of laws against theft, and likewise, sexual exploitation is not the result of the state's underenforcement of laws against rape. By conflating the problem of exploitative and expropriated sexuality with the problem of rape, we engage not only in conceptual confusion but also strategic misdirection. Much of third-wave feminism—the Take Back the Night rallies, self-defense and antirape education initiatives on high school and college campuses—although arguably vital to ensuring women's safety on the street, might be oversold as a means to ensuring women's equality and an end to their sexual exploitation. We *do* need to address the conditions, states of mind, and social structures that so overwhelmingly prompt, suggest, or compel women to consent to sex they don't desire or want: That is the deepest, most vital, and most profoundly historic claim at the heart of MacKinnon's reconstruction of radical feminism. That sex, however, is not rape, and we don't come any closer to addressing it by calling it what it is not.

Let me turn to the very different—in fact, quite opposite—objections to liberal understandings of rape, and the role of consent within it, put forward more recently by queer theorists. The queer theoretic critique of the liberal reliance on consent as the demarcation between sex and rape is not that by so doing liberals understate the amount of wrongful sex in the world. Rather, the worry is that by so doing, they overstate it: They are led to overregulate, condemn, or punish what ought to be noncriminal and deregulated sexual conduct. Thus, and in a modern echo of a very old argument—that rape is too easily alleged, too difficult to disprove—queer theorist Janet Halley has argued over the last half decade that in a culture such as ours that is overtly hostile to sexual variation and unduly hostile to sex itself, claims of nonconsensual sex—claims of rape—are often the product of a "sex panic" rather than an actual assault.[23] The claim that some particular sexual encounter is "rape" masks the likely truth of the matter, which is that the sex was in fact both desired by, but also abhorred by, the complainant. The "victim" calls the sex a "rape" so as to negate any possible suggestion that she may have enjoyed it. Nonconsent is an unreliable marker of rape from nonrape, then, simply because in a sex-phobic culture it is too often falsely claimed. Somewhat more broadly, Michel Foucault argued toward the end of his life that even a child's lack of consent to sex ought neither to be presumed, nor should an affirmative declaration of consent be even required, so long as the child does not actively resist the adult's sexual advance.[24] Presumably, if even a *child's* lack of express consent should not trigger an accusation of rape, the same should hold with respect to adult women. In the context of U.S. understandings of rape, then, it is not unfair to infer that Foucault implicitly advocated a return to a "perpetrator's force plus victim-resistance"—rather than lack of consent—definition of actionable rape. Lastly and most sweepingly, Law Professor David Kennedy suggested in the wake of the Lewinsky-Clinton scandals from the 1990s that in the world of sexuality (perhaps unlike elsewhere), such liberal banalities as "consent," choice, and autonomy are all just not as important as we have believed.[25] Nonconsensual sex, in this telling, like sadomasochistic sex or sex within hierarchies, is simply another form of unconstrained sex, and unconstrained sex—whether nonconsensual, sadomasochistic, hierarchic, or thoroughly vanilla—is of such great hedonic value that it simply should not be sacrificed to legal niceties. We should, in effect, quit fetishizing consent. Sex, and more particularly the sexualized, eroticized power that drives it, is good, not to be lightly tossed aside. We don't need consent to police it.

To generalize: All three of these theorists share a deeply positive stance toward all forms of sexual expression, including those often abhorred as aberrant, those often mistakenly viewed as coercive or nonconsensual, and those (such as sadomasochism) that overtly or covertly employ, require, celebrate, or revel in the hedonic uses of power, a deeply skeptical stance toward claims of both self-identified victims and adults speaking on behalf of children that the sex imposed by a stronger party on a weaker party was unwanted, unwelcome, undesired, and not enjoyed—and certainly that it should ever be presumed to be such— and a belief that the harms of truly nonconsensual sex are not particularly grave. They all accordingly share a skeptical stance toward sexual regulation, and a skeptical stance toward "consent" as the marker of much of anything. Hot, transgressive sex, particularly sadomasochistic transgressive sex, has all the markings of nonconsensuality. From there, it's a short step to the conclusion that perhaps nonconsensual sex itself is an overrated harm, and a too-often prosecuted crime. This is the view I'm labeling, I hope not unfairly, as "queer theoretic."

The queer theoretic critique of the role of consent as the marker of illegality has attracted some feminist response (although not much of a liberal one): To summarize what will no doubt be a growing cottage industry, the idea of a "sex panic" motivating false rape claims might be little but an urban myth, the proposed deregulation of sex crimes and the trivialization of sexual injury on which it rests threaten second- and third-wave feminist gains, and the denial of the importance of consent and choice to our assessment of the relative costs and benefits of laws governing sexuality simply ignores women's and gay men's experiences of rape, which have not been transgressively ecstatic.[26] Here again, though, I want to focus on a different problem with the queer critique, and one that it shares with radical feminism, for all its dramatic and much proclaimed oppositional stance to that movement. The queer theoretic critique, like the feminist, *also* obscures the distinction between consensual and nonconsensual sex, and like the radical feminist argument it attacks, it does so by ignoring the experience of victims, and focusing instead on the power inherent in both consensual and nonconsensual sex. The difference between radical feminism and queer theory—and it is indeed a dramatic one—is that queer theorists do this *not* toward the end of asserting the wrongness and ubiquity of oppressively sexualized power regardless of consent or its lack, but, rather toward the end of asserting, and then valorizing, the ubiquitous transgressiveness of sexualized power—and therefore its value. But the shared ground is considerable. Like feminists, the queer critic sees in all sex, both consensual and nonconsensual, the presence of a power imbalance—although this time to applaud the power imbalance rather than condemn it. As the radical feminist conflates consensual sex with sex infused with power, so as to condemn it all, so the queer theorist conflates nonconsensual sex likewise with sex infused with power, so as to affirm it all.

This parallelism is much noted (and lauded) by queer theorists themselves.[27] Not so noted, though, is the flimsiness of the shared premise: Just as there is nothing to sustain the radical feminist identification of a power imbalance between parties with a lack of consent, and therefore sex with rape, here, likewise, there's nothing to sustain the lack of consent that might define rape with the power imbalance that might define hot and desired sex. Even if it is true, in other words, that sex (to many, obviously not all, but not an insignificant number either) is pleasurable, ecstatic, and transgressive precisely because of the power—and power imbalances—that infuse it, it doesn't follow that nonconsensuality likewise is inconsequential or pleasurable, just because it too involves an imbalance of power. A rape victim is not a bottom. The experiences aren't comparable. Sadomasochistic sex is not rape, regardless of the presence of handcuffs, rope, chains, and the like in the former and the lack of all that in the latter. The affirmation of the transgressive pleasures of sadomasochism does not imply that we give rape a pass—unless we just blithely ignore these differences.

Put more generally, a benign, desired, and consensual power imbalance in a sexual relationship is not the same thing as the coercion in a nonconsensual rape, any more than a *non*benign power imbalance between actors in a consensual but hierarchic relationship is coercive, and therefore rape. Neither hot, desired, transgressive sadomasochism nor the dreary, dull "compulsory heterosexuality" in hierarchic relationships is rape. They aren't rape, furthermore, whether the rhetorical point of the conflation is to condemn it all as rape or praise it all as hot. The experience of rape is shot through with an unwilled invasion of the body, fear for one's own imminent death, and the pain of nonconsensual physical touching; none of that is present in either consensual sadomasochistic or hierarchic sex whether hotly desired or not. One could conflate or confuse these drastically different subjective experiences only by ignoring, willfully or not, the experience of the rape victim. There's no good reason to do that, and plenty of good reasons not to.

At the heart of this odd convergence between feminism and queer theory, I believe, is not simply (as is claimed by queer theorists who have noted the same convergence) a shared objective view of the nature of sex with then different affective stances toward it. Or it is not only that. Rather, what radical feminists and queer theorists share (or also share) is a philosophical premise: They both overendow sexual power (and perhaps power itself) with hugely exaggerated normative significance, and for just that reason, they both downplay—or forthrightly deny—the normative significance of subjective experiences of harm. Thus, radical feminists tend to see coercion wherever they see sexual power, and accordingly give it a negative valence, regardless of whether or not the sex it produces is consensual, regardless of whether or not it is accompanied by desire or pleasure, and regardless of whether its participants experience it as harmful or injurious. Consent, then, pales as a marker of coercion and autonomy, and hence of legality and illegality, and the subjective experience of harm or injury pales as the trigger of both legal intervention and justified communal concern. Sexual inequality, and hence unequal sexual power, and hence the expression of sexual power, is bad per se, so to speak, with or without attendant harm. Queer theorists identify transgressive pleasure—almost definitionally—with sexualized power, and therefore give it a positive valence, with or without attendant harm, generally dismissed by queer theorists as either imagined or trivial. The experience of all that sexualized power as either welcome or not, desired or not, consensual or not, and harmful or not is inconsequential. From either perspective, then, consent fades in significance as power looms: For radical feminists, sexual power is coercive with or without consent, and for queer theorists, sexual power is transgressive and pleasure enhancing, with or without it. The consequence of all of this is a misdescription of the experience of rape and a misappraisal of the seriousness of its harm—as well as a misapprehension of its boundaries. Radical feminists tend to overstate the importance of rape and rape law in the perpetuation of patriarchal regimes, while queer theorists understate rape's destructive power in the individual lives of the women so victimized. Against the implications of these critiques, the now old-fashioned—but nevertheless still quite liberal—reliance, by liberals and liberal feminists, on consent as the demarcation of criminal and noncriminal sexual conduct looks, basically, right.

Consensual Sexual Harms

What doesn't look right, though, is what is too often inferred by that liberal reliance: that because consensual sex is and should be noncriminal, it is also, thereby, harmless and should be shielded from all forms of legal or even communal regulation likewise. As a moment's reflection should show, a transaction that is consensual, and with no third-party negative effects, doesn't imply that it is therefore harmless, or good for both parties, or in their interest, or good for the world, or just good, period. The consensual transaction with no third party effects might well be *pareto superior*, or efficient, or wealth maximizing (one can and normative legal economists often do typically define those terms in such a way as to make all of that tautologically true[28]), but that doesn't make it good or harmless in anything remotely resembling our ordinary usage of either word. At most, the consensuality of the transaction implies *only* that *if* the transaction is harmful or bad, it is so for reasons other than the harmful or bad consequences that flow from the exercise of coercion or force.

In nonsexual contexts, this is not so difficult for most of us to see. An exchange of labor for wages—or even a gift of that labor for nothing in return—if consensual, is not "slavery," so if it's harmful, it's harmful for reasons that are different from whatever it is that makes slavery bad. It doesn't follow from the fact that it's not slavery that it is therefore good. It might be a good deal or a bad one; it might be harmful, or harmless; if harmful, it might be trivially or profoundly so. That it is consensual doesn't tell us that it is harmless, or good, or beneficial. All we know from the fact that it is "consensual" is that *if* it is bad, it is bad for reasons other than coercion. It still might have been exploitative, alienating, or grossly unfair. The trade itself might be, for the laborer, only the next best thing to starvation—not good at all, and quite harmful indeed, but nevertheless better than the alternative. It might infect the laborer with cancer-causing asbestosis. It might be unsafe, endangering life and limb. It might be grueling and unpleasant and monotonous and alienating. The noise alone might be so loud and repetitive as to numb his brain and deafen him. It might be underpaid and sap too many hours, days, weeks, or years of a man's life. It might require tedious motion for long hours at low wages. It might also be harmful to the laborer in more subtle ways. It might, for example, have the effect of legitimating in the minds of the worker and the employer both a larger injustice, as numerous critical legal scholars have maintained—it might make both feel that the world, and their place within it, is a moral and good place, and thus squelch both the sympathetic and reformist instincts of the more powerful and the organizing instincts of the less powerful.[29] If any of this is true, then even if the transaction is consensual, the consensual labor contract might well do more harm than good, might undermine progress, and so on. If consensual, it doesn't enslave anyone. If consensual, it might indeed create wealth—we can define wealth in such a way that it does so by definition. But it isn't therefore good, and the world it leaves is not necessarily an improved one.

The same can be said of the sale of a thing for money. The consensual sale, for example, of a kidney for life-saving purposes, or of skin to a skin graft bank for cosmetic purposes, or of eggs to an infertile couple for reproductive purposes, if consensual, is not a theft. The seller or donor is not the victim of a theft, and the buyer or donee has not perpetrated one. It doesn't follow, though, that the sale of body parts is good for the parties or for the rest of us. Such sales—or gifts—might unduly alienate the seller from parts of his or her body that are and should remain so integral to personhood as to be inalienable. Alienating body parts for sale might constitute a serious injury to personal integrity. Likewise, the sale or purchase of a service—say, a medical procedure—may be consensual, but it clearly is not therefore good. Virtually every consensual surgery is by virtue of the consent therefore not a battery; it doesn't follow that it was medically indicated, that it was a wise decision, that it was well performed, that it wasn't profoundly injurious, or that it was what the patient needed. Plenty of consensual surgeries are negligently performed, some fatally so.

Surely the same is true, roughly, of sex: that a sexual transaction is consensual and with no third-party repercussions doesn't imply that it is harmless, or good for either party, or good for both of them, or good for the world. For various reasons, however, even the logical possibility of some of these harms is broadly denied, in law and in culture, and as I will argue in the next section, in queer and feminist legal theory likewise. But first, what are they? Consensual labor can be exploitative, consensual sales of that which should not be commodified might be alienating, and so on. What is the harm in consensual sex?

Let me begin my answer by highlighting an ambiguity, and hence a complexity, in the phrase "consensual sex," and then distinguishing between two very different sorts of harm that consensual sex, depending on how the ambiguity is resolved, might carry. The ambiguity is this: "Consensual sex" might be desired or wanted (whether or not ultimately enjoyed or pleasurable), or it might not be. Sometimes, maybe more often than not, maybe less often than not, women consent to sex that we want or desire, and entirely for its own sake. We consent to sex, in other words, because we actively desire the sex. Sometimes, though, we consent to sex that we don't want at all, and some women and girls, and some men and boys as well, might do that quite a bit.

Why would anyone do such a thing? Think first of married women. For years—centuries—married women have consented to sex that they do not want with their husbands either out of a sense of religious obligation, out of fear of their husbands' violence, or from their understanding of the requirements of their wifely role. Until well into the twentieth century, in this country alone, a married woman's consent was not required by law—forcible sex without consent between a man and his wife was not rape—and her pleasure and desire likewise were either irrelevant or their importance minimized by social norm. It was her *availability* that was expected of her, and that defined her sexual being, not her rapturous participation. This state of affairs obviously did not turn on a dime when married men lost the legal power of chastisement, in the nineteenth century, or when they lost the legal immunity to rape prosecutions with the abolition of marital rape exemptions in the last quarter of the twentieth; as a casual perusal of advice columns and women's magazines from the mid- to late twentieth century will show (or just ask your mother), married women continued to consent to unwanted marital sex out of a learned conviction that their lack of desire evidenced their own problematic and neurotic frigidity, an alienation from their own suppressed desires, or just a selfish unwillingness to get along. What lack of sexual desire within marriage did *not* constitute, for married women, was a good reason to resist the imposition of invasive, undesired penetration of their bodies by their husbands. Married, mid-twentieth-century women consented to undesired sex, in other words, well after they were formally and legally entitled to say "no," in part because a chorus of advice from well-meaning or not-so-well-meaning friends, family members, marriage counselors, advice columnists, and religious advisors urged them to do so.

What of unmarried women? Why might unmarried heterosexual women and girls consent to sex they don't want? Here's just a laundry list, speculative and anecdotal, of familiar enough reasons. Heterosexual women and girls, married or not, consent to a good bit of unwanted sex with men that they patently don't desire, from hook-ups to dates to boyfriends to cohabitators, to avoid a hassle or a foul mood the endurance of which wouldn't be worth the effort, to ensure their own or their children's financial security, to lessen the risk of future physical attacks, to garner their peers' approval, to win the approval of a high-status man or boy, to earn a paycheck or a promotion or an undeserved A on a college paper, to feed a drug habit, to survive, or to smooth troubled domestic waters. Women and girls do so from motives of self-aggrandizement, from an instinct for survival, out of concern for their children, from simple altruism, from friendship or love, or because they have been taught to do so. But whatever the reason, some women and girls have a good bit of sex a good bit of the time that they patently do not desire.

So, where's the harm in all of this? First, note a contrast: *Wanted* consensual sex carries with it risks of harms that are fairly well understood, and for various reasons often exaggerated, in our law, in our theory, and in our culture—we acknowledge them, we discuss them with our partners and with our children, we take precautions against them, and we worry a lot over whether or not to regulate against them. Lately, we regulate against them less and less, but we don't deny their existence. Fully desired consensual sex might be harmful for a good number of reasons. Wanted sex might lead to an unwanted pregnancy or to disease, and in either case it might be injurious or even life threatening. The pregnancy, if itself unwanted and carried to term, might curtail a girl's adolescence or young adulthood and lay the path for a difficult, quite possibly impoverished, limited, and pleasure-deprived midlife. If engaged in with an inappropriate partner, such as a high school or college teacher or work supervisor, wanted sex might result in her expulsion and his dismissal, in which case it might curtail a promising academic career or remunerative employment. Or, it might have negative long-term conse-quences not so readily tallied: Hot desired sex between a graduate student and professor might lock a girl into first an eroticized, but eventually a dreary domestic role. Rather than become a teacher, scholar, or employable adult citizen, that graduate student who was so taken by her teacher might instead become a lover, wife, and mother—which might be just great, or it might ultimately prove to be tedious, boring, unchallenging, and not hot at all. Sex between supervisors and workers or presidents and interns might be even-tually harmful over the long haul for similar reasons, even if fully desired by both parties. If consensual, all of this ultimately harmful sex is clearly not rape. If the sex is welcome, it is not sexual harassment either. It might nevertheless be harmful, though, even though it is neither rape nor harassment. It might be harmful even though it is consensual, legal, nontortious, nonharassing, and much desired by both parties.

Obviously, these harms might attach to unwanted sex likewise. Are there any distinctive harms, though, that attach to unwanted sex? Although it is hard to prove—and understudied—I believe that participation by many women and girls, in unwanted but consensual opposite-sex sex, particularly over time, carries with it harms that are different from those that attend to wanted consensual sex, are often serious, and are not only unregulated by law but also largely *unrecognized.* Consider a relationship extending over weeks, months, years, or decades—perhaps an entire adulthood—in which a girl or woman repeatedly engages in unwanted and unpleasing sex. That sex is, first, physically invasive. It may also be emotionally abusive; repetitive sex wanted by one party but undesired by the other, night after night for months, years, or an entire adulthood, carries with it the message that her subjective hedonic life—her pleasures, pains, and interests—are of no consequence. They don't figure into the equation of what to do. That is damaging to a person's self-sovereignty as well as one's sense of self-sovereignty: A woman who endures unpleasant invasive sex over time has implanted in her body, so to speak, the truth that her subjective pleasures and interests don't matter. Her will does (the sex is consensual), but her pleasures don't; they are not determinants of her body's actions. Rather, the subjective pleasures of another determine the use to which she puts her body.

Such sex is likely to be alienating, and in something like the original sense of that word: It alienates a girl or woman from her own desires and pleasures, and from that sense of unified identity that comes from acting in the world on the basis of one's own desires and pleasures. She internalizes, literally, the message that her body is for the pleasure of another rather than herself—a self-image that will not serve her well in an individualistic society that presupposes actors who choose on the basis of self-regarding preferences. Put in less political terms, she trivializes her self, her injuries, and her importance in the world when she accepts as an existential truth that her own pleasures and pains will not determine her choices or her actions. If the sex that results becomes a central, defining part of a way of life, the reason for her continued existence and for the material support of her partner becomes a threat to the largeness of her self and ambitions. And, if it becomes a central part of a life that ties her existence, survival, and hence her interests to that of another—if unwanted sex is the *raison d'etre* for a way of life that limits her mobility, her ambition, and the development of her talents or remunerative skills—it constitutes a threat to her autonomy, likewise.

Of course, unwanted consensual sex is not *always* harmful in any of these ways. Obviously, we consent to do things we don't really want to do for all sorts of benign reasons. I see movies I don't want to see to please my children's or husband's tastes, rather than my own, to say nothing of the social events, household chores, and so on that I not so cheerfully tolerate. Likewise with sex: Women and men both might consent to undesired sex on occasion—even on many occasions—for benign or harmless reasons. A woman might, on occasion, rather watch television, read, or sleep but agree to sex she doesn't particularly desire, because she loves her partner, because she's accustomed to trade-offs of this sort that benefit both, because she doesn't feel it as a burden, because she knows that her lack of desire may give way to desire, and so on. But that some undesired sex is harmless hardly means that it all is.

Is there a way to capture, descriptively, the subclass of unwanted consensual sex that is harmful from that which is not? I'm not sure, but a (highly contested) concept borrowed from the law regulating sexual harassment on the job and in schools may help. Unwanted sex or sexual advances at work or school are actionable harassment if they are not only unwanted, as I've used the term above, but also *unwelcome*.[30] It is not simply *all* sex, welcome or not, that occurs between persons differently situated on various hierarchies—presidents and interns, CEOs and secretaries, professors and students, generals and privates—that is actionable sexual harassment (although many people mistakenly believe it to be). Such sex between unequals at work or school, *if welcome*, may or may not violate a firm's or a school's antifraternization polities, but it is not sexual harassment simply by virtue of the existence of a hierarchic relation. Rather, to constitute sexual harassment, the sex or the sexual advance must be unwelcome. The "unwelcomeness" requirement in law has proven difficult and vague, and has elicited quite a bit of criticism.[31] Nevertheless, it is unwelcome sex, sexual advances, or sexual innuendo at work or school—not sex within hierarchy—that is the gravamen of a sexual harassment complaint.

My suggestion is that something like the "unwelcomeness" requirement borrowed from sex harassment law might also help us to see when unwanted sex might be harmful and when not, apart from work or school. When we consent to undesired or unwanted sex that is nevertheless *welcome*, we typically don't suffer the harms attendant to unwanted consensual sex (we might, of course, suffer the harms that attend to all consensual sex—disease, unwanted pregnancy, and so on). When we consent to unwanted sex for friendship, for love, as a favor, to cement trust, or to express gratitude, none of this is necessarily harmful. Unwanted sex to which we consent for these reasons might also be, and I suspect often is, welcome—we don't want it, but we welcome it anyway, as a part of a relationship that is in its whole constructive, healthy, and pleasing. But when undesired consensual sex is also unwelcome, it is likely to carry the harms to self-sovereignty spelled out previously, and it is those harms which, I believe, are seriously underreckoned by liberal valorizations of consensuality. We don't tend to notice them, we don't dwell on them, we certainly don't use law's regulatory apparatus so as to deter or compensate for them, we don't (much) make movies or write novels about them, and we don't warn our young sons and daughters against them. We also don't theorize much about them, even in those radical traditions where we might expect to. Unlike the role of the exploitative but consensual sale of labor or the alienating but consensual sale of body parts in various strands of neo-Marxism, the unwanted but consensual sexual transaction plays a *de minimus* role in radical feminism and virtually no role in liberal feminism, and its coherence as well as its importance is quite aggressively denied in queer theory. Culturally, theoretically, and critically, we don't much worry about all of this one way or the other.

Invisible Harms

The harms occasioned by wanted and welcome consensual sex are by no means invisible to either law or culture. Quite the contrary. Until relatively recently they have long been the subject of intense legal regulation: Unintended pregnancies outside of marriage, the degradation of family relations that might attend adulterous sex, the various real or imagined harms attendant to underage sex, the damage to reputation and the institution of marriage that might be done by sex for pay, and, of course, the moral corruption attendant to all forms of sexual deviance have all been targeted by laws regulating and to some degree criminalizing fornication, adultery, abortion, contraception, prostitution, teenage sex, illegitimacy, and sodomy. Much—most—of this regulation is fading fast: Some of it has been struck as unconstitutional. We are now aware not only of the risks attendant to wanted or welcome sex but also of the risks attendant to regulating in such a fashion as to minimize them. Nevertheless, even as we forego legal regulation as a way to combat them, we are more than aware of their existence. We weigh them in our own minds, we write novels and make movies about them, we study them endlessly, we rehearse them with our teenage children, and we create school curricula intended to drive the message home. Consensual, wanted, welcome sex, we all know, and we teach our children, comes with risks of quite serious harms, whether they are regulated by law or not—of disease, unintended pregnancies, unwanted abortions and unplanned births, poverty, domestic misery, stunted or altogether missed childhoods, and interrupted career paths. Pleasure has its traps, the familiar message goes, so watch out.

By contrast, and with the important exception of some of the harms attendant to unwelcome sex in the workplace and at school,[32] the harms of *unwelcome* consensual sex outlined previously are almost entirely invisible to law, and for the most part, always have been. We don't regulate against them, we don't attempt to deter them, and we don't compensate for them when they occur. This is not likely to change: The Supreme Court's groundbreaking decision in *Lawrence v Texas* striking antisodomy laws seemingly holds that virtually all consensual sex is now not only presumptively legal but also constitutionally *protected* against regulation—as Justice Scalia, perhaps a bit too bitterly, but correctly, complained.[33] There's no reason not to think that the constitutional protection now accorded the full-fledged right to consensual sex by *Lawrence* wouldn't include the unwelcome as well as the welcome kind, same-sex or otherwise. Now of course, law isn't the whole story, here or elsewhere. With the sexual liberation and women's liberation movements of the 1960s and 1970s (and with the dismantling of marital rape exemptions), social expectations regarding unwelcome sex have shifted somewhat: Many women are now more likely to regard themselves and their sexual desires as of equal importance and their sovereignty over their bodies as something not to be foreworn lightly in the absence of desire. Nevertheless, the cultural expectation that wives will submit to husbands' sexual advances and that girls and women outside of marriage will likewise comply to some unknown degree remains in place for large swaths of the population. Law has done nothing to interrupt this expectation. These harms simply have no legal salience. Law's authorities—whatever might be true of cultural authority—are silent with respect to them.

Why, though, have our critical scholarly movements—liberal, feminist, and queer, movements that do not, as a rule, make a habit of embracing the logic of Supreme Court decisions—*also* been silent with respect to these legitimated harms? With respect to liberal legalism, I think the reasons are transparent. As noted at the outset, liberal-legalists, albeit for different reasons, tend to confer consensual transactions across the board—economic, political, sexual—with presumptive value that largely overshadows, if not negates, the possibility that those transactions might also create harm. Liberal aversion to moralistic legislation that interferes with sexual choice is indeed considerably more intense, and sweeping, than liberal aversion to legislation that interferes with economic choice. But this, too, is not hard to explain. The closeted, privatized, indeed sequestered invisibility of these harms—in women's bodies, inside homes, and inside intimate relationships—in spaces where privacy is revered plays a heavy and explicit role, as does a host of cultural factors, not so explicitly acknowledged: the continuing effect of religious traditions that count female asceticism and sacrifice in all things sexual as both a virtue and a duty, the overhang of a fairly brutal family law history that negated or minimized even severe manifestations of these harms, and, we might surmise, a healthy dollop of men's sexual self-interest. If we put all this together—the liberal regard for individual choice, the presumptive nexus between consent and value central to economic forms of liberal legalism, the hard-fought-for constitutional and liberal regard for familial and sexual privacy that now surrounds both abortion decisions and same-sex sexual activity, a general hostility to paternalistic and morals legislation, and a host of cultural factors to boot—the liberal-legalist blindness to the harms of unwanted sex is not so surprising. If anything, it's overdetermined.

The story is much more complicated, I think, with respect to radical legal scholarship, and particularly both radical feminism and queer theory. I'll start with feminism. Radical feminism is hardly wedded to an excessively rosy-eyed view of consensual sex, but nevertheless, it too has failed to attend to the distinctive harms of unwelcome consensual sex outside of the school or workplace. I think there are two reasons. The first is quasi-logical and suggested by the previous discussion: Radical feminism has been committed for some time now to an extraordinarily broad view of coercion, by which whatever is demonstrably bad for women that seemingly follows from consensual choices women make within conditions of inequality is viewed as necessarily coercive. Therefore, for radical feminists, the category of "consensual harms" is vaguely oxymoronic. If something is harmful, it must be the result of inequality, and if unequal, then coercive, and if coercive, then not consensual. The category of "consensual harms" disappears.

There is, though, a second and I think deeper reason for the invisibility of these harms in radical feminist scholarship and writing, which goes not to their skepticism regarding the viability of consent in conditions of inequality, but rather to skepticism regarding the distinction between welcome and unwelcome sex. Central to radical feminism for at least the last 30 years has been what is now called a "critique of desire": Sexual desires across the board, according to radical feminist critique, are as socially constructed as anything could ever be.[34] Women's sexual desires, furthermore, are particularly suspect: They are politically and socially constructed by pernicious and patriarchal forces and are then aimed, like a weapon, against women's interests, autonomy, dignity, and equality.[35] As a consequence, women often desire sex that is on its face debasing, humiliating, and submissive, and, whether known to the woman who harbors the desire or not, the sex so desired is injurious, unequal, and subordinating. This was—and is—an audacious claim, and its stark clarity in many ways accounts for the strength and staying power of the feminist movement it in part defined. The willingness to hold on to it in the wake of the total uproar it elicited from all corners, when it first hit the public scene in the 1980s, is a lasting testament to the tenacity of those, but primarily Catherine MacKinnon, who held it.

Nevertheless, it might have been a misguided claim, and if it was, one consequence is that its target—women's actual sexual desires, particularly for submissive or sadomasochistic sex—might have been ill-chosen. I've argued elsewhere that it was, that these desires are largely inconsequential and harmless. What I want to suggest here is that it also had an unfortunate and generally unnoticed implication: The radical feminist claim that women's felt sexual desires are harmful to women's interests and equality overshadows—and in many ways undercuts—the claim (made here) that *undesired* sex might sometimes cause harms, precisely because it is undesired. The former claim, after all, rests on a thoroughgoing skepticism regarding the normative significance of desire—if you desire something, nothing whatsoever follows about whether or not what you desire might be good for you—while the latter rests on an affirmation of desire, and a worry about the choices made against it. The problem with which feminism must centrally reckon, according to radical feminist argumentation, is *not* what is suggested here—that women often consent to sex that they do not welcome, and that when they do so the sex is sometimes injurious, precisely because it is unwelcome. Rather, the problem is the desires women have, and with the sex women actually welcome—not that they have sex they don't want. The deepest harm, so to speak, occasioned by patriarchy upon women's psyches, according to radical feminism, is the contorted nature of female desire, not that we consent to sex against the counsel of our desire. The problem, in short, is our desires, not our choices. The relative invisibility of the harms done by unwelcome sex, then, is one cost extracted by the theoretical insistence on the harmfulness of the objects of our felt desires.

And lastly, queer theory. Queer theorists likewise fail to see any harm in unwanted sex, and for a simple reason: They deny the existence of the category, or more precisely, they tend to regard it as a null set. As with purportedly nonconsensual sex, purportedly unwanted sex is (often, or usually) not really unwanted at all; the claim that sex is unwanted is the result of a "sex panic," undue repression, or displaced shame. Therefore, claims of unwelcome sex, in sexual harassment actions, for example, should be viewed skeptically.[36] Sex is awfully desirable, apparently, even when it's not desired: The claim that it isn't desired is what should be viewed critically, not the sex itself. Whether or not sex is welcome can't be read off of objective facts about the sex itself: Welcome sex can be painful, humiliating, shameful, and of course transgressive. But nor can it be read off of victims' protestations: Victims just protest too much, as we used to say. The result is a highly circumscribed (if that) law of sexual harassment—and no room at all for a critique of sex that proceeds in the absence of desire, and of course no reason to abstain from sex on the basis of its lack.

Here again the unnoted parallelism, and not just the much noted contrast, with radical feminism is telling. Radical feminist and queer theoretic understandings of unwanted sex differ in almost all particulars, but they converge on this point: They both fail to lend normative significance to felt desires. Neither desire, for feminists, nor its lack, for queer theorists, is a trustworthy guide to the interests, the well-being, or simply the subjective pleasures and pains of the person who does or doesn't hold it. For both, desire is not a meaningful distinction within the larger category of consensual sex, just as consent itself is not a meaningful distinction within the larger category of sex. Thus, radical feminists are skeptical of the authenticity of women's sexual desires, and particularly of nonvanilla sexual desires, the content of which seemingly runs contrary to objective interest and substantive equality. That women have a desire for it has no normative significance: There is no harm in frustrating women's desires, and plenty of good reason to do so. Again, the problem with which feminism must contend is that women have desires that are contrary to their interest in equality, not that they choose to engage in sex they don't desire. Queer theorists, on the other hand, are skeptical of the authenticity of heterosexual women's felt or expressed *lack* of desire: A felt or proclaimed lack of desire that runs contrary to the transgressive pleasure to be had from sexual power is most likely inauthentic. The specific harm, then, that might follow from consenting to sex one does not desire or does not welcome just fails to register.

So, note the common ground: Radical feminists critique desire, while queer theorists critique its lack—but both camps build political perspectives on the basis of their devaluation of the veracity and coherence of desire, and I would say more broadly of women's (and some men's) subjective experience. That skepticism, on both sides, carries with it pernicious consequences. Most obviously, but perhaps least consequentially, the radical feminist critique of desire targets sexual desires—particularly desires for sadomasochistic sex—that are largely harmless and politically meaningless. Second, though, and I think more important, the feminist critique of desire leads to a deeply regrettable blindness to a particular form of harm, of which radical feminists in particular ought to be acutely aware—harm caused by women's consent to sex that is in point of subjective fact unwelcome and contrary to what they desire. It may be that some of our sexual desires are inauthentic in the way argued by radical feminists, and that, when acted upon, they are harmful to us. I don't mean to deny that; I just don't know. But whether our desires are inauthentic or not, many women, very often, choose to participate in consensual sex that they quite strongly do not welcome or desire. We ought to be concerned that the choice to do so might itself be harmful precisely because it is so alienating—precisely because it is contrary to desire. We can't even consider the possibility if we are mightily distracted by the claim that it is the desires themselves that are suspect.

Queer theorists, in what can charitably be described as an overcorrection, have put forward what we could call, following Gowdri Ramadachian's helpful suggestion,[37] a "critique of the lack of desire": When women (or men) claim not to want or welcome sex, we should be skeptical, particularly where those claims in turn are the motivators of claims of rape or sexual harassment. Sexual desire, by the teachings of queer theory, is what is ubiquitous: The claim that one does not feel it is just not believable. We have had too long a history, in this country and virtually all others, of rampant and often vicious denials of sexual desire to simply accept such protestations. This skepticism of course is not pulled from thin air: Indeed there are false rape claims, as there are false claims of all sorts. But not much of interest follows from that. There's no evidence that those false claims result from ambiguously felt *desire,* or that the legal system does a worse job here than elsewhere of ferreting them out. When women express a lack of desire for sex, there's no good reason to assume that expression is a panicked response to repressed sexual desire. If the sex is imposed anyway, in the face of her lack of consent, it's a rape, and if provable, ought to be prosecuted as such. If she consents in the absence of desire, she may have done so for good reason or ill—the unwanted sex might be welcome or not. If it's welcome, more power to both of them. If not, we should treat that as the canary in the mine it surely is. If unwelcome sex is a constant in a woman's life, for weeks, months, years, and decades, it is likely to be alienating and oppressive—in a word, injurious. We might decide for all sorts of reasons that we cannot imagine a legal response to such a private injury. It doesn't follow, though, that we should deny or ignore it.

Conclusion

Liberal, feminist, and queer theoretic arguments for failing to attend to the harms of consensual but unwelcome sex are unconvincing. Liberals have been rightly faulted for half a century now for casting a veneer of legitimacy around consensual states of affairs in nonsexual spheres of life, both political and economic. The consent of the governed can be produced by pernicious forces and with disastrous consequences; the consent of buyers of goods or sellers of labor can likewise. Consensual transactions can unduly commodify that which should not be bought and sold, and can worsen rather than enrich our relations with ourselves, each other, and the natural planet we inhabit. Surely, the same is true in our sexual lives: The sex to which we consent, when it is contrary to our desires and when within the context of relationships that are less than welcome in our lives, can alienate us from our bodies, our subjective pains and pleasures, our needs, our interests, our true preferences, our histories, and our futures. Unwelcome sex can carry all of these harms, yet be fully consensual. We don't see this if we mistakenly accept "consent" as a reliable marker for well-being. Consent may well be a good marker for the divide between the criminal and noncriminal in sex as elsewhere; I believe it is. It's not a good proxy for well-being. We should not treat it as such.

Feminism and queer theory both, no less than liberalism, have also overrelied on proxies for well-being—but different proxies. For radical feminists, the proxy is the power imbalance. Power imbalances poison all transactions that occur within them—desired and undesired both—so the distinctiveness of harms caused by undesired consensual transactions gets subsumed within a larger problem: desires that run contrary to interest. Thus, both desired and undesired consensual sex (as well as consensual and nonconsensual sex) is damned by the imbalance that underscores it all. Inequality becomes the proxy for harm. For queer theorists, power, and particularly sexual power, is the proxy for pleasure and value both. The consequence is a pervasive skepticism regarding the veracity and even the coherence of claims of sexual aggression of all sorts. The result is a complacency at best and complicity at worst, with a good deal of sexual violence and oppression both.

We could reverse this tide in one fell swoop by simply honoring the authenticity of women's felt desires, and their lack. And, we could do so while consistently maintaining an openly critical stance toward the possibility that the sexual choices women make, when those choices are contrary to felt desires, are harmful. Thus, when consensual sex is fully desired, there's not much reason to question the authenticity of the desire or the value to its participants, no matter how nonvanilla the flavor. We could, and I think should, abandon the "critique of desire" without losing any of the quite real strengths of radical feminism. On the other hand, when conditions prompt women to consent to sex that they do not desire, there is no reason not to name and contend with the harms to integrity and self-sovereignty to which those choices, and that consensual sex, might lead. We don't need to construct fanciful explanations for that lack. We could drop the critique of the "lack of desire" without losing what might be an important insight at the heart of so much queer theory: that power imbalances in sexual acts are exciting, pleasurable, and largely benign. We should drop, in sum, both the critique of desire developed by the radical feminism of the 1980s and the critique of its lack developed by queer theory of the last decade. If we do so—and maybe only if we do so—we might then bring into focus what is otherwise thoroughly obscured by both, and that is the harms occasioned by the unwelcome sex to which women consent, in the absence of any desire of their own. We should at least open an inquiry into the value of the unwanted sex to which we consent, as well as the harms occasioned by the rapes to which we decidedly don't.

Notes

1. See, e.g., Stephen Shulholfer, *Unwanted Sex: The Culture of Intimidation and the Failure of Law* (Cambridge, MA: Harvard University Press, 1998); Susan Estridge, *Real Rape* (Cambridge, MA: Harvard University Press, 1987); Donald Dripps, "Beyond Rape: An Essay on the Difference Between the Presence of Force and the Absence of Consent," *Columbia Law Review* 92 (1992): 1780–1806; Michelle Anderson, "Negotiating Sex," *Southern California Law Review* 78 (2005): 1401–38; "What Is Rape?" *St. John's Law Review* 79 (2005): 625–44; "Marital Immunity, Intimate Relationships, and Improper Inferences: A New Law on Sexual Offenses by Intimates," *Hastings Law Journal* 54 (2003): 1464–1557.

   The liberal claim that consent should define the boundary between sex that is a crime (either rape or something less serious) and sex that is not remains a reform proposal. It still does not accurately reflect virtually any state's law, although it is widely and correctly understood as the sensible endpoint of the overall direction of the changes that have occurred in rape law over the last couple of centuries. It has also attracted a substantial body of internal friendly critical attention from legal reformers, legal scholars, and moral and legal philosophers, much of which is concerned with boundary issues: is sex consensual when it is the product of various sorts of promises, threats, or misrepresentations; is it consensual if induced by fear not of imminent bodily harm but eventual bodily harm; how much duress is required to render consent only apparent rather than real; should nonconsensual sex with unconscious or for some other reason incapacitated victims be criminalized to the same degree, if there is no evidence of physical injury; and so on. These issues are all important, and as Alan Wertheimer correctly notes, their resolution requires real-world deliberation and moral reasoning, and not simply elaboration of various possible definitions of consent. Alan Wertheimer, "Consent and Sexual Relations," in *The Philosophy of Sex*, ed. Alan Soble (Lanham, MD: Rowman and Littlefield; 2002). They can also, I believe, be resolved consistently with an insistence on lack of consent as the primary marker of criminal sexual behavior. They are not, however, the focus of this paper.

2. John Stuart Mill, *The Subjection of Women*, ed. Sue Mansfield, (Arlington Heights, IL: AHM Publishing, 1980). For an excellent history of feminist

political reform movements on issues pertaining to sexual violence within marriage during the Victorian era, see Mary Shanley, *Feminism, Marriage, and the Law in Victorian England, 1850–1895* (Princeton, NJ: Princeton University Press, 1989).

3. See Shulhofer, note *supra*, Anderson, note *supra*, Estridge, note *supra*.

4. See Nadine Strossman, *Defending Pornography: Free Speech, Sex, and the Fight for Women's Rights* (New York: NYU Press, 2000); see also Nan D. Hunter and Sylvia Law, "Brief Amici Curiae of Feminist Anti-Censorship Task Force, et al. in American Booksellers Association v. Hudnut," *University Michigan Journal of Law Reform* 21 (1987–88): 69–136.

5. See Barry Lynn, "Civil Rights' Ordinances and the Attorney General's Commission: New Developments in Pornography Regulation," *Harvard Civil Rights-Civil Liberties Law Review* 21 (1986) 27–125.

6. See Igor Primoratz, "What's Wrong With Prostitution," in *The Philosophy of Sex* (New York: Rowman and Littlefield, 2002), 451–73; Lars Ericsson, "Charges Against Prostitution: An Attempt at a Philosophical Assessment," *Ethics* 90 (1980): 335–66.

7. See David A. Richards, *Women, Gays and the Constitution: The Grounds for Feminism and Gay Rights in Culture and Law* (Chicago: University of Chicago Press, 1998).

8. For a discussion and critique of these liberal arguments for same-sex marriage and against sodomy laws, see generally Chai R. Feldblum, "Gay Is Good: The Moral Case for Marriage Equality and More," *Yale Journal of Law & Feminism* 17 (2005): 139–84.

9. For a history see David Garrow, *Liberty and Sexuality: The Right to Privacy and the Making of Roe v. Wade* (New York: Macmillan, 1994; updated paperback edition, Berekeley: University of California Press, 1998).

10. See Eugene Volokh, "How Harassment Law Restricts Free Speech," *Rutgers Law Journal* 47 (1995): 561; "Freedom of Speech and Workplace Harassment," *UCLA Law Review* 39 (1992): 1791–1872; "Workplace Harassment and the First Amendment, I," *Encyclopedia of the U.S. Constitution*, ed. Leonard Levy and Kenneth Karst (New York: Macmillan Reference, 2000), 2925.

11. See, e.g., Randy Barnett, "Justice Kennedy's Libertarian Revolution: *Lawrence v. Texas*," *Cato Supreme Court Review* 2002–2003 (2003): 21–41; Barnett and Douglas Rasmussen, "The Right to Liberty in a Good Society" in "Symposium on the Constitution and the Good Society," *Fordham Law Review* 69 (2001): 1603–15.

12. See generally, Tom Grey, "Eros, Civilization, and the Burger Court," *Law and Contemporary Problems* 43:3 (1980): 83–100; Jed Rubenfeld, "The Right of Privacy," *Harvard Law Review*, 102 (1989): 737–807.

13. Richard Posner, *Sex and Reason* (Cambridge, MA: Harvard University Press, 1992), 388; and Posner, *Economics of Justice* (Cambridge, MA: Harvard University Press, 1981), 60–61.

14. Strossman, note *supra*; see also Carole S. Vance, ed., *Pleasure and Danger: Exploring Female Sexuality* (1st ed., Boston and London: Routledge & Kegan Paul, 1984), (2nd ed., with new introduction, London: Pandora, 1992, 1994).

15. See, e.g., Catherine MacKinnon, *Feminism Unmodified* (Cambridge, MA: Harvard University Press, 1987), 81–93; MacKinnon, *Toward a Feminist Theory of the State* (Cambridge, MA: Harvard University Press, 1989), 146, 174; Robin Morgan, *Going Too Far: The Personal Chronicle of a Feminist* (New York: Random House, 1977), 165–66 ("rape exists any time sexual intercourse occurs when it has not been initiated by the woman, out of her own genuine affection and desire.... How many millions of times have women had sex 'willingly' with men they didn't want to have sex with?... How many times have women wished just to sleep instead or read or watch the Late Show?... Most of the decently married bedrooms across America are settings for nightly rape"). See generally Carole Pateman, "Sex and Power" [Review of *Feminism Unmodified* by Catharine A. MacKinnon], *Ethics* 100:2 (1990): 398–407, and "Women and Consent," *Political Theory* 8:2 (1980): 149–68. Reprinted in *The Disorder of Women: Democracy, Feminism, and Political Theory* (Cambridge: Cambridge University Press, 1989), 71–89.

16. MacKinnon, *Toward a Feminist Theory*, 1.

17. See, e.g., Kathy Abrams, "Sex Wars Redux: Agency and Coercion in Feminist Legal Theory," *Columbia Law Review* 95 (1995): 304–76.

18. See Robin West, "Law's Nobility," *Yale Journal of Law and Feminism* 17 (2005): 385–458.

19. Adrienne Rich, *Compulsory Heterosexuality and Lesbian Existence, in Blood, Bread and Poetry* (New York: W.W. Norton, 1986).

20. See Catharine A. MacKinnon, "Pornography Left and Right," *Harvard Civil Rights-Civil Liberties Law Review* 30 (1995): 143–68 at 143–47.

21. See, e.g., MacKinnon, *Feminism Unmodified*, 54 (arguing that it is difficult to sustain the customary distinctions between sex and rape); MacKinnon, *Toward a Feminist Theory*, 146.

22. MacKinnon, *Toward a Feminist Theory*, at 1.

23. Janet Halley, "Sexuality Harassment," in *Directions in Sexual Harassment Law*, ed. Catharine MacKinnon and Reva Siegel (New Haven, CT: Yale University Press, 2003), 182, 193–98. See also Janet Halley (writing under the name Ian Halley), "Queer Theory by Men," *Duke Journal of Gender Law and Policy* 11 (2004): 7–52; Halley, "The Politics of Injury: A Review of Robin West's Caring for Justice," *Unbound* 1 (2005): 65–92.

24. Michel Foucault, *Politics, Philosophy, Culture, Interviews and Other Writings, 1977–84,* ed. Lawrence D. Kritzman (New York: Routledge, 1988), 204–05.

25. David Kennedy, "The Spectacle and the Libertine," in *Aftermath: The Clinton Impeachment and the Presidency in the Age of Political Spectacle,* ed. Leonard V. Kaplan and Beverly I. Moran (New York: NYU Press, 2001), 279, 289.

26. I have addressed these problems and others with queer theory elsewhere. See Robin West, "Desperately Seeking a Moralist," *Harvard Journal of Law & Gender* 29 (2006): 1–50. For a recent and related critique of queer theory on the grounds that it embraces a sexualist ideology that privileges the valorization of sex over life itself, and the tragic repercussions of that ideology during the AIDS crisis of the 1980s, see Marc Spindelman, *Sexuality's Law,* Columbia J. of Law and Gender (forthcoming 2009).

27. *Id.* at 37–38; Bersani, "Is the Rectum a Grave," *AIDS: Cultural Analysis/Cultural Activism,* 43 (Winter, 1987): 197–222 at 213–15.

28. Posner, *Economics of Justice,* 60–61.

29. See the essays collected in *The Politics of Law: A Progressive Critique,* ed. David Kairys (New York: Basic Books, 1998); Roberto Unger's classic essay, "The Critical Legal Studies Movement," *Harvard Law Review* 96 (1983): 561; and Robert Gordon, "Unfreezing Legal Reality: Critical Approaches to Law," *Florida State University Law Review* 15 (1987): 195–220 for strong examples of this critical point.

30. *Meritor Savings Bank v. Vinson,* 477 U.S. 57 (1986).

31. See Louise Fitzgerald, "Who Says? Legal and Psychological Constructions of Women's Resistance to Sexual Harassment," and Kathryn Abrams, "Subordination and Agency in Sexual Harassment Law," and Jane Larson, "Sexual Labor," in *New Directions in Sexual Harassment Law,* 94–137.

32. See generally, Catherine MacKinnon, *The Sexual Harassment of Working Women* (New Haven, CT: Yale University Press, 1979); *Meritor Savings Bank v. Vinson,* 477 U.S. 57 (1986).

33. For a related critique of *Lawrence,* see Marc Spindelman, "Surviving Lawrence v. Texas," *Michigan Law Review* 102 (2004): 1615–67.

34. MacKinnon, *Feminism Unmodified,* 54; *Toward a Feminist Theory,* at 129–31.

35. *Id.*

36. Halley, "Sexuality Harassment," 197.

37. In conversation in a workshop at Georgetown Law Center.

10

Contracts

Brian H. Bix[1]

Introduction

As many commentators have pointed out,[2] consent, in terms of voluntary
choice, is—or at least appears to be or purports to be—at the essence of
contract law.[3] Contract law, both in principle and in practice, is about allowing
parties to enter arrangements on terms they choose, each party imposing
obligations on itself in return for obligations another party has placed upon
itself. This "freedom of contract"—an ideal by which there are obligations to
the extent, but only to the extent, freely chosen by the parties—is contrasted
with the duties of criminal law and tort law, which bind all parties regardless of
consent. We do not individually choose the legal obligations we have not to
murder and not to defraud, but we have an obligation to pay Acme Painting
$400 to paint our fence if and only if we choose to take on that duty.[4]

At the same time, one might argue that consent, in the robust sense
expressed by the ideal of "freedom of contract," is absent in the vast majority
of the contracts we enter into these days, but its absence does little to affect the
enforceability of those contracts. (Consent to contractual terms in this way
often looks like consent to government: present, if at all, only under a
fictional—"as if"—or attenuated rubric.) By an absence of consent in the
robust sense, I mean that parties to contracts are often unaware of the terms
of their agreements (including the default terms and remedial terms not
expressly stated in the transaction documents or verbal exchanges, but provided
by state and federal law), and even where aware of the terms, may not fully

understand their significance. Additionally, there is a relative lack of consent in the sense that there may be no reasonable alternatives to entering the transactions in question. (And during the rare circumstances when the parties are aware of terms, and understand them, there are issues relating to consent that arise from cognitive biases and other forms of bounded rationality.)

Even those who recognize the significant shortfall in consent in contractual relations disagree about how to respond to it. If one concludes that a contract was entered into with insufficient consent on one side (or on both sides), or if one reaches that conclusion as regards individual terms within the contract,[5] what is the recourse? One option is to refuse to enforce the agreement in total or, if possible, to refuse enforcement only to the offending provisions. Alternatively, the court might rewrite an offending term to one it considers fairer to both parties. However, as Richard Craswell points out, courts rewriting terms cannot solve the problem of unconsented-to terms: At best, they can substitute a court-imposed (and, one hopes, fair) term for a party-imposed (and frequently one-sided) term.[6]

In any event (and as will be discussed later), there are obvious benefits to enforcing at least a significant portion of the agreements that parties enter into with less than complete consent. There is too much at stake—to those seeking to enter agreements as well as to third parties—to set the bar too high too often on contractual consent. Among other problems, making too many commercial transactions subject to serious challenge on consent/voluntariness grounds would undermine the predictability of enforcement that is needed for vibrant economic activity.

This chapter will explore many of the issues relating to consent in contract law (while necessarily falling far short of any sort of comprehensive guide).[7] Part I offers an overview of the nature of consent, before considering in general terms the elements of consent in contract law. Part II reviews the way that questions of consent are dealt with in Anglo-American contract law doctrine. Part III considers how recent principles and practices have raised new consent-related problems, and what the response has been from legislatures and courts. Finally, Part IV samples theories of contract law that focus on consent, before concluding.

I. Consent

A. Nature of Consent

It is sometimes argued that consent[8] can be understood either at an internal or subjective level (state of mind, preferences, volition) or at an external or objective level (performatives),[9] or some combination of the two. While contract law discussions may sometimes point to the internal aspects of consent, the actual doctrinal tests focus on externals: what was said, written, and signed. This is just a specific instance of a more general focus on external criteria, and objective tests, within contract law.[10]

As others have noted,[11] if one treats the presence or absence of consent as an empirical matter, there remain normative questions in moral and legal inquiries to determine the effect of the consent in question. Though consent is itself a morally loaded term (we are more likely to "find consent" in situations where we believe that a promise *is* morally binding or that the transaction *should* be enforced), it is always open for a commentator (or judge) to conclude that even though there *was no* consent (or no consent in the fullest sense), the transaction *should be* enforced, or that even though there *was* consent, the transaction *should not* be enforced.[12] At the least, there are questions of proof and trust on one hand,[13] and issues of third-party effects on the other,[14] that may lead us to enforcement decisions that go the opposite way of our most considered judgment regarding the presence of consent. Equally important, the term "consent" can be used for a wide range of attitudes, actions, and circumstances, and the level or kind of consent that might be sufficient to ground enforcement in one type of situation may not be sufficient in another.[15]

This gap between the assertion that there had (not) been consent and the conclusion that the agreement should (not) be binding is often hidden by use of terms like "*full* consent" or "*valid* consent," which indicate, at the least, that there are different types or different extents of consent or, alternatively, that consent needs to be combined with other factors for it to transform the moral or legal effects of some action.

B. Elements of Consent in Contract Literature

It is commonplace, going back at least to Aristotle, to think of consent (or "voluntariness," a sister concept) as a function of some combination of understanding and freedom from coercion.[16] In the contract context, this is often rephrased in terms of "knowledge" and "reasonable alternatives," and these will be considered in turn.

1. Knowledge

One cannot consent to terms, in any robust sense of consent, without knowledge of the terms. Of course, there are different levels of knowledge (or, looking from the other direction, there are different levels of ignorance) possible. In contracting, one may be ignorant that there are terms that apply (or even ignorant that one has entered a contractual relationship). This may be common in the downloading of computer software (a topic discussed further later). One can be aware in principle that there are terms but be ignorant of the existence or content of some or most of the ones that apply to the transaction in question.[17] This occurs frequently with long, standardized forms, not least when these forms are provided some time after the purchase. And one can know of specific terms but be ignorant of (or misread) the meaning of the terms (understandable, when documents are full of legal or business jargon).

Contracting parties' ignorance of terms has been a prominent issue in discussions on electronic contracting and, in prior generations, other forms of "contracts of adhesion."[18] Even sophisticated parties often choose not to read all the fine print, as it is more reasonable to use the time and efforts on other tasks, and it is likely that the tendency to "skip the terms" is even more pronounced in Internet commerce.[19] One could see these decisions not to read both as a background fact that may justify greater regulation of terms or as a factor pointing the other way—that the choice not to read is itself an aspect of autonomous choosing that should be respected as part of a general inclination to let parties shape their own (commercial) interactions.

2. Reasonable Alternatives

A standard element in analyses of contractual consent—seen in doctrinal discussions of both unconscionability and duress (both discussed below)—is the question of what alternatives the party had entering the contract. Reference to alternatives can point to choice in at least three different directions. First, how free was the party not to enter this contract (or a similar contract with another party) at all? That is, what would have been the cost of not contracting? Second, was a comparable agreement available with this contracting partner, or a suitable alternative party, with different terms? That is, were there choices relating to particular terms? Third, even if the party had little choice but to contract, and with this partner, was there a reasonable chance to negotiate alternative terms to the one offered?

One can lack choice regarding a term if there is only one (monopoly) party with which one can deal on this matter (as may be the case with certain utilities or other services).[20] Equally common, one can lack choice regarding a term if one had a choice of contracting parties, but all use the same term (and are not willing or not allowed legally to negotiate changes in that term).[21] This happens with insurance policies—sometimes when state legislatures or insurance agencies dictate terms—and also with many commercial providers (as when all providers of a given good disclaim warranties and consequential damages, or when all employers in a field impose mandatory arbitration of employment disputes).

3. Other Factors

In considering the extent of a party's consent to a proposal (or, if one prefers a different terminology, the extent to which the choice was [fully] voluntary), one might consider a variety of factors beyond those (knowledge and existence of reasonable alternatives) already considered.[22] For example, (1) is the other party threatening to harm the proposal recipient (make the situation worse relative to the status quo) if the recipient does not accept the proposal, or will the recipient be left at its original status quo? and (2) would accepting the proposal be rational in terms of the recipient's stable, long-term preferences? (we will return to the question of bounded rationality below).[23]

The first factor pointed toward lack of consent, relating to threats that involve a change to the status quo, often comes up in "modification" cases, cases where one party asks for a one-sided change of terms (for example, extra pay for the same amount of work already agreed to). In bad faith "hold-up" cases, the party seeking the changed terms has no good reason for doing so, and will threaten unjustified nonperformance if the requested changes are not agreed to. So the contractor will "request" additional pay and suggest that nonperformance (or significantly slowed or sloppy performance) will result if the extra sums are not promised and paid.[24] The second factor pointing toward lack of consent is present in different contexts, including circumstances where one party's dire economic circumstances forces that party to consider proposals it would otherwise consider demeaning or oppressive.

C. Consent and Validity

As Wertheimer points out,[25] it serves neither autonomy nor welfare to demand the fullest form of consent before we treat the relevant moral or legal threshold as being met. This has, perhaps, been most frequently and prominently discussed in relation to the doctrine of duress (discussed further below), where the doctrinal rule allows a party to void a contract if it can show an appropriate combination of wrongful threat on the part of the other contracting party and a lack of reasonable alternatives to entering the contract on its own part. In considering when such a defense should be allowed, Judge Richard Posner pointed out that reading the doctrinal standard to allow rescission of the contract[26] whenever contracting parties are in such dire economic circumstances that they have no practical alternative to entering the agreement is actually contrary to the interests of parties in bad economic circumstances.[27] If a poorly situated party could always get out of such agreements, few other parties would enter agreements with it.[28]

II. Doctrinal Treatment of Consent

A. Objective Versus Subjective

As noted, consent or autonomous choice has, for a long time, been considered at the core of contract law—at least back to the early English Writ of Assumpsit, claiming a cause of action based on obligations that a party had "assumed and faithfully promised" (*assumpsit et fideliter promisit*)[29]—as contrasted with obligations that parties have regardless of their choices.[30]

Some commentators and judges took the idea of "freedom of contract" quite seriously: viewing it as a legal principle, and not just a rhetorical justification, that people should be bound only to the extent that they subjectively so chose. Under this subjective theory of contract law (more precisely, the subjective theory of contract formation[31]), there would only be contractual agreement when each party's subjective understanding of the agreement matched the other's exactly ("meeting of the minds"). This is *Raffles v. Wichelhaus*,[32] where the parties agreed to pay for cotton being sent from Bombay on a ship called "Peerless." However, unknown to the parties, there were two ships called "Peerless" carrying cotton from Bombay, and one contracting party intended the earlier ship, and the other the later ship. The court held that there was no contract because the parties' minds did not meet.[33]

While this subjective approach to contract formation seems to give due regard to freedom of contract and the importance of a kind of "informed consent" to contractual terms, the suggested legal standard would lead to too much uncertainty in the enforceability of agreements. Anglo-American contract law soon settled instead on an objective standard for formation issues.[34] An objective approach focuses on the reasonable understanding of public acts or the words spoken and written, rather than on the parties' (sometimes idiosyncratic) understanding of those acts and words. If one party signs another party's proposed contract, there will be a valid contract, even if the two parties understood the terms differently.

Another example of the contrast between subjective and objective approaches to consent can be found in the well-known case of *Lucy v. Zehmer*, where the Zehmers claimed that their offer to sell their farm to Lucy for $50,000 had been a joke (made while drinking), but Lucy claimed not to have known that the offer was intended in jest. The court held that, from an objective standpoint, the offer was valid and could be accepted to form a valid contract.[35]

B. Absence of Express Consent

There are a number of contract law doctrines that make agreements void or voidable in circumstances where there are significant doubts about the consent of one of the parties. These include duress, undue influence, minority, mental incapacity, intoxication, and unconscionability.

1. Duress and Undue Influence

Duress and undue influence involve "improper pressure in the bargaining process...."[36] Duress involves obtaining a party's assent to an agreement by an improper threat. The doctrine was originally confined to threats of physical violence, but has been extended, in most jurisdictions, to economic threats (sometimes called "duress of goods"). Under traditional treatments of duress, the question had been whether the other party's will had been overborne. This traditional approach was abandoned long ago, not merely because of the difficulty of determining when a will had been (or, if one preferred an objective test, should have been) overborne, but also because such a test seems to exclude too many cases where nonenforcement seemed justified on moral or policy grounds.[37]

Under the modern approach, the party claiming duress needs to prove some wrongful act by the other party combined with a lack of reasonable alternatives. In some circumstances or in some jurisdictions, the party must also show that the other party caused the lack of reasonable alternatives[38] or in bad faith took advantage of that situation.[39] As one commentator puts it, there is a sense in which the modern doctrine of duress is more about "wrongness or unfairness" than about "freedom and voluntariness...."[40]

Under the doctrinal test for duress, "wrongful acts" include illegal actions, but extend beyond that to some immoral acts, including threats of criminal prosecution and claiming a right or failing to perform on a contract when one does not (subjectively) believe that one is legally justified.[41] In principle, litigation for breach of contract is a reasonable alternative, unless the party's business circumstances make the costs or delays of litigation unsustainable.[42]

Some commentators have suggested that the rules of what does (and does not) constitute duress can best be seen as a set of collective choices regarding what sort of "advantage taking" or "strategic behavior" we will condone (or even encourage) in transactions: for example, that getting the better bargain through greater intelligence or diligent research or crafty persuasion (short of misrepresentation of facts) is acceptable, but that obtaining a better bargain through, say, superior strength is not.[43]

Undue influence involves a combination of overpersuasion by one party and vulnerability or susceptibility by the other party.[44] While it is a notion perhaps more at home in the law of wills and estates (with family members trying to persuade those weakened by age or disease or clergy using fear of the afterlife to receive more favorable terms in a will or other legal document), it is a doctrine accepted in contract law to rescind certain agreements. The cases usually involve parties who are competent, but perhaps barely so, often weakened by age, physical exhaustion, grief, or the like—parties who could not protect their interests in the face of significant pressure, or parties who might be susceptible to particular sorts of persuaders (like, those with whom they have relationships of trust: for example, clergy, lawyers, trustees).[45]

2. Minority, Mental Incapacity, and Intoxication

There are a series of contract law doctrines dealing with parties who are not (or are not considered to be) competent to protect their own interests: These involve those who are below the age of majority (the doctrine of minority, or infancy) and those who are not (or no longer) competent due to mental disease or defect (mental incapacity) and intoxication.

In each case, the lack of competency gives the affected party the right to rescind the agreement, at least under certain circumstances. The legal rule, however, sharply differs between incompetency on the basis of age—an objective standard, in principle easily checkable—and forms of incompetency that are not as easily discerned or tested.

Children under the age of majority have the power to rescind their agreements up to, and slightly beyond, obtaining that age.[46] (If they wait any significant period of time beyond the age of majority, they will be held to have tacitly ratified the agreement.) There are different statutory-based exceptions in some states (allowing minors to enter valid agreements, for example, for some medical procedures); in some states a minor may be liable for benefits received or depreciation of the subject of a rescinded contract, and the parents or guardians of a minor will be obligated to pay the fair market value of any object the minor purchased if the object was a "necessity."[47]

With intoxication and mental incapacity, the afflicted party generally has the right to rescind an agreement if the other party knew (or should have known) of the incapacity.[48] Additionally, some states allow mentally incapacitated parties to rescind agreements, without regard to the knowledge of the other party, if the parties can be returned to the status quo.

3. Unconscionability

Unconscionability has its roots in the Roman doctrine of *laesio enormis*, under which a contract could be rescinded if a party had to pay more than twice an object's market price.[49] Under the English common law, unconscionability covered cases where the terms were so one-sided that the agreement was one "such as no man in his senses and not under delusion would make on the one hand, and as no honest and fair man would accept on the other."[50]

This picks up an ongoing theme in discussion of unconscionability, that it combines concerns about acceptable levels of (un)fairness with suspicions that there may have been some important defect in the formation process. Richard Epstein, though no supporter of governmental paternalistic intervention, defended unconscionability as a doctrine that would allow a defense to enforcement in circumstances where there likely had been some issue of duress, undue influence, or fraud, but where these elements could not be proven sufficiently for the use of those doctrines.[51]

Contemporary American contract law[52] does seem to go further than this, though the standards for this doctrine's application remain notoriously amorphous, and its application in cases highly inconsistent. The doctrine is usually held to include a requirement of significant defects on both procedural and substantive levels,[53] though one can find occasional cases that seem to deal only with significantly one-sided terms. In the cases where unconscionability is found, there is often an underlying theme of exploitation[54] (for example, Wertheimer 1996, 36–76).

Courts have found, or at least strongly indicated, unconscionability in cases involving cross-collateral agreements with poor consumers and luxury goods,[55] a provision giving a clothing retailer the right to cancel its order at any time for any reason,[56] arbitration provisions that constrained employees but not employers,[57] and the sale to a poor consumer of a freezer for three times its fair market value.[58]

One may need to know more about particular transactions or sets of transactions to evaluate whether prohibitions of agreements on certain terms is purely paternalistic or serves other functions. The question is what the effect would be of the prohibition. In some cases, the only alternative to transacting on extremely one-sided terms may be no transaction at all (some have argued that this is the case with certain consumer sales contracts with consumers who have little resources and poor credit).[59] In other cases, however, the alternative to an agreement on extremely one-sided terms may well be an agreement on more reasonable terms: The potential husband might be interested in marrying even if the terms of his proposed premarital agreement must be made more fair; the boat captain offering rescue might be willing to act on market terms if extortionate terms are unenforceable; and the employer may settle for a 2-year and local restrictive covenant if a 5-year and nation-wide covenant would be struck down. In such cases, restrictions strengthen the bargaining position of the weaker party without foreclosing its ability to enter an agreement on the matter in question.[60]

4. "Duty to Read"

It is the general rule that one cannot avoid contractual obligation by reporting that one had not read the terms of an agreement, or even that one was unable to read the terms because one was illiterate.[61] Though one might raise questions about the existence or the quality of the consent if one party did not read a form, could not read a form, or was unable to understand the form's language, contract law prefers to put the onus on the parties to read a document, or have it read to them, and to understand it, or have it explained to them.

5. Consideration

The doctrine of consideration separates enforceable bargained-for exchanges from unenforceable gift promises.[62] The doctrine itself is both intricate and controversial, and a number of different justifications have been offered for it, so the connection between that doctrine and consent is never going to be straightforward. In rough and general terms, an agreement is only enforceable when something of value is given or promised by both sides. "Something of value" includes an agreement not to sue[63] and an agreement to refrain from some activity one has a legal right to do (my promising never to run a marathon or never to visit Siberia would be consideration, even if these were things I would never be interested in doing in any case).[64] For the purposes of consideration, there is no requirement that what one party gives or promises be of comparable value to what the other party gives or promises.[65]

Among the arguments offered for the doctrine of consideration is that as a kind of formal requirement it distinguishes agreements on which parties have given serious thought from those that might have been entered into impulsively.[66] At the same time, like technical formal requirements, the doctrine of consideration can result in the nonenforcement of transactions where both parties firmly intended and expected enforcement (and there was no strong reason to doubt the voluntariness of the parties' actions or the fairness of the transaction).[67]

C. Implied Terms and Hypothetical Consent

Implied terms are terms that are not expressly part of the parties' agreement, but which nonetheless are enforced. Courts and commentators frequently distinguish terms "implied by law" and those "implied in fact." The former are terms not grounded on the parties' shared preferences, but instead based on legislative or judicial judgments of fairness, policy, or efficiency.[68] These will be discussed later, under "Mandatory Terms."

Terms "implied in fact" sometimes refers to terms, or assent to terms, that can be read off someone's behavior (as pumping gas at a self-serve gasoline station is held to be acceptance of purchase at the price listed on the pump). More interesting, for our purposes, are the terms implied into a contract on the basis that these are provisions on which the parties would have agreed if they had been asked at the time they entered the agreement. This is an argument from hypothetical consent. Often terms are implied into a particular contract in the course of resolving a dispute regarding that agreement. "Implied in fact" terms also include doctrinal rules that could be justified on the basis that these terms are what parties would likely have agreed upon if they had been asked at the time of execution.[69]

Justice Oliver Wendell Holmes, Jr., had argued for a "tacit agreement" test for consequential damages that went beyond usual levels of damage: that recovery should only be available where the special circumstances had been brought to the defendant's attention and the other party had directly or indirectly assented to the higher level of liability.[70] This is a somewhat stricter standard than the *Hadley* test of foreseeability that is in fact doctrinal law in most American jurisdictions, and the tacit agreement test has been expressly rejected by most courts and commentators.[71]

There are a number of equitable doctrines that allow parties to rescind an agreement under extraordinary circumstances that have arisen since the execution of an agreement. These doctrines include impracticability, impossibility, and frustration of purpose. Though highly exceptional in their application, they are established parts of the contract law landscape, and are often understood as claims of implied agreement: that certainly the parties could not have expected performance if certain very unusual and unexpected circumstances were to arise.[72]

In limited circumstances, a party can rescind an agreement, or at least avoid its enforcement, on the basis of a mistake of fact made at the time the agreement was entered.[73] The equitable relief is more easily available if the mistake was shared by both parties at the time of the agreement, but in extreme circumstances relief may be available even for unilateral mistake.

Some commentators view the doctrines of mutual and unilateral mistake as basically general statements regarding implied terms: that these are circumstances in which parties to a contract would normally expect that performance would be excused. This view may be supported by the doctrinal rules that state that the agreement will not be subject to rescission if the party seeking rescission has, in some sense, accepted the risk of the mistake.[74]

D. Mandatory Terms and Rules
1. Background Rules

While contract law emphasizes the freedom of parties to choose their own terms, there are two prominent sets of exceptions: background rules and mandatory rules. I will deal with background rules in this section, and mandatory rules in the next.

By "background rules," I mean the formation and remedial rules of contract—the "rules of the game" as it were—which the parties have not chosen,[75] and most of which are not within the powers of the parties to contract around. For example, despite strong criticism from many commentators, parties cannot (enforceably) agree to extracompensatory liquidated damages, punitive damages, or emotional distress damages,[76] or to the waiver of the requirement of consideration.

These are only indirectly consent issues, mostly showing the limitations of "freedom of contract": that there are terms that the state will not enforce, even though the parties have consented to them. Not only terms, of course, but whole types of agreements are held to be unenforceable, from agreements in restraint of trade (now mostly covered by federal antitrust legislation) to agreements to procure illegal drugs, killers for hire, or prostitutes services, and the like.[77]

2. Mandatory and "Implied in Law" Terms

There are some terms that are implied into agreements—some terms implied into all agreements, others into only certain categories of agreements. And the source of the mandatory terms can range from common law judicial rules to state or federal statutes.

Such terms include the nonwaivable duty of good faith[78] and the provisions of various state and federal consumer protection statutes.

Additionally, there are default terms that the parties can circumvent by express agreement, but which otherwise apply to the parties even when they have not consented to them (though here, in particular, the distinction between waivable terms implied in fact and waivable terms implied in law may be hard to discern). These may include terms relating to termination of an ongoing commercial relationship and duties of "best efforts" one party has toward forwarding the interests of another within a contractual relationship.[79]

III. Recent Challenges to Contract Law's Treatment of Consent

A. Promissory Estoppel and Other Grounds for Recovery

In the twentieth century, promissory estoppel developed as an alternative ground for recovery within, or related to, contract law. Though it (and the other contract-like grounds of recovery discussed in this section) has roots in the case-law that go back a long ways, recent expansions in use have caused some to see it as a challenge to contract law's consent-based approach.[80]

Promissory estoppel is liability on a promise even where the traditional requirements of offer, acceptance, and consideration are not present. This equitable remedy is available where a promise has been reasonably relied upon and injustice can only be avoided by enforcing the promise.[81] While some might argue that liability in such contexts is contrary to the consent-based ideal of freedom of contract, the ultimate complaint goes more to the relative fuzziness of the standard (a promise on which the other party could *reasonably* rely), a complaint that can be brought against most equitable remedies. There is a sense in which a party consents to potential liability as much by making a promise on which the other party might reasonably rely as by making an offer that the other party might accept.

There are other exceptional grounds for recovery for circumstances where the parties have not reached a valid agreement (or a previously valid agreement has been legally rescinded) but justice seems to warrant granting some right to recovery. For example, there is promissory restitution, where a "promise made in recognition of a benefit previously received . . . is binding to the extent necessary to prevent injustice."[82] Additionally, there are circumstances where a party can seek restitution for the unjust enrichment of another party, for example, where a contract has been rescinded after payments were made or services rendered, or where emergency services are provided in circumstances where an agreement was not possible.[83] Such rights and obligations are not grounded in consent, but in claims of justice and fairness.

B. Standardized Forms and Electronic Contracting

Standardized forms are also not especially new, though (again) relative to the common law development of contract law doctrine (arm's length negotiation between equals), they are contrary to the paradigm that underlies much of the doctrine, and thus raise distinct challenges.[84]

Karl Llewellyn's response to the problem of standardized forms was to argue that one could not reasonably see one party as having assented to the boiler-plate provisions of the other party's standardized forms, as it is unlikely that such provisions were read, and even less likely that they were understood even if read.[85] Instead, he argued that the courts should treat parties as offering "blanket assent . . . to any not unreasonable or indecent terms the seller may have on his form, which do not alter or eviscerate the reasonable meaning of the dickered terms."[86]

Randy Barnett has made a similar argument, comparing assent to terms in form contracts (including those in electronic contracting) to agreeing to do whatever a friend has written in a paper now sealed in an envelope.[87] Such assent would not be seen to be plenary, but would include, in the contract context, an intention "to be bound by the terms I am likely to have read [for example, those involving price and quantity] (whether or not I have done so) and also by those unread terms in the agreement . . . that I am not likely to have read but that do not exceed some bound of reasonableness."[88]

In this context, it is interesting to watch the contests regarding the regulation of electronic contracting[89] in the United States, especially as they have developed in the course of the battles over proposed revisions to Article 2 of the Uniform Commercial Code, UCITA (Uniform Commercial Information Transactions Act), and the proposed American Law Institute's *Principles of Software Contracts*. Those who sell computers and those who sell or lease software have argued, under the rubric of "freedom of contract," for the right to have terms incorporated into contracts even if the terms appear through "clickware" or "browseware" or are sent later "in the box." On the other side, consumer advocates have argued for more prominent notice to consumers that there are relevant terms, and perhaps for a requirement that such terms be posted on Internet sites or available in stores that sell the goods.[90] Unsurprisingly, the two sides also disagree about the extent to which the doctrine of unconscionability or consumer protection legislation should limit possible terms or impose mandatory terms.[91]

One standard argument for allowing the enforcement of terms in electronic contracting, despite issues with the timing of the terms' presentation, and despite doubts about the likelihood of the terms having been read, is that more stringent requirements would create an unworkable situation, or at least a situation significantly less attractive for consumers and providers alike.[92] Additionally, while recent empirical work has found that software license agreements tend, almost universally, to have pro-seller provisions (relative to default rules), there appears to be little evidence that the agreements were any more pro-seller in dealings with consumers than they were with larger business and corporate buyers.[93]

In Arthur Leff's suggestive analogy, contracting on standardized forms (and, one would now add, electronic contracting) is, in contrast to a much earlier paradigm of contract, more product ("thing") than process.[94] As the contractual terms become less subject to negotiation, there is, in a sense, a "collapse of the terms into the product."[95] One might add that there is more attention to the general social benefits of easy and enforceable transactions than there is to how full or informed the assent is to terms. This is not necessarily a bad thing, and it may be that no richer sense of autonomy is available in the context of modern commercial interactions.

C. Bounded Rationality and Cognitive Biases

Modern debates about consent in contract law have been enriched, or at least complicated, by recent discussions of "bounded rationality" and "cognitive biases." These are challenges to the rationality assumption of much of economic analysis—and much of contract law—challenges based on experimental research.[96]

Among the experimental results were that parties value objects more when they own them than when they do not (the "endowment effect") and, analogously, treat perceived losses as far more serious than "opportunity costs" (gains they would have had, had they acted or chosen differently); people's preferences among alternatives A and B may depend on other alternatives (C, D, and E), particularly where the additional alternatives make an option seem either moderate or extreme; and we tend to suffer from self-serving biases, overoptimism, and an underestimation of the possibility of lower-frequency events.[97]

Many of these differences from modeled rationality have effects on consent arguments. For example, commentators often argue that consent to a term can be derived from the failure to object to a term, or to demand alternative terms. The endowment effect can counter the argument that parties must not want more protective contract terms because they never (or rarely) negotiate for them: If parties sufficiently valued a protective term, the argument goes, they would trade off some other good (perhaps low price in a consumer good, or higher wages in an employment contract) to get it.[98] However, if the valuation of the good varies according to whether it is initially assigned to the consumer or employee or not, then the derivation from failure to negotiate is, at best, not so simple. Also, Melvin Eisenberg has written convincingly of how many rules imposing limits on particular kinds of agreements—liquidated damages, express conditions, form contracts, waiver of fiduciary obligations, prenuptial agreements,[99] and limiting terms in employment contracts—can be seen as responding to our cognitive limits.[100]

Both premarital agreements and employment agreements with restrictive covenants[101] are good examples of contracts that may raise special concerns about consent. Someone about to marry, fully in love, may not be well positioned to think reasonably about which rights to demand and which to waive, regarding alimony and property division, for a future divorce that he or she, at that moment, cannot imagine occurring. Similarly, an employee taking up a job may not be able to think clearly about posttermination rights when the current relationship between employee and employer is at its most positive. And many commentators have raised questions regarding the assent in a surrogacy agreement[102] to giving up parental rights to a child (especially if the woman in question has never before been pregnant and has not experienced the bond many pregnant women feel with the children they carry).[103]

Some theorists in the area have used arguments grounded in bounded rationality theory to advocate more use of mandatory contract terms (and a broader application of unconscionability doctrine).[104] And there is a long tradition of imposing "cooling off periods" (a period after signing an agreement during which time the party can change its mind and no longer be legally bound)—for transactions ranging from door-to-door sales to giving up a child for adoption—grounded on similar concerns regarding consent.

IV. Consent Theories of Contract

It may be worth adding, for the sake of completeness, the role that consent plays in contract law, for theories above the doctrinal level. While there are many important theories of contract law that do not focus on consent (in particular, the law and economics theories of contract law[105]), there are two prominent approaches that focus, directly or indirectly, on consent: the promise theory of Charles Fried and the consent theory of Randy Barnett.[106]

For Fried, the "promise principle" is the "moral basis of contract law," connected with the idea that "contractual obligations [are] essentially self-imposed...."[107] A promise itself is an obligation consented to by the party making the promise, and Fried also would have a requirement that the promise be in some sense assented to by the promisee before there would be an obligation.[108]

Standard criticisms of Fried's theory include (1) that it operates at too general a level to be able to explain detailed contract doctrine or remedial rules (which, critics claim, can be better explained by economic analysis[109]) and (2) that it excludes, by fiat, significant portions of what is conventionally considered part of contract law and practice.[110]

In Barnett's "consent theory," "legal enforcement [of an agreement] is morally justified because the promisor voluntarily performed acts that conveyed her intention to create a legally enforceable obligation by transferring alienable rights."[111] A basic difference between Barnett's theory and Fried's lies in Barnett's greater acceptance of objective approaches to assent. Barnett's theory might be called an "appears to consent" theory of contract, or a reasonable reliance theory.[112]

Conclusion

Law is full of standards imposed with little or no consent of those affected— from the criminal law and tort law restrictions on our liberty to the obligations parents owe their children—yet most of the time we think that such standards might nonetheless be legitimate and fair. If we are especially concerned about consent in contract law, it is because it is an area of law that is built on the idea, or ideal, of parties choosing the standards by which they will be bound. Though contract practice clearly falls far short of the ideals of "freedom of contract" and full consent,[113] it remains one of the few areas of law where the question of consent is taken very seriously, and re-examined regularly.

Likely, the contract law (and contract theory) rhetoric of "freedom of contract" and "meeting of the minds" never matched contracting practice in more than a small percentage of agreements, even if that small percentage is now getting even smaller.[114] And if we often consent in only the weakest sense to the terms that bind us (as we consent in only a weak sense to the laws that bind us and the government that governs us), there are important interests of the contracting parties themselves, as well as societal interests, that justify giving the full force of law to the vast majority of such agreements.

Notes

1. Frederick W. Thomas Professor of Law and Philosophy, University of Minnesota. I am grateful for the comments and suggestions of Peter A. Alces, Curtis Bridgeman, Jeffrey M. Lipshaw, David McGowan, Franklin G. Miller, and Alan Wertheimer.

2. E.g., Barbara H. Fried, "What's Morality Got to Do With It?" *Harvard Law Review Forum* 120 (2007): 53–61, http://www.harvardlawreview.org/forum/issues/120/jan07/bfried.pdf.

3. This view goes back many centuries. Consider this quotation from Pufendorf's 1672 "On the Law of Nature and of Nations": "But the things which I owe another from pacts and agreements, these I owe for the reason that he has acquired a new right against me from my own consent." Samuel Pufendorf, "On the Law of Nature and of Nations," Book III, ch. 4, reprinted in *The Political Writings of Samuel Pufendorf,* edited by Craig L. Carr (Oxford: Oxford University Press, 1994), 166.

4. Of course, even consent in its fullest sense does not guarantee that the other party has not done us wrong in entering into (an unjust) contract with us. At best, consent only removes one sort of complaint that we can reasonably make about that agreement. See Joseph Raz, "On the Authority and Interpretation of Constitutions: Some Preliminaries," in *Constitutionalism,* edited by Larry Alexander (Cambridge: Cambridge University Press, 1998), 152–93, at 163.

5. As Andrew Robertson points out, in contract law, the issue is as often about the consent or voluntariness of limitations of rights accepted as it is about performance obligations undertaken. Andrew Robertson, "The Limits of Voluntariness in Contract," *Melbourne University Law Review* 29 (2005): 179–217, at 187.

6. Richard Craswell, "Property Rules and Liability Rules in Unconscionability and Related Doctrines," *University of Chicago Law Review* 60 (1993): 1–65, at 34–37; see also Robertson, "The Limits of Voluntariness in Contract," 196–201.

7. The focus of my paper will be on U.S. contract law. While the details of contract law differ somewhat in other common law countries, and more markedly in some civil law countries, it is my best guess that much of the analysis that follows holds true across legal systems—in general argument, even if not in detail.

8. There may be grounds for questioning the assumption (that I will carry over in this paper) that consent is basically the same matter across quite different contexts (for example, informed consent to medical treatment, consent to government,

consent to sexual relations, contractual consent, etc.), but such an inquiry must await another occasion or another author.

9. For a defense of the performative perspective, see Alan Wertheimer, "What is Consent? And Is It Important?" *Buffalo Criminal Law Review* 3 (2000): 557–83; on the subjective approach, see Heidi M. Hurd, "The Moral Magic of Consent," *Legal Theory* 2 (1996): 121–46, and Larry Alexander "The Moral Magic of Consent (II)," *Legal Theory* 2 (1996): 165–74.

10. Of course, a focus on external, observable behavior is common to law generally.

11. E.g., Wertheimer, "What is Consent?"

12. See Wertheimer, "What is Consent?"; Alan Wertheimer, *Coercion* (Princeton, NJ: Princeton University Press, 1987), 46–53.

13. That is, the criteria of consent may involve issues of knowledge, opportunity, and options that are difficult to prove or disprove in court.

14. Third parties may rely on the validity and enforceability of agreements, and if those agreements can be undermined on grounds not easily observable by those third parties, predictability would be significantly undermined.

15. This is the problem of "equivocation" in the term, discussed in Alan Wertheimer, "Remarks on Coercion and Exploitation," *Denver University Law Review* 74 (1997): 889–906, at 892–94.

16. Aristotle, *Nicomachean Ethics*, Book III, 1, in *The Complete Works of Aristotle*, edited by Jonathan Barnes. (Princeton, NJ: Princeton University Press, 1984), vol. 2, 1729–1867, at 1752–55.

17. For an overview of the literature on how often (or, more to the point, how rarely) parties read either their own standardized forms or the forms of the parties with whom they are dealing, see Robertson, "The Limits of Voluntariness in Contract," 188–90.

18. E.g., W. David Slawson, "Standard Form Contracts and Democratic Control of Lawmaking Power," *Harvard Law Review* 84 (1971): 529–66.

19. Robert A. Hillman, "Online Boilerplate: Would Mandatory Website Disclosure of E-Standard Terms Backfire?" *Michigan Law Review* 104 (2006): 837–56, at 840–42, 849–52 . It is commonly argued that the failure to read contractual terms is "rational," but the rationality (understood narrowly) may frequently be overstated, as the choice not to read could be based on a desire not to offend, a belief that the terms will always be fair, a belief that courts would not enforce unfair terms, an undue optimism that the circumstances covered by restrictive terms would not arise, etc. Robertson, "The Limits of Voluntariness in Contract," 190–93.

20. It should be noted that there is evidence that monopolies are as responsive to consumer preferences as companies in more competitive situations. Alan Schwartz, "A Reexamination of Nonsubstantive Unconscionability," *Virginia Law Review* 63 (1977): 1053–83, at 1071–76.

21. See, e.g., *Ting v. AT&T*, 182 F. Supp.2d 902, 914, 929 (N.D. Cal. 2002) (lack of variety of dispute resolution terms in available long-distance telephone service providers in California).

22. This discussion is based largely on Alan Wertheimer, "Remarks on Coercion and Exploitation," *Denver University Law Review* 74 (1997): 889–906, at 900–02.

23. Wertheimer lists other factors that would be relevant for an exploration of the question of whether a proposal was "exploitative": for example, whether the terms are fair, the extent to which the recipient's situation is "desperate," the extent to which the recipient's situation is due to unjust background conditions, and whether the proposal involves commodification of goods that are usually not commodified. Wertheimer, "Remarks on Coercion and Exploitation," 900–02. Though all of these factors are relevant to an overall moral or legal judgment regarding enforcement of a contract or promise, some are less directly relevant to questions of consent.

24. By contrast, in the "good faith" forms of modifications, a party seeks a modification of terms only because it must, because of unexpected changed circumstances (for example, unexpected price increases from its suppliers, labor trouble, or unexpected complications in performance), and does not threaten nonperformance unless it sincerely believes that it has a legal justification.

25. See Wertheimer, "What is Consent?"

26. The cases often involve a party trying to avoid enforcement of a settlement agreement, in which that party accepted less than its full claim to resolve a breach-of-contract dispute.

27. *Selmer Co. v. Blakeslee-Midwest Co.*, 704 F.2d 924, 928 (7th Cir. 1983) (Posner, J.).

28. Wertheimer gives a comparable example regarding informed consent to a medical procedure, where a patient's consent might have been said to have been less than fully voluntary, because of the dire health consequences of not going forward. In such circumstances, it certainly does not benefit patients suffering from severe medical conditions for them to be unable to validly consent to medical procedures. Wertheimer, "What is Consent?" 564.

29. David J. Ibbetson, *A Historical Introduction to the Law of Obligations* (Oxford: Oxford University Press, 1999), 131.

30. On the history of the Writ of Assumpsit, see A. W. Brian Simpson, *A History of the Common Law of Contract: The Rise of the Action of Assumpsit* (Oxford: Clarendon Press, 1975); Ibbetson, *A Historical Introduction to the Law of Obligations*, 126–51.

31. There is a related but distinct subjective approach to interpretation of terms within a contract. See, e.g., E. Allan Farnsworth, *Contracts*, 4th ed. (New York: Aspen Publishers, 2004), 445–54.

32. (1864) 159 E.R. 375, 2 Hurlstone & Coltman 906 (Ct. Exch.).

33. The standard reading of *Raffles v. Wichelhaus* is, as discussed, as a paradigm case of the subjective approach. E.g., Grant Gilmore, *The Death of Contract*, 2nd ed. (Columbus, OH: Ohio State University Press, 1995), 39–47. A few commentators, including, prominently, Justice Oliver Wendell Holmes, Jr., have tried to construe the case as consistent with an objective approach. For example, Robert L. Birmingham, "Holmes on 'Peerless': Raffles v. Wichelhaus and the Objective Theory of Contract." University of Pittsburgh Law Review 47 (1985): 183–204. In any event, it is not crucial that this particular case be read in this way, as there seem to be numerous other cases where the subjective approach is exemplified. Gilmore, *The Death of Contract*, 44.

34. E.g., Gilmore, *The Death of Contract*.

35. *Lucy v. Zehmer*, 84 S.E.2d 516 (Va. 1954).

36. American Law Institute, *Restatement (Second) of Contracts* (1981), Topic 2, Introductory Note.

37. Wertheimer has a good general discussion of contract law's historical treatment of consent in the context of duress. Wertheimer, *Coercion*, 19–53. On the particular point in the text above, see Ibid., 23, 32–34.

38. See, e.g., *Northern Fabrication Co. v. UNOCAL*, 980 P.2d 958 (Alaska 1999).

39. See, e.g., *Rich & Whillock, Inc. v. Ashton Development, Inc.*, 204 Cal. Rptr. 86 (Cal. App. 1984); *Butitta v. First Mortgage Corp.*, 578 N.E.2d 116 (Ill. App. Ct. 1991). One might, if one prefers, describe the intentional taking advantage of another party's distress more as "exploitation" than "duress," Wertheimer, *Coercion*, 40, but "exploitation" is not an available doctrinal defense. Also, the cases one might be inclined to describe as "exploitation" tend generally to be analyzed under the rubric of "unconscionability," a defense courts are even more reluctant to recognize than "duress."

40. See Wertheimer, *Coercion*, 53.

41. *Restatement (Second) of Contracts* §§ 175, 176. Using a subjective, not an objective, standard here is important, among other reasons, to encourage parties to enter binding agreements settling legal disputes. It would make such agreements too easy to attack collaterally if it were sufficient to argue later that, *objectively speaking*, one of the parties had no valid legal claim. Additionally, a subjective test picks up the "bad faith" aspect of parties insisting on legal positions they themselves do not believe to be justified, simply in order to gain bargaining leverage.

42. E.g., *Totem Marine Tug & Barge, Inc. v. Alyeska Pipeline Service Co.*, 584 P.2d 15 (Alaska 1978).

43. E.g., Anthony J. Kronman, "Contract Law and Distributive Justice," *Yale Law Journal* 89 (1980): 472–511, at 478–83.

44. *Restatement (Second) of Contracts* § 177. The paradigmatic case for applying undue influence to a contract (or, at least, contract-like) case is *Odorizzi v. Bloomfield School District*, 246 Cal. App. 2d 123, 54 Cal. Rptr. 533 (1966).

45. E.g., *Moore v. Moore*, 81 Cal. 195, 22 P. 589 (1889) (invalidating on grounds of undue influence a transfer of land procured by family members from widow immediately after funeral of husband who had been shot, widow had been hampered by grief, lack of sleep, and pregnancy; no reason was given why transaction needed to be done right after funeral other than to take advantage of widow's condition).

46. See *Restatement (Second) of Contracts* § 14; Farnsworth, *Contracts*, §§ 4.3–4.5.

47. See Farnsworth, *Contracts*, § 4.5, at 225–26; American Law Institute, *Restatement of the Law: Restitution and Unjust Enrichment, Tentative Draft No. 1*, April 6, 2001, § 16, at 270–71.

48. On mental incapacity, see *Restatement (Second) of Contracts* § 15; Farnsworth, *Contracts*, §§ 4.6–4.8. On intoxication, see *Restatement (Second) of Contracts* § 16; Farnsworth, *Contracts*, § 4.6, at 230.

49. Reinhard Zimmermann, *The Law of Obligations: Roman Foundations of the Civilian Tradition* (Oxford: Oxford University Press, 1990); J. B. Thayer, "*Laesio Enormis*," *Kentucky Law Journal* 25 (1937): 321–41.

50. *Earl of Chesterfield v. Janssen*, 2 Ves. Sen. 125, 155, 28 Eng. Rep. 82, 100 (ch. 1750) (per Lord Hardwicke).

51. Richard A. Epstein, "Unconscionability: A Critical Reappraisal," *Journal of Law and Economics* 18 (1975): 293–315, at 294–305.

52. *Uniform Commercial Code* § 2-302; *Restatement (Second) of Contracts* § 208; Farnsworth, *Contracts*, §§ 4.27–4.28.

53. See, e.g., *Williams v. Walker-Thomas*, 350 F.2d 445, 449–450 (D.C. Cir. 1965); *Davis v. O'Melveny & Myers*, 485 F.3d 1066, 1072 (9th Cir. 2007) (summarizing California law).

54. See Alan Wertheimer, *Exploitation* (Princeton, NJ: Princeton University Press, 1996), 36–76.

55. *Williams v. Walker-Thomas Furniture*, 350 F.2d 445 (D.C. Cir. 1965).

56. *Gianni Sport Ltd. v. Gantos, Inc.*, 391 N.W.2d 760 (Mich. App. 1986).

57. *Armendariz v. Foundation Health Psychcare Servs.*, 6 P.3d 669 (Cal. 2000).

58. *Jones v. Star Credit Corp.*, 298 N.Y.S.2d 264 (Sup. Ct. 1969).

59. E.g., Epstein, "Unconscionability: A Critical Reappraisal," 306–08.

60. See Wertheimer, *Exploitation*, 72–73.

61. See, e.g., Farnsworth, *Contracts*, § 4.26, at 287.

62. Modern American contract law creates some exceptions to consideration doctrine, making a few categories of promises enforceable without consideration. The most prominent exception, promissory estoppel, is discussed below.

63. Refraining from bringing a lawsuit constitutes consideration only if one sincerely believes that one has a colorable legal claim; the fact that one's belief may be unreasonable and without foundation in the law is not relevant.

64. Discussions of consideration often refer to "benefit" and "detriment," but these terms are meant in a sort of abstract or logical way. "Detriment" just means giving up something that one has a legal right to do or have; a promise to do something or to refrain from doing something remains consideration even if the promised act or omission arguably benefits the promisor. See, e.g., *Hamer v. Sidway*, 27 N.E. 256 (N.Y. 1891) (promise not to smoke, swear gamble, or drink until 21 years old is consideration).

65. However, any one-sidedness in the bargain may help to prove unconscionability, or be evidence of misrepresentation, duress, undue influence, or mistake.

66. E.g., Lon L. Fuller, "Consideration and Form," *Columbia Law Review* 41 (1941): 799–824. A different, if still related argument is that consideration distinguishes "market transactions," with their mentality of rational actor analysis, from social promises, with their more informal and altruistic tendencies. See Roy Kreitner, "The Gift Beyond the Grave: Revisiting the Question of Consideration," *Columbia Law Review* 101 (2001): 1876–1957.

67. For an example of a case of this sort, see *Dougherty v. Salt*, 125 N.E. 94 (N.Y. 1919).

68. On implied terms generally, see Farnsworth, *Contracts*, §§ 7.15–7.17.

69. One sign that a doctrine or equitable exception is justified on "implied in fact" grounds would be an exception allowing parties to waive or circumvent the terms of that standard by express agreement. See, e.g., *Uniform Commercial Code* §§ 2-314, 2-316 (describing the default implied warranty of merchantability, and the process for excluding or modifying it).

70. *Globe Refining Co. v. Landa Cotton Oil Co.*, 190 U.S. 540, 544–546 (1903) (Holmes, J.).

71. See, e.g., *Restatement (Second) of Contracts* § 351, Comment a; UCC § 2-715, Comment 2; *Rexnord Corp. v. DeWolff Boberg & Assoc. Inc.*, 286 F.3d 1001 (7th Cir. 2002).

72. See, e.g., Farnsworth, *Contracts*, 623–624, 630–632, 636–637.

73. See *Restatement (Second) of Contracts* §§ 151–158; Farnsworth, *Contracts*, 599–619.

74. See *Restatement (Second) of Contracts* § 154.

75. Randy Barnett writes: "In assessing the enforceability of form contracts, we must never forget that contract law is itself one big form contract that goes unread by most parties most of the time." Randy E. Barnett, "Consenting to Form Contracts," *Fordham Law Review* 71 (2002): 627–45, at 644. He goes on to argue that there is a sense in which parties consent to the default rules of contract

law. Ibid., see also Randy E. Barnett " . . . And Contractual Consent," *Southern California Interdisciplinary Law Journal* 3 (1993): 421–44.

76. There is a quite limited category of contracts (slightly larger in England than in the United States) where emotional distress damages are available for breach of contract. See *Restatement (Second) of Contracts* § 353; Farnsworth, *Contracts*, 808–10. The limitation described in the text refers to the vast majority of contracts, where such damages are not available. On liquidated damages and punitive damages, see *Restatement (Second) of Contracts* §§ 355–356; Farnsworth, *Contracts*, 760–64, 811–20.

77. On these "public policy" restrictions, see *Restatement (Second) of Contracts* §§ 178–179; Farnsworth, *Contracts*, §§ 5.1–5.9.

78. *Uniform Commercial Code* § 1–203.

79. See generally Farnsworth, *Contracts*, §§ 7.15–7.17.

80. See Gilmore, *The Death of Contract.*

81. *Restatement (Second) of Contracts* § 90(1). "The remedy granted . . . may be as limited as justice requires." Ibid.

82. *Restatement (Second) of Contracts* § 86.

83. See, e.g., Farnsworth, *Contracts*, § 2.20.

84. E.g., Arthur Allen Leff, "Contract as Thing," *American University Law Review* 19 (1970): 131–57.

85. See Karl N. Llewellyn, *The Common Law Tradition: Deciding Appeals* (Boston: Little, Brown and Company, 1960), 362–71.

86. See Llewellyn, *The Common Law Tradition*, 370.

87. See Barnett, "Consenting to Form Contracts."

88. Barnett, "Consenting to Form Contracts," 638.

89. "Electronic contracting" covers the somewhat different legal contexts of (1) the sale of computers and sale or lease of software, where the provider of the goods has inserted terms in the packaging that cannot be scrutinized until long after the item has been purchased; and (2) the downloading of software, where the provider's terms are posted on an Internet site, and the consumer may ("clickware") or may not ("browseware") be required to click a box to indicate assent to those terms.

90. See Hillman, "Online Boilerplate."

91. EU legislation tends toward significant use of mandatory terms and restrictions on allowable terms in consumer contracts, while U.S. law tends toward allowing party choice and market pressures to be the primary, and often the sole, constraint on contract terms. Jane K. Winn and Brian H. Bix, "Diverging Perspectives on Electronic Contracting in the US and EU," *Cleveland State Law Review* 54 (2006): 175–90.

92. See, e.g., *ProCD, Inc. v. Zeidenberg*, 86 F.3d 1447, 1452 (7th Cir. 1996) (Zeidenberg's position, if accepted, "would drive prices through the ceiling or

return transactions to the horse-and-buggy age"); *Hill v. Gateway* 2000, 105 F.3d 1147, 1149 (7th Cir. 1997) (requiring disclosure of full terms prior to purchase would be impractical and would serve little purpose).

93. See Florencia Marotta-Wurgler, "What's in a Standard Form Contract? An Empirical Analysis of Software License Agreements," *Journal of Empirical Legal Studies* 4 (2007): 677–713.

94. See Leff, "Contract as Thing"; cf. Margaret Jane Radin, "Boilerplate Today: The Rise of Modularity and the Waning of Consent," in *Boilerplate: The Foundation of Market Contracts,* edited by Omri Ben-Shahar (Cambridge: Cambridge University Press, 2007), 189–99, at 192–94.

95. Radin, "Boilerplate Today," 195.

96. See Daniel Kahneman, Paul Slovic, and Amos Tversky, eds., *Judgment Under Uncertainty: Heuristics and Biases* (Cambridge: Cambridge University Press, 1982); Cass R. Sunstein, ed., *Behavioral Law & Economics.* (Cambridge: Cambridge University Press, 2000).

97. See Cass R. Sunstein, "Behavioral Analysis of Law," *University of Chicago Law Review* 65 (1997): 1175–95.

98. E.g., Lucian A. Bebchuk and Richard A. Posner, "One-Sided Contracts in Competitive Consumer Markets," *Michigan Law Review* 104 (2006): 827–36.

99. In premarital agreements (also known as "antenuptial" and "prenuptial" agreements), the parties enter an agreement right before getting married, in which one or both parties waives rights relating to property or alimony upon divorce.

100. See Melvin Aron Eisenberg, "The Limits of Cognition and the Limits of Contract," *Stanford Law Review* 47 (1995): 211–59.

101. With restrictive covenants, employees agree to restrict where they work after their present employment is terminated, restrictions usually in terms of not working in the same industry/field, and covering some geographical range and duration.

102. In surrogacy agreements, a woman agrees to carry a child for other intended parents. Surrogates are often divided into "gestational surrogates," who are not genetically related to the children they carry, and "traditional surrogates," who are egg donors for the resulting children as well as carriers. Statutes and case-law are somewhat more inclined to enforce the parental rights of intended parents against surrogates when the carrier is a gestational surrogate.

103. This is separate from the objections some raise to enforce surrogacy contracts based on the alleged exploitation involved. E.g., Wertheimer, *Exploitation,* 96–122; Alan Wertheimer, "Exploitation and Commercial Surrogacy," *Denver University Law Review* 74 (1997): 1215–29.

104. E.g., Russell Korobkin, "Bounded Rationality, Standard Form Contracts, and Unconscionability," *University of Chicago Law Review* 70 (2003): 1203–95.

105. Economic theories are not entirely indifferent to consent, but tend to be satisfied by the "hypothetical consent" they claim for wealth (or utility) maximization and the "revealed preferences" based on actual choices. See, e.g., Richard A. Posner, *The Economics of Justice* (Cambridge, MA: Harvard University Press, 1981), 88–103.

106. Charles Fried, *Contract as Promise: A Theory of Contractual Obligation* (Cambridge, MA: Harvard University Press, 1981); Randy E. Barnett, "A Consent Theory of Contract," *Columbia Law Review* 86 (1986): 269–321.

107. Fried, *Contract as Promise*, 1, 2. Fried does not deny the value or validity of imposing (what he would consider) noncontractual liability, for example, when "people . . . give assurances that cause foreseeable harm . . . ." He continues: "Justice often requires relief and adjustment in cases of accidents in and round the contracting process . . . ." Ibid., 24.

108. Fried, *Contract as Promise*, 42–43.

109. See Richard Craswell, "Contract Law, Default Rules, and the Philosophy of Promising," *Michigan Law Review* 88 (1989): 489–529, at 511–29.

110. See Jody S. Kraus, "Philosophy of Contract Law," in Jules Coleman and Scott Shapiro, eds., *The Oxford Handbook of Jurisprudence & Philosophy of Law* (Oxford: Oxford University Press, 2002), 687–751, at 705–06 and n. 38.

111. See Barnett, "A Consent Theory of Contract," 269.

112. See, e.g., Robertson, "The Limits of Voluntariness in Contract," 203–04. For the argument that Barnett's theory is susceptible to many of the same criticisms as Fried's theory, see Craswell, "Contract Law, Default Rules, and the Philosophy of Promising," 523–28.

113. This point has been made by a number of other commentators. For an excellent recent article on the topic, see Robertson, "The Limits of Voluntariness in Contract."

114. In the lament of one commentator, the idea of contract as the "voluntary exchange . . . between autonomous individuals" has become "vestigial." Radin, "Boilerplate Today," 196. That commentator continued: "The idea of voluntary willingness first decayed into consent, then into assent, then into the mere possibility or opportunity for assent, then to merely fictional assent, then to mere efficient rearrangement of entitlements without any consent or assent." Ibid.

Bibliography

Alexander, Larry. "The Moral Magic of Consent (II)." *Legal Theory* 2 (1996): 165–74.

American Law Institute. *Restatement of the Law: Restitution and Unjust Enrichment, Tentative Draft No. 1*, April 6, 2001.

——, *Restatement (Second) of Contracts* (1981).

Aristotle. *Nicomachean Ethics.* In *The Complete Works of Aristotle,* edited by Jonathan Barnes. Princeton, NJ: Princeton University Press, 1984, vol. 2, 1729–1867.

Barnett, Randy E. "A Consent Theory of Contract." *Columbia Law Review* 86 (1986): 269–321.

——, "...And Contractual Consent." *Southern California Interdisciplinary Law Journal* 3 (1993): 421–44.

——, "Consenting to Form Contracts." *Fordham Law Review* 71 (2002): 627–45.

Bebchuk, Lucian A. & Richard A. Posner. "One-Sided Contracts in Competitive Consumer Markets." *Michigan Law Review* 104 (2006): 827–36.

Benson, Peter. "Contract as a Transfer of Ownership." *William and Mary Law Review* 48 (2007): 1673–1731.

Birmingham, Robert L. "Holmes on 'Peerless': Raffles v. Wichelhaus and the Objective Theory of Contract." University of Pittsburgh Law Review 47 (1985): 183–204.

Craswell, Richard. "Contract Law, Default Rules, and the Philosophy of Promising." *Michigan Law Review* 88 (1989): 489–529.

——, "Property Rules and Liability Rules in Unconscionability and Related Doctrines." *University of Chicago Law Review* 60 (1993): 1–65.

Eisenberg, Melvin Aron. "The Limits of Cognition and the Limits of Contract." *Stanford Law Review* 47 (1995): 211–59.

Epstein, Richard A. "Unconscionability: A Critical Reappraisal." *Journal of Law and Economics* 18 (1975): 293–315.

Farnsworth, E. Allan. *Contracts,* 4th ed. New York: Aspen Publishers, 2004.

Fried, Barbara H. "What's Morality Got to Do With It?" *Harvard Law Review Forum* 120 (2007): 53–61, http://www.harvardlawreview.org/forum/issues/120/jan07/bfried.pdf.

Fried, Charles. *Contract as Promise: A Theory of Contractual Obligation.* Cambridge, MA: Harvard University Press, 1981.

Fuller, Lon L. "Consideration and Form." *Columbia Law Review* 41 (1941): 799–824.

Gilmore, Grant. *The Death of Contract,* 2nd ed. Columbus, OH: Ohio State University Press, 1995.

Hillman, Robert A. "Online Boilerplate: Would Mandatory Website Disclosure of E-Standard Terms Backfire?" *Michigan Law Review* 104 (2006): 837–56.

Hurd, Heidi M. "The Moral Magic of Consent." *Legal Theory* 2 (1996): 121–46.

Ibbetson, David J. *A Historical Introduction to the Law of Obligations.* Oxford: Oxford University Press, 1999.

Kahneman, Daniel, Paul Slovic, and Amos Tversky (eds.), *Judgment Under Uncertainty: Heuristics and Biases.* Cambridge: Cambridge University Press, 1982.

Korobkin, Russell. "Bounded Rationality, Standard Form Contracts, and Unconscionability." *University of Chicago Law Review* 70 (2003): 1203–95.

Kraus, Jody S. "Philosophy of Contract Law." In *The Oxford Handbook of Jurisprudence & Philosophy of Law,* edited by Jules Coleman and Scott Shapiro. Oxford: Oxford University Press, 2002, 687–751.

Kreitner, Roy. "The Gift Beyond the Grave: Revisiting the Question of Consideration." *Columbia Law Review* 101 (2001): 1876–1957.

Kronman, Anthony J. "Contract Law and Distributive Justice." *Yale Law Journal* 89 (1980): 472–511.

Leff, Arthur Allen. "Contract as Thing." *American University Law Review* 19 (1970): 131–57.

Llewellyn, Karl N. *The Common Law Tradition: Deciding Appeals.* Boston: Little, Brown and Company, 1960.

Marotta-Wurgler, Florencia. "What's in a Standard Form Contract? An Empirical Analysis of Software License Agreements." *Journal of Empirical Legal Studies* 4 (2007): 677–713.

Posner, Richard A. *The Economics of Justice.* Cambridge, MA: Harvard University Press, 1981.

Pufendorf, Samuel. *The Political Writings of Samuel Pufendorf,* edited by Craig L. Carr. Oxford: Oxford University Press, 1994.

Radin, Margaret Jane. "Boilerplate Today: The Rise of Modularity and the Waning of Consent." In *Boilerplate: The Foundation of Market Contracts,* edited by Omri Ben-Shahar. Cambridge: Cambridge University Press, 2007, 189–99.

Raz, Joseph "On the Authority and Interpretation of Constitutions: Some Preliminaries." In *Constitutionalism,* edited by Larry Alexander. Cambridge: Cambridge University Press, 1998, 152–193.

Robertson, Andrew. "The Limits of Voluntariness in Contract." *Melbourne University Law Review* 29 (2005): 179–217.

Schwartz, Alan. "A Reexamination of Nonsubstantive Unconscionability." *Virginia Law Review* 63 (1977): 1053–83.

Simpson, A. W. Brian. *A History of the Common Law of Contract: The Rise of the Action of Assumpsit.* Oxford: Clarendon Press, 1975.

Slawson, W. David. "Standard Form Contracts and Democratic Control of Lawmaking Power." *Harvard Law Review* 84 (1971): 529–66.

Sunstein, Cass R. "Behavioral Analysis of Law." *University of Chicago Law Review* 65 (1997): 1175–95.

——, ed., *Behavioral Law & Economics.* Cambridge: Cambridge University Press, 2000.

Thayer, J. B. "*Laesio Enormis.*" *Kentucky Law Journal* 25 (1937): 321–41.

Wertheimer, Alan. *Coercion.* Princeton, NJ: Princeton University Press, 1987.

——, *Exploitation.* Princeton, NJ: Princeton University Press, 1996.

——, "Exploitation and Commercial Surrogacy." *Denver University Law Review* 74 (1997): 1215–29.

——, "Remarks on Coercion and Exploitation." *Denver University Law Review* 74 (1997): 889–906.

——, "What is Consent? And Is It Important?" *Buffalo Criminal Law Review*, 3 (2000): 557–83.

Winn, Jane K. and Brian H. Bix. "Diverging Perspectives on Electronic Contracting in the US and EU." *Cleveland State Law Review* 54 (2006): 175–90.

Zimmermann, Reinhard. *The Law of Obligations: Roman Foundations of the Civilian Tradition.* Oxford: Oxford University Press, 1990, 259–70.

Consent With Inducements: The Case of Body Parts and Services

Janet Radcliffe Richards[1]

Introduction

Some years ago, when news of kidney selling by live vendors first broke in the West, politicians from all points of the political compass rushed to declare it illegal, and medical organizations were equally quick to pronounce their professional anathema. The reaction was so immediate as to allow hardly any time for debate, but as challenges appeared to this first response justifications for prohibition of organ sales began to proliferate, and many of the arguments depended on claims about invalidity of consent. Analysis of these arguments can throw light on the matter of consent in general, as well as on the broader issue of payment for the use of bodies and body parts.

Consent derives its importance from the fact that law and convention place a circle of presumptive inviolability around individuals. There is, of course, endless scope for difference of opinion about how wide and how impregnable that circle should be, and societies differ in their judgments about where the rights of the individual should end and where those of other individuals or the wider society should begin. In some societies many individuals may lack full rights even over such fundamental matters as bodily integrity (for instance, there may be no such thing as rape within marriage), while in others the range of individual rights stretches far beyond this. But wherever the boundary of individual control is established, consent is presumptively necessary for its transgression. And, specifically to the point here, it is also generally sufficient. Because the purpose of the boundary is to protect the bounded individual, the consent of that individual for any breach generally settles the matter of its acceptability. To whatever extent the law gives you a right to privacy within your own home, others may not intrude without your consent; but if you do consent, that provides exemption from whatever blame or penalties their intrusion would otherwise incur, and makes legitimate what would otherwise be an offense against you.

There are, however, a few contexts where this *prima facie* sufficiency of consent seems to be regarded as breaking down. Even though some matter looks as though it should come well within the accepted circle of individual control, and even though apparently valid consent has been given for its breach, it may be illegal, or regarded as unacceptable or wrong, for others to act on this consent.[2]

The most familiar cases of this kind concern actions that would not involve illegality if you did them yourself, but which others may not do to you even with your consent. So, for instance, suicide and attempted suicide ceased to be criminal offenses in the United Kingdom when the 1961 Suicide Act was passed, and they were to that extent moved out of the area of public interest and returned to the circle of individual control. But the same act explicitly stated that "aiding, abetting, counselling or procuring" the suicide of another remained criminal offenses, and it also left untouched the classification of euthanasia as murder even if the person killed had consented to, or even pleaded for, death. Similarly, self-harm is not generally regarded as a criminal offense, unless its purpose is to commit some other offense such as avoiding conscription or defrauding an insurance company, and to that extent the law regards individuals' treatment of themselves as a matter for personal decision. But there are still limits to the amount of harm others legally can do to you, even with your consent. This shows in legal rulings about harm caused during consensual sadomasochistic activity[3] and in the uncertain legal situation of surgeons who operate on patients seeking the amputation of normal but unwanted limbs. Even willing organ donation for the benefit of others is restricted. Surgeons refused to accept the consent of a man whose first kidney donation to his son had failed and who then wanted to sacrifice his second kidney for another attempt,[4] and the sacrifice of an organ essential for life is legally out of the question. "A man may declare himself ready to die for another, but the surgeon must not take him at his word."[5]

There are well-known problems of principle about such matters. Should they be regarded as remnants of paternalism, arguably out of place in a liberal society that regards individuals as the appropriate judges of what constitutes their own interests, or can they be given some other justification in terms of public interest? Interesting as this problem is, however, I shall not discuss it here, because the subject of this chapter is an even more puzzling one. It concerns contexts where it is already accepted, in general, that consent should be sufficient to allow what has been consented to, but where the situation is regarded as radically changed by the involvement of payment.

This is what makes the kidney-selling issue so interesting. Although some kinds of organ donation are forbidden outright by law, living kidney donation does not come into that category. You may give one of your kidneys to a friend or relative who needs one, because your other kidney will be able to take over the function of the missing one, and the law has accepted that the minimal risk of long-term harm is justified by the gain to the recipient. In most countries, however, consent to the very same operation may not be accepted if money is involved in the transaction. And although this issue provides a particularly striking illustration of the matter, it is part of a much wider controversy about payment for body parts or services involving bodies. It arises in debates about organ, tissue, and blood donation, as well as gamete donation, surrogacy, prostitution, and nontherapeutic medical research.

It is difficult to discuss the problem in a general way, because there is a huge range of both opinion and legislation about all these issues. About most of them there are differences of opinion about whether the procedure in question should be allowed at all, whether it should be allowed only without payment, or whether there is nothing wrong with payment. The variation is expressed partly in laws and partly in feelings, and there is variation within societies as well as between them. Individuals who feel strongly about payment in some of the areas may feel less strongly, or have no objection at all, to payment in others. Tracking these complexities would be an enormous project.

Fortunately, however, the variations are not relevant to the central problem here, which is one of general principle. It can be understood as concerning a particular kind of conditional. *If* you regard it as appropriate that some matter (for example, living kidney donation) should normally be regarded as lying within the circle of individual decision, so that the individual's consent is both necessary and sufficient for the appropriate action by others (the surgeon may proceed on its basis), *but* you also think that payment should not be allowed (the surgeon may not accept the consent if payment is involved), how can you justify the distinction?

It will be useful to concentrate the discussion on the sale of kidneys by living vendors, because this is the context in which there is most unanimity of feeling and where the debate has been most intensively developed. The discussion should, however, be regarded as applicable to all these topics.

The Problem

Once it had been established that a kidney could be removed with minimal risk of lasting harm to the donor, and immunosuppression had solved the problem of rejection, it was only a matter of time before commercial opportunities were spotted. Since anything that can be given can also be sold, and most things that are ours to give are also ours to sell, the rapid development of a trade between people who were desperate for kidneys on the one hand and money on the other should probably have been anticipated from the start. Apparently, however, it was not, and when the issue first came to widespread public attention in the West, the reaction was one of horror. In the United Kingdom this happened in 1991, when it was revealed that two Turkish peasants had come to Harley Street—the London abode of expensive doctors with correspondingly affluent patients—to sell kidneys for patients in need of transplants. There was no law against such transactions at the time, but the immediate reaction, from both politicians and the medical profession, was one of outrage. The exchange was immediately halted, the doctors concerned were struck off the medical register even though there had been no explicit policy to prevent their acting in this way, and legislation to ensure it never happened again was rushed through the UK Parliament with almost unprecedented speed. Professional bodies rapidly declared their absolute opposition, and soon payment for kidney donation was illegal in most of the world.

But what exactly was the objection? The rhetoric was about the greedy rich and exploited poor, but although the Harley Street connection provided a plausible connection with the rich, not many people would say that using whatever money you had to try to save your life—or even to escape the crushing constraints of life on dialysis—constituted a paradigm case of greed. Most people would probably scrape together everything they had for the chance of escaping death; and anyway, if greed were the issue, the objection should apply equally to all the treatments the rich can buy in Harley Street and other private clinics throughout the world. The real objection was obviously not about the access of the rich to treatment, but the poor as the source of the organs.

The trouble was, it was about the poor themselves who had made the decision to sell. Later, when people became aware of the commercial value of transplant organs, rumors began to spread about kidnapping and murder, or people who had come to rich countries for jobs and then woken up in hospital with a kidney missing. But even if it had been reasonable to credit all these stories, they were about people whose kidneys had been stolen or taken by force. The Turkish men in London had not been murdered or kidnapped, or even, as far as we know, put under pressure by the intended recipients or their agents. They had volunteered their kidneys, and we even knew why—or at least, the reasons they gave. One of them had a daughter with leukemia, and was trying to save her life. He could not begin to afford the necessary treatment at home, and selling a kidney seemed to provide his only hope.

Furthermore, if his daughter had herself needed a kidney, there would have been no problem about accepting his consent to donate one of his. In trying to sell his kidney to provide treatment for her, he was making exactly the same offer with exactly the same motivation. Why, then, was it regarded as obvious that the transplant doctors should have known they should not accept his consent? Why was there such widespread support for the new laws prohibiting payment? How can the involvement of money justify distinguishing between the acceptability of consent for procedures that are otherwise identical?

Feelings about the matter were strong, and a great many attempts have been made to justify the prohibition of payment for organ donation. I have dealt with many of these elsewhere.[6] Most of this article is specifically concerned with claims that the problem about payment lies in its invalidating the vendors' apparent consent.

Invalid Consent

The requirement that consent should be valid is an essential element of its being required at all. Since someone with your consent to act within your protected circle may do what would otherwise be an offense against you, a necessary element of protecting your rights is making sure that anyone who claims to have your consent really has it. The standards of validity required are themselves a substantive part of any society's specification of the extent of individual rights.

The overall challenge is to find a justification for rejecting consent to transactions that involve payment, when consent to the same transaction without payment would be acceptable. It is now generally accepted that, in order to be valid, consent must be given by a competent person, that it must be freely given, and that it must be informed. The consent-based arguments against organ selling make the connection with payment by claiming that the poverty of would-be vendors results in the failure of one or more of these criteria.

Competence

The first line of argument uses poverty as the basis for doubt about prospective vendors' competence. "Since paid organ donors will always be relatively poor, and may be underprivileged and undereducated, the donor's full understanding of [the] risks cannot be guaranteed."[7]

In clinical practice, the requirements for mental competence (capacity) are that the consenter should be able to understand, retain, and weigh up the treatment information in order to reach a decision. At present, those requirements are interpreted as weighted strongly in favor of crediting the individual with capacity. Adults must be presumed competent until demonstrated otherwise, and the level of competence required must be no higher than is required for understanding the issue at hand. People of borderline competence should be helped to achieve as much understanding as possible. The requirements for understanding have themselves also become increasingly minimal. There are no requirements that beliefs should be true, or the weighing-up process regarded as rational.[8]

Nobody seriously applying these standards could defend a noncompetence justification of prohibition. The requirements allow no escape from the need to assess people individually, and the vast majority of potential vendors would certainly reach the required standards. And anyway, people from the same uneducated groups are routinely treated as competent to consent in all other contexts—including unpaid organ donation. However, criteria for the assessment of competence are not morally neutral. They are themselves expressions of moral views, and the standard currently accepted reflects a particularly strong version of the liberal idea that all individuals should be free to determine both what constitutes their own good and how best to achieve it. But many people of broadly liberal inclinations think that even though individuals should always determine what *constitutes* their interests, it may be justifiable to go against their immediate wishes if a mistaken or inadequate understanding of the workings of the world results in mistaken beliefs about *how to achieve* those interests. It is arguable that such "weak paternalism" may often be justified, and many doctors admit to sometimes acting without consent in order to achieve what patients themselves would count as their long-term interests. And, they claim, those patients are grateful afterwards.

Suppose, then, the noncompetence argument against organ selling is interpreted as intending a claim that the criteria for competence should be narrowed, to the extent that a serious lack of education and knowledge may result in noncompetence and justify paternalist intervention. There would still be a considerable leap to the conclusion that we should treat everyone who wanted to sell an organ as coming into this category, but could this at least be the first step, of showing that anyone noncompetent in this way should not be allowed to consent to organ selling?

This seems to be the intention behind the noncompetence claim. The trouble is, however, that a judgment of noncompetence can never in itself entail that whatever was noncompetently consented to should actually be prevented from happening. All it entails is that *consent* cannot be used as part of the justification of whatever action is proposed, and that the decision must be made on some other basis. And whereas in general it is accepted that "the absence of consent has much the same effect as a refusal,"[9] this is not so in the case of the noncompetent. If they are not able to decide for themselves, someone else must decide for them. The generally accepted principle is that the decision must be made in their best interests.

This may not seem to make much difference. It is widely believed that kidney selling cannot possibly be in anyone's interests, and the impression is reinforced by frequent reports from campaigning organizations and investigative journalists who expose exploitation, cheating, shoddy operations, lack of counseling and follow-up, and a train of vendors with damaged health and no lasting benefit to compensate. Whether the would-be vendors recognize it or not, it may well be argued, the course they are trying to pursue is far too dangerous to be reasonable. We, who know better, must save them from themselves for (what we hope they will eventually agree is) their own sake. "State paternalism grounded in social beneficence dictates that the abject poor should be protected from selling parts of their bodies to help their sad lot in life."[10]

One difficulty about this line of argument is that there are problems about the claimed evidence. Even if there is little reason to doubt individual stories about harm to vendors, what is less clear is how representative they are. It is easy to find evidence if you look only on one side, and most of the research seems to have been done by people strongly opposed to organ selling. As far as I know there is no systematic research into how many vendors are satisfied with the transaction—though there is anecdotal evidence to suggest that many are.

But even if most of the vendors do end up worse off, why exactly is this? Living organ donation is now so safe that many surgeons actively recommend it, which they would hardly do if they expected a string of dead or damaged donors. The only intrinsic difference between paid and unpaid donation is that the vendor receives something in return—which, to all appearances, is a positive advantage. This suggests that if kidney vendors are in practice disproportionately harmed, the reasons must lie not in the loss of a kidney in itself, but in the surrounding circumstances. No doubt these are complex, but it is striking that all the harms alleged—cheating, careless medical practice and the rest—are exactly the ones you would expect of a black market. In a black market there can be no controls on standards of care. Vendors at present cannot rely even on assessments of their competence to consent, let alone on the care with health and well-being currently given to most unpaid donors or the financial and life-planning advice that could be enforced if their activities were legal.

There is, of course, some minimal risk in kidney donation, whether paid or not. Whether any risk is worth taking, however, depends on the reward balanced on the other side, and if the rewards are the amounts of money that could transform a family's life, it is hard to see why the minimal risk of a properly performed nephrectomy should not be well worth taking. This chapter is being written during the financial crisis of 2008–09, and it is easy to imagine that many of its victims might willingly sacrifice a kidney to prevent something as catastrophic as the repossession of their homes. (You might consider what price would induce you to part with your own kidney.) The expected benefits would be even greater to the desperately poor, who might see in selling a kidney the only hope of making anything of their wretched lives, and perhaps even of surviving, than to the relatively rich with mortgage problems. You might rather think, contra Dossetor and Mackinavel, that the poorer you were, the more rational it would be to risk selling a kidney, and that even if you were not competent to make that decision yourself, a benevolent paternalist might well, in principle, push you in that direction.

This is why the noncompetence case for prohibition could not be made even if it were conceded that the appropriate standard of competence was that of the weak paternalist, and even if some reasonable way could be found of making the leap from widespread noncompetence to total prohibition. Prohibition prevents many people—both donors and recipients—from making an exchange that could in principle be enormously beneficial to both. The only thing that prevents these benefits from being realized is the illegality that abandons both sides to the mercies of the black market and results in the harms that the campaigners report.

Prohibition has not stopped the trade, and it never will: as long as there are people who are desperate for kidneys on the one hand and money on the other, the two sides will get together somehow. This means that illegality does not have only the negative harm of obstructing individuals in the pursuit of what they may rationally perceive as their own good, but also the positive harm of exposing people who pursue that good in spite of the law to quite unnecessary levels of risk. Whether or not a coherent justification can be found for prohibition, the argument from invalidity of consent through incompetence certainly cannot provide it.

Voluntariness

The second requirement for valid consent is that it should be voluntarily (freely, autonomously) given. Arguments claiming that consent for kidney selling fails to meet this standard depend on the idea of coercion, and they take two main forms: coercion by unrefusable offers and coercion by poverty.

Unrefusable Offers

In another of his early papers on the subject, Robert Sells objects to any "externally applied constriction of an individual's right to choose not to donate," and includes in this category "all cases where a person sells one of his organs during life," because "here the financial benefits have such an impact on the life of the donor and his family as to be irresistible: the element of voluntariness of donation must be at least compromised, or, in extreme cases, abolished."[11] The idea that a good enough offer constitutes a kind of coercion appears in many contexts where payment is at issue.[12]

It is important to distinguish this line of argument from the previous one, about noncompetence. The argument as presented here emphasizes the amount of money offered relative to the incomes of the people who might be tempted to sell, and one concern might be that the poor would be so dazzled by the prospect of riches as to become incapable of rational thought. If so, the appropriate kind of discussion would be the one outlined in the previous section. The argument here must be regarded as distinct, applying to people already deemed competent.

If significant financial benefits constitute a compromise or abolition of voluntariness in some sense, what is that sense? Presumably the idea is something along these lines. If you are a prospective vendor, you do not actually *want* to lose your kidney; you are proposing to do it *only because* of the prospect of payment. If the offer is impressive, it leaves you with *very little choice* about whether to accept it, and if it is impressive enough, it leaves you with *no choice* at all. (This seems to catch Sells's intuitions about the difference between compromising and abolishing voluntariness.) All of these are, indeed, perfectly good colloquial descriptions of such a situation, which is why it may seem that the voluntariness criterion cannot be met. The relevant question here, however, is not whether the choice is in *some* sense nonvoluntary, but whether it is so in any sense that would work as a general criterion for invalidity of consent.

Consider first the idea that your consent is not truly voluntary because you do not really want to lose your kidney. If this is understood as a claim that you find the prospect of losing your kidney intrinsically undesirable, it is almost certainly true: nobody actually relishes the idea of being opened up and having organs cut out. But the whole point of offering any inducement, such as payment, is to get you to agree to something you do not like *in itself* by making it part of a package that is, *all things considered*, preferable to simply avoiding the element you do not like. If you dislike the idea of parting with your kidney, but are willing to do it in return for enough money to start a business or send your children to school, you have already decided that doing without the school or the business is *worse* than doing without the kidney. It would be extraordinarily perverse for anyone to claim, on the basis of a concern for voluntariness, that because you disliked one element of the package your consent should be declared invalid, and you should be left in a situation whose elements you liked even less. And, of course, our criteria for valid consent obviously imply nothing of the sort, or they would prevent our accepting dreary jobs in return for good salaries, or selling anything that we did not positively want to get rid of. If the argument seems to work, it is only because of an equivocation between wanting something *in itself* and wanting *all things considered* a package that contains it.

What about the other idea, then, that a good enough offer cannot count as voluntary, because it leaves you with no choice about whether to accept it? Once again, however, ordinary English is unhelpful as a guide, since—oddly enough—the expression is never used except when there is in fact a choice. If you are asked why you jumped into a raging torrent and your choice did not come into the matter, you do not say, "I had no choice": you deny the implication that you made a choice and say, "I didn't jump; I slipped"—or whatever. If you say, "I had no choice; my child had fallen in," you obviously did have a choice: what you mean is that the option of not jumping in was unthinkable. Similarly, if you say, "I had no choice about selling the kidney; they offered me enough money to get my family out of poverty," what you mean is that it would have been ridiculous for you to take the option—still open to you—of keeping your kidney and remaining in poverty. If having no choice in this sense compromised or abolished voluntariness in a way that invalidated consent, it would follow that valid consent could occur only when there was hardly anything to choose between the available options. You could not validly consent to marry the suitor whose merits were out of sight of those of his rivals: your consent to accept one of the available candidates would be valid only if they were so much of a muchness that there was nothing to choose between them.

This would actually be quite a useful line of argument for opponents of organ selling. It would mean that the only way to make consent voluntary and therefore valid would be to reduce the price until it was unclear that the transaction was worthwhile, by when the deal would have become so pointless that no one would consent to it anyway. But this is obviously a non-starter as a serious account of voluntariness and validity of consent. The whole point of inducements is to make people willing to consent, and the more unrefusable the inducement, the more reason there would be to suspect any *other* choice of being invalid.

Coercion by Poverty

It is really pretty obvious, as soon as the matter is addressed directly, that increasing someone's range of options—which is what an offer of payment always does—could not in itself constitute any kind of coercion or restriction of freedom. The next line of argument against organ selling—not usually differentiated, but in fact radically different—avoids this problem by seeing the coercion as lying not in *the offer of money,* but in *the background poverty* that makes the offer attractive. "Surely abject poverty . . . can have no equal when it comes to coercion of individuals to do things – take risks – which their affluent fellow-citizens would not want to take? Can decisions taken under the influence of this terrifying coercion be considered autonomous? Surely not . . . ."[13] "A truly voluntary and noncoerced consent is also unlikely . . . . [T]he desperate financial need of the donor is an obvious and clear economic coercion."[14] And, it is implied, since coerced consent is not genuine, the choice should not be allowed.

Coercion by circumstances, so described, involves a situation in which you consent to something intrinsically undesirable because it is the best of a severely limited range of options. Once again, however, this would be hopeless as a general criterion for invalidity of consent. It does not normally occur to us that people coerced by circumstances into doing things they would not otherwise do should have their consent regarded as invalid. If you have cancer, with the choice between risking its unchecked progression and putting up with pretty nasty treatments, nobody would think of arguing that the narrow range of options made your consent to the treatment invalid. Nor, closer to the point here, would anyone regard as invalid your consent to donate a kidney to your sister on the grounds that you had been as-it-were coerced into making the offer by the misfortune of her kidney failure. Once again, it is obvious why a voluntariness criterion could not work as an invalidator of consent in such situations. If you are concerned by someone's being forced by constricted circumstances into making an intrinsically unwelcome choice, you cannot improve the situation by taking away the best of their options and leaving them with something even less welcome. (And if it is argued that the constriction of circumstances leaves people incapable of making rational decisions, the issue is once again competence and paternalism, not voluntariness.)

However, there obviously remains a puzzle. If none of these suggested interpretations of the voluntariness criterion for validity makes any sense, how should it be interpreted? A full understanding of what is going wrong in these (and many other) spurious coercion-by-circumstances arguments is probably best achieved through analysis of contexts in which coercion does properly support a judgment of invalidity.

Paradigm cases of consent invalidated by coercion involve deliberate coercers who deliberately curtail the options of their victims until the best one left is the one the coercers want them to take. So, for instance, consider a girl on her way to school at the beginning of term, carrying her carefully finished summer project, and also her bag of marbles. A couple of boys from the same school waylay her, grab the project, and threaten to throw it into the river unless she agrees to hand over her marbles. Before this incident she could keep both the work and the marbles; now her options have been lessened, and she has to choose between them. She chooses to keep the work and gives the boys the marbles. But if she can persuade the teacher of what happened, the teacher will say her agreement to hand them over was not valid, and insist on their being restored.

Or suppose your daughter is kidnapped and the kidnapper says he will shoot her unless you sign a document agreeing to sell your house, for next to nothing, to a company that wants the site for building. Beforehand, you had the child and the house; now you have to choose between them. After the child is restored the company denies any knowledge of the kidnap and wants to enforce your signed agreement to sell, but if you can convince the judge of what happened, your consent to the sale will be declared invalid and your house returned to you. Or, if it is too late and the demolition has already gone ahead, you will be given compensation.

What is the essence of these cases that justifies the decision that the consent is invalid and should not be accepted? How do they differ from the spurious arguments so far discussed? First, note that they have nothing whatever to do with the overall range of options available. Maybe the girl was rich and the boys had hardly any toys; maybe you had dozens of houses and the developers wanted to build a much-needed clinic for a deprived area. Such facts would be entirely irrelevant to the question of whether the consent was valid. The essence of the paradigm cases is the involvement of actual coercers who set about a deliberate restriction of options in order to get their victims' consent to what they (the coercers) are trying to achieve, and which they could not achieve without that consent. Furthermore, restriction of options alone is not enough to invalidate the resulting consent: the restriction must also be illicit. If the boys had got the marbles by saying the girl could not come to their party unless she agreed to hand them over, or the developers persuaded you to sell by threatening to lower the value of your house even further by building a supermarket next door, they would have been within their accepted rights and there would have been no grounds for declaring the consent invalid. In other words, the essence of these cases is not the overall range of options or even the reduction of an existing set, but coercion in contravention of accepted standards by the person obtaining the consent.

This is quite unlike the matter of metaphorical coercion by poverty, for many reasons. For one thing, the declaration of invalidity in the paradigm cases refers to the existing standards of the relevant society, whereas the claim that society as a whole has left someone with too few options demands justification in terms of appropriate, highly contested, political theories. For another, the declaration of invalidity in the paradigm cases is intended as a means of restorative justice against the person who used illicit coercion to achieve consent, which is quite different from general claims about an unfair situation for which the beneficiary of the resulting consent is in no way responsible.

Still, it may be argued, even if the situation of the poor is different from that of the people who have been wrongfully coerced in the paradigm cases, both do involve the unjust deprivation of options. If the coercion that leads to judgments of invalid consent involves lessening your range of options until the best one left is the one the coercer wants you to take, surely it is clear why poverty, although having no intentions of any kind, might count in an extended, metaphorical sense as a coercer. Poverty, it may be claimed, is like the bullies and the kidnapper, in making the victim choose what other people, "affluent fellow-citizens" with a wider range of options, would not choose. That is why the consent of the poor to sell their organs should be regarded as invalid, just as your consent to sell your house and the girl's to hand over her marbles should be.

However, the relevant issue here is not just whether there is injustice of some sort in the situation, but the specific matter of invalidity: the *point* of declaring consent invalid. Once again, the concept of invalidity is an integral part of the requirement of consent. Anyone who acts within your protected boundary without consent has committed an offense against you, which—as an implication of society's giving you that set of rights in the first place—will incur sanctions. Someone who wants to act within your boundary therefore has an interest in getting your consent, or at least giving others the impression that your consent has been given. The kidnapping syndicate wanted a document with your signature on it, authorizing their taking over your house, which without your consent they would not be allowed to do. What the court does in declaring your consent invalid is say that since the coercion that brought about your consent was illicit, the situation must be treated *as though the consent had not happened.* Society will support your keeping of the house and will probably also punish the coercer for wrongful pressure or, if the house has already been demolished, will treat it as a wrongful taking of what was rightfully yours and demand restitution. The consent is discounted, your original range of options is (more or less) restored, and the illicit coercer, who was trying to benefit from it, is thwarted.

This may not seem enough to break down the analogy with coercion by poverty. Surely if people have been forced by wrongful poverty to make unwelcome choices, we should count their consent as invalid too? If this seems plausible, note two further points about the paradigm cases of coercion. First, because the root of the issue is the contravention of individual rights, the recognition of invalidity is sought by or on behalf of the people whose consent has been wrongfully obtained. They agreed to something they would not have agreed to but for the coercion, and they now want that agreement recognized as void. Second, this will happen only when the situation has changed and the clutches of the coercer have been escaped. Once your child is free of the kidnapper you want to withdraw your consent to the sale of your house, *but until that happens you do not.* Suppose the police appeared on the kidnapping scene and prevented you from signing the document, perhaps with the outcome that your child was shot. They might have good public policy reasons for doing this—they might want to demonstrate to other would-be kidnappers that they could not get away with their nefarious plots—but it would be preposterous for them to claim that they were doing it because the consent you were trying to give would be invalid. Once again, the whole point of declaring invalidity is to protect the alleged consenter, and here the police would actually be compounding the wrong done to you by constricting still further the range of options already constricted by the kidnapper. The point of the invalidity declaration arises only later, when the coercers want society to hold you to the agreement you made when your options were unfairly constricted, and you want society to refuse and restore the status quo ante.

This shows why, even if you stretch to its limits the already tortured analogy between coercion by poverty and coercion by a wrongly acting individual who is trying to get your consent by illicit means, you still cannot reach the conclusion that poverty-coerced consent should not be accepted. Since the metaphorical coercer (poverty) is still present, and the individual is making the best choice among a still-constricted range of options, disallowing the choice is like preventing you from meeting the demands of the kidnapper while he still has your child.

This is why it is quite wrong to say that the poor should be protected from selling their kidneys, "preferably, of course, by being lifted out of poverty,"[15] but otherwise by the complete prevention of sales. It implies that prohibition and lifting out of poverty are unequally desirable variations on the same general theme, whereas they are, in the relevant sense, direct opposites. Protecting the poor from kidney selling by removing poverty works by increasing the options until something more attractive is available—the equivalent of getting rid of the bullies or kidnapper. Prevention of sales, in itself, only closes a miserable range of options still further, which is like your being prevented by the police from making the choice that will save your child's life. To the metaphorical coercion of poverty is added the coercion of the supposed protector, who comes and takes away (what the prospective vendor sees as, and what may indeed well be) the best option that poverty has left.

There is also one final point to make about the voluntariness criterion for validity of consent, this time in contrast with the requirement of competence. Although the threshold for competence may be a matter of contention, the procedure for deciding whether some consent meets the relevant standard is more or less clear: you look at the person consenting and assess (some aspects of) their mental state. It may therefore be easy to slip into thinking that the second criterion for validity, of voluntariness, involves a kind of external version of the same process: you look at how many constraints there are in a person's circumstances and see whether there is enough freedom to count as reaching the threshold for valid consent. But the analysis of the paradigm cases shows that the issue is radically different in kind. The matter to be assessed is not *the situation of the person consenting*, but *the behavior of the person obtaining the consent*. There are certain things you must not do in your attempts to get consent, and if you do them you will be deemed to have acted without it. The complaint involved is specifically about a wrong action that requires restitution rather than about a less than ideal state of affairs, and the two are irreducibly different. Furthermore, the argument about coercion by poverty shows the positive harm that can result from conflating them. To argue that consent to payment for such things as organ selling is invalidated by the poverty of the sellers, and therefore should not be accepted, is to make matters even worse for people whose range of options is alleged to be already too constrained while giving the appearance—because the requirement of validity is a protection of individual rights—of actually helping them.

In ordinary circumstances, of course, this problem does not arise. When medical and other practitioners learn about valid consent, they learn that they should not put certain kinds of pressure on patients in order to get their consent. Claims that the voluntariness criterion justifies overriding the choices of competent people whose circumstances are less than ideal are, in practice, made only when justifications are being sought for disallowing decisions that are really objected to on quite other grounds. That is obviously what is going on in these debates about payment for body parts and services involving bodies.

Information

In light of this distinction between complaints about states of affairs and complaints about the actions of particular agents, it is also worth commenting briefly on the final condition for validity of consent, the information requirement—even though it does not seem to appear in the organ-selling debate. The idea of adequate information, too, is capable of two interpretations, supporting two quite different kinds of possible complaint. One question is about *how much someone ought (ideally) to know*, the other is about *how much the person seeking the consent ought to tell them.*

Again, these are irreducibly different. You could know a great deal about some matter but still not have been told something that someone else had a duty to tell you; conversely, the person receiving your consent could have told you all that was known about, say, the effects of some very new drug, and you would still know very little about it. And, as in the case of coercion, it is only the first that results in invalidity of consent. Obviously you can consent to something that nobody knows much about—going on expeditions to unexplored places, agreeing to innovative operations, and so on—and anyone determined to prevent you from taking risks of these kinds would need to justify doing so on the basis of some other ground than invalidity of consent. The relevant matter is not how much the consenter knows, but how much information the person receiving the consent should have given.

This again is well known in practice, and clear in law. "The patient is free to decide whether or not to submit to treatment recommended by the doctor and therefore the doctor impliedly contracts to provide information which is adequate to enable the patient to reach a balanced judgment...."[16] If a patient consents to, and is harmed by, treatment that would not have been consented to if the information had been given, compensation will be due. But if the two are confused, someone might be tempted to think that consent was invalid in cases where the consenter did not know enough, rather than when not enough information had been given. This happens quite often in the case of new treatments. For instance, "The most compelling argument against face transplants involves the risk factors. As with any new procedure, it's difficult to anticipate or calculate all the risks, which has caused some to question the validity of the informed consent process."[17] But once again, it is crucial to recognize that the purpose of declarations of invalidity is to protect the allegedly consenting individual. Individuals are entitled to decide about which risks they want to take, and to declare consent invalid on the grounds that nobody knew much about the matters in question would be a denial of that very entitlement.

It is interesting to note, given the failure of the competence and voluntariness criteria to establish any general invalidity of consent to body selling, that by the information criterion a good deal of the consent currently given by organ sellers may indeed be invalid. We know that vendors are often given inadequate support and counseling, and if such cases came to court their consent might well be judged invalidly given. But even if so, this could not be part of the overall argument for prohibition because it is, once again, the very illegality of organ selling, and its being confined to a black market, that means we cannot regulate the provision of information and cannot provide restitution when not enough is given.

The Roots of the Problem

To return again to the beginning, the problem being addressed in this chapter concerns the puzzling matter of attitudes to payment where bodies, body parts, and certain uses of bodies are concerned. In contexts where it is accepted that individuals may freely consent to the unpaid giving of these parts or services, there may nevertheless be objections to their consenting to exactly the same procedures where payment is involved. States vary in their laws—and individuals in their opinions—about which procedures come into this category, but the question here is just about the general conditional: *if* you think it is legitimate to give the body part or service in question, *but* you think it is not legitimate if money is involved, how can you justify the distinction?

In the context of organ selling, one set of attempts tries to make payment relevant by claiming that would-be vendors are bound to be poor and underprivileged, and that this makes their consent invalid. However, these arguments fail for the reasons already given, and this means that another justification must be sought for disallowing the sufficiency of consent by vendors when it is acceptable for donors. That presumably means showing either that the money somehow turns the matter into one of public interest rather than individual rights or that it puts the matter into the category of harms that are not allowable even with the person's full consent.

As already mentioned, I have gone into most of these other attempts elsewhere.[18] However, they do all seem to run into the difficulty described previously, of involving mistakes of reasoning that nobody would make in ordinary circumstances.[19] They are offered only in contexts where people are already convinced of the conclusions they want to defend and are hunting around for justifications. The whole debate falls into a pattern described (in another context) by John Stuart Mill:

> [If an opinion] were accepted as a result of argument, the refutation of the argument might shake the solidity of the conviction; but when it rests solely on feeling, the worse it fares in argumentative contest, the more persuaded its adherents are that their feeling must have some deeper ground, which the arguments do not reach; and while the feeling remains, it is always throwing up fresh entrenchments of argument to repair any breach in the old.[20]

The arguments in the organ-selling debate are presented ambiguously between *explanations* of why opponents feel so strongly that it should not be allowed and *justifications* of that opposition. The implication is that opponents were actually led to their conclusion by the application of the principles to which they appeal. But as one attempted justification after another is shown to fail—and to fail in a way that could not be overlooked without prior conviction of the rightness of the conclusion—it becomes clear that even if a justification of the policy of prohibition can eventually be found, the *explanation* of the impulse to ban organ selling must be different. It is also interesting not only that the feeling persists through the demolition of all the attempts at justification, but also that it is largely shared and understood even by people who think that prohibition cannot be justified. They may (as I do) accept that a properly regulated market could do a great deal of good for both recipients and vendors, and regard it as essential to regulate the trade to protect the inevitable participants, while still feeling that there is something deeply disturbing about the whole business.

This suggests another line of enquiry. Most of the familiar debate concentrates on candidate *justifications* for prohibition, but if those have nothing to do with the causes of the feeling that there is an enormous difference between giving and selling, what are those causes? *Why* do people—at least in Western societies—seem to feel that there is such a great difference between the two, and that there is something seriously unpleasant about the idea of organ selling? What difference between the selling and giving situations actually prompts these feelings? If that could be pinned down, it might throw light on the moral question of whether there was indeed some justification for prohibition.

Such an enquiry could at one level be a full-scale investigation in the social sciences, calling for comparisons of different groups with different cultural and religious backgrounds. But a similar kind of enquiry can be conducted, personally, by anyone who has these feelings. Because the debate has consisted of attempts at justification, it has concentrated on trying to make the differentiation in morally plausible terms; but the investigation of causes is not constrained in that way. We can consider *any* differences between the two situations and then construct thought experiments to see whether that difference produces the same feelings in other contexts of selling as opposed to giving.

So, for instance, we might try the hypothesis that we respond differently to the two kinds of cases because giving involves generosity and altruism, and selling does not. But if that were the case, why do we not have similar feelings about all cases of selling as opposed to giving? We applaud giving, but do not generally feel uncomfortable about selling. And, furthermore, withholding is just as much a failure of generosity as is selling, but we do not feel revulsion about the fact that most of us never make a living kidney donation. Anyway, if generosity is the issue, why do we feel differently—as most of us intuitively do—about a father who donates a kidney to his daughter and one who sells it to buy other treatment she needs just as urgently? From the point of view of his motivation, there is no difference.

Perhaps, then, the feeling might have to do with the lack of personal connection between donor and recipient that characterizes selling: perhaps we have deep, possibly evolved, intuitions about giving parts of ourselves only when there are already connections. But that, again, does not match the pattern of most people's feelings. For instance, the idea of so-called Samaritan donation—where living people offer kidneys to strangers—seems to generate quite different kinds of response from that of organ selling. Nor can this theory account for the apparent acceptability of "paired donations," where A wants to donate a kidney to B but is insufficiently well matched, and the same is true of C and D. If A matches D and C matches B, the two pairs may agree to do simultaneous, crossover donations. Such donations are conducted anonymously, and are therefore to strangers, but everyone seems to feel that the case is radically different from what it would be if A sold a kidney in order to buy treatment for B. If so, a direct connection between donor and recipient cannot be what prompts the feeling.

These suggestions represent only the beginning of a complicated enquiry; but it does seem that, over and over again, attempts to explain the involvement of money in terms of other aspects of the situation cannot account for the feelings. It does seem as though money as such is the problem. But why, when we normally regard money as a necessary, sensible, everything-improving aspect of ordinary life, facilitating complex exchanges that would otherwise not be possible?

Here is what seems to me the only possibility. The essential difference is that from the point of view of the unpaid kidney donor, the harm and risk to the donor are being accepted because a kidney is *the only thing that will meet the need*. But if you sell your kidney, it has become simply a means of getting money, and *anything else might in principle fulfill the same function*. That is true whatever your reason for wanting the money—even saving your daughter's life. Why should that cause such a horrified reaction? Presumably because it looks like a desperate, last-ditch attempt to find the essentials of life. We presume that people will find any other way they can of getting money before submitting to the deliberate infliction of bodily harm as a means. Even if there is no moral degradation involved, there is desperation, and its visibility may (depending on context) involve deep social degradation. It may be this that causes the disgusted response.

This suggestion needs enormously more detailed analysis. If it is on the right lines, I would expect the reaction to be proportionate to the intuitively perceived harm (not necessarily actual harm), and also the existing position of the vendor. It should account for differences of attitude to payment for different kinds of body parts and services, and also for other kinds of conspicuous harm undertaken for money. It might also imply that most (Western?) individuals' own willingness to sell a kidney for an attractive price would depend on how likely it was that anyone else would find out. There are also deeply interesting questions about the precise nature of the feelings of revulsion. Such emotions could be a morally based revulsion for suffering, but they could also be, for instance, a kind of aesthetic turning away from degradation. There are all kinds of possibilities, and the matter is potentially sensitive and contentious as well as difficult.

However, the moral question of what attitude to take to the feelings can probably be addressed irrespective of their precise diagnosis. The deeply uncomfortable feelings most of us seem to have about the idea of organ selling may be manifestations of morally praiseworthy sensibilities, as are impulses to turn away from other kinds of pain and suffering. But even though it is better to be appalled by suffering than to look at it indifferently, it does not follow that the actions intuitively prompted by those sensibilities must be praiseworthy by the same standards.

Consider, for instance, one conference participant whom I heard defending prohibition by saying, "I don't want to live in a society where people sell their organs to live." An expression of this sort can be interpreted in different ways. It might mean something like, "It is terrible that people are so poor that sacrificing a kidney for money is their best option." But if the situation of the poor is the speaker's concern, prohibition—as already argued—should be recognized as making their position worse. The only thing that would improve matters would be (the far more difficult matter of) "lifting them out of poverty" until they had no temptation to sell. (And if that happened there would be no need for prohibition because no one would want to sell. The whole point of prohibition—of anything—is to prevent people's doing what they would otherwise choose to do.) But a quite different interpretation of the statement is something like, "I personally find the knowledge of people's selling their organs repulsive, and that is why I want it banned." In that case, prohibition is being advocated for the benefit of the person whose sensibilities are being offended by awareness of such unpleasant goings-on—*at the cost of making things worse* for the badly off. If these two interpretations are not distinguished, the assertion may succeed in advocating what is really for the benefit of the feelings of the speaker, while giving the impression that it is for the benefit of the badly off—who will, in fact, be paying the cost. It may be bad to live in a world where people sell their organs, but it is surely better than living in one where the rich make themselves feel more comfortable by further restricting the limited options of the poor, while claiming to do it out of concern for them.

There is also another matter to bear in mind, which is the proportionality of our visceral reactions. For most of history opening people up and taking out their organs was both brutal and usually fatal, so it is not surprising that our intuitive disgust for the idea is strong. But the advance of medicine has completely changed the situation. Kidney donation is now far less dangerous than other things we routinely do, but our emotions have simply not caught up. If the situation of the badly off is considered impartially, we should be far more horrified by the working conditions in which most of the world struggles for less than adequate incomes than by their resorting to kidney selling.

There is much more work to be done on these subjects, but whatever the eventual outcome, it is clear that our intuitive responses to payment for body parts represent a quick fix for uncomfortable feelings. The issue as a whole is still in a state of intellectual, and therefore moral, confusion.

Notes

1. Uehiro Centre for Practical Ethics, Faculty of Philosophy, University of Oxford.
2. I shall not distinguish between legal, conventional, and moral unacceptability, as the differences between them are not relevant to the argument here.
3. E.g., *R v Brown* (1993) 2 All ER 75.

4. Josefson, "Prisoner wants to donate his second kidney."

5. Extrajudicial comment by Edmund Davies LJ (cited Dworkin, "The law relating to organ transplantation in England").

6. E.g., Radcliffe Richards, "From Him that Hath Not," "Nephrarious Goings On," "A Dangerous Superstition", "Feelings and Fudges," "Is It Desirable to Legitimize Paid Living Donor Kidney Transplantation Programmes?", "Selling Organs, Gametes and Surrogacy Services," "Paid Legal Organ Donation: Pro: The Philosopher's Perspective," and others.

7. Sells, "Resolving the Conflict in Traditional Ethics."

8. See, e.g., the current guidelines issued by the UK Department of Health, at http://www.dh.gov.uk/en/Publichealth/Scientificdevelopmentgeneticsandbioethics/Consent/index.htm.

9. Lord Donaldson MR, *Re T (Adult: Refusal of Treatment)* 1992 4 All ER 649, CA.

10. Dossetor and Manickavel, "Commercialization."

11. Sells, "Voluntarism of Consent."

12. E.g., Council for International Organisations of Medical Science (CIOMS) Guidelines 2002: "Payments in money or in kind to research subjects should not be so large as to persuade them to take undue risks or volunteer against their better judgement. Payments or rewards that undermine a person's capacity to exercise free choice invalidate consent."

13. Dossetor and Manickavel, "Commercialization."

14. Abouna, "The Negative Impact of Paid Organ Donation," 166.

15. Dossetor and Manickavel, "Commercialization," 63.

16. L.J. Templeman, *Sidaway v. Board of Governors of the Bethlem Royal Hospital and the Maudsley Hospital* (1985) AC 871; 1 All ER 1018, HL.

17. Greenwald, *Heroes with a Thousand Faces.* I am grateful to Sarah Edwards for this illustration.

18. See note 5.

19. Radcliffe Richards, "Nephrarious Goings On," 400 ff.

20. John Stuart Mill, *The Subjection of Women* (1869; widely reprinted), first page.

Bibliography

Abouna, G.M., Sabawi, M.M., Kumar, M., and Samhan, M. (1991) "The Negative Impact of Paid Organ Donation." In *Organ Replacement Therapy: Ethics, Justice, Commerce,* edited by W. Land and J.B. Dossetor. Berlin: Springer-Verlag, 1991, 164–72.

Dossetor, J.B., and V. Manickavel. "Commercialization: The Buying and Selling of Kidneys." In *Ethical Problems in Dialysis and Transplantation,* edited by C.M.

Kjellstrand and J.B. Dossetor. Dordrecht: Kluwer Academic Publishers, 1992, 61–71.

Dworkin, G. "The law relating to organ transplantation in England." *MLR* (1970): 33.

Greenwald, L. *Heroes with a Thousand Faces: True Stories of People with Facial Deformities and Their Quest for Acceptance.* Cleveland Clinic Press, 2007.

Josefson, D. "Prisoner wants to donate his second kidney." *BMJ* (1999): 318.

Radcliffe Richards, J. "From Him that Hath Not." In *Organ Replacement Therapy: Ethics, Justice, Commerce,* edited by W. Land and J.B. Dossetor. Berlin: Springer-Verlag, 1991, 191–97.

Radcliffe Richards, J. "Nephrarious Goings On. Kidney Sales and Moral Arguments. *The Journal of Medicine and Philosophy* 21 (1996): 375–416.

Radcliffe Richards, J. (1998) "A Dangerous Superstition." *Clinical Transplants* (1998): 345–47.

Radcliffe Richards, J. "Feelings and Fudges: The State of Argument in the Organ Selling Debate." *The Medico-Legal Journal* 71 (2003): 119–24.

Radcliffe Richards, J. "Is It Desirable to Legitimize Paid Living Donor Kidney Transplantation Programmes? Part 1: Evidence in Favour." In *Living Donor Kidney Transplantation: Current Practices, Emerging Trends and Evolving Challenges,* edited by R. Gaston and J. Wadstrom J. London: Taylor and Francis, 2005, 171–81.

Radcliffe Richards, J. "Selling Organs, Gametes and Surrogacy Services." In *The Blackwell Guide to Medical Ethics,* edited by R. Rhodes, L.P. Francis, and A. Silvers. Oxford: Blackwell, 2007, 254–68.

Radcliffe Richards, J. "Paid Legal Organ Donation: Pro: The Philosopher's Perspective." In *Living Donor Organ Transplantation,* edited by W.G. Gruessner and E. Benedetti. New York: McGraw Hill, 2008, 88–94.

Sells, R.A. "Voluntarism of Consent in Both Related and Unrelated Living Organ Donors." In *Organ Replacement Therapy: Ethics, Justice, Commerce,* edited by W. Land and J.B. Dossetor. Berlin: Springer-Verlag, 1991, 18–24.

Sells, R.A. "Resolving the Conflict in Traditional Ethics Which Arises from Our Demand for Organs." *Transplantation Proceedings* 25 (1993): 2983–84.

12

Political Obligation and Consent

A. John Simmons

I. Consent Theory

Throughout the history of thought about political obligation, the genesis of that obligation in *consent* has been a constant theme (either as a conclusion or as a target). Indeed, for Americans it is especially hard to think of political obligation as other than consensual in origin. The Mayflower Compact of 1620 was a voluntary agreement to submit only to that government (and those governors) chosen by "common consent"; The U.S. Declaration of Independence argues that the just powers of government derive solely from "the consent of the governed"; and *Federalist* No. 85 maintains that the United States was founded on "the voluntary consent of a whole people." It is consequently almost second nature for U.S. citizens to begin thinking about political obligation in terms of popular consent. But, as we will see, the appeal of the consent theory of political obligation extends far beyond such a contingent heritage of public political philosophy.

To begin, let us loosely define "political obligation" as the general moral obligation of a citizen to obey the laws (or, at least, the satisfactorily just laws) and support the (just) legal and political institutions of her or his country. And we can characterize "consent" as naming any of a variety of kinds of voluntary undertakings (including promises, contracts, authorizations, and so forth) whose point is to allow people to freely transfer rights to others and undertake obligations with respect to those others. In thus undertaking new obligations and conveying to others new rights, acts of consent create special moral *justifications* for conduct by others toward us that would normally be unjustified. In the political context, the idea is that, in consenting to be governed, citizens agree to obey the laws of the land (and so forth) and convey to their government (governors, fellow citizens, political community) the right to govern them (by, for example, making and enforcing law), thus justifying or legitimating (with respect to them) the actions of their government.[1] While, as we will see, there are several ways in which consent and political obligation can be connected, the clearest and most direct connection is the one advocated by the *consent theory* of political obligation: The actual, personal consent of each citizen is *necessary* for that citizen's political obligations, and that consent is also (at least within limits) a *sufficient* ground of political obligation.

In trying to understand consent theory, we can be a bit more precise about both the nature and the appeal of consent as the ground of political obligation. Let us say, more precisely, that consent is the deliberate (and communicatively successful[2]) performance of acts or omissions whose conventional or contextual point is to communicate to others the agent's intention to undertake new obligations and/or convey to others new rights (with respect to the agent). Consent, so understood, is a kind of *act*, not—as in so-called "subjective" theories of consent—an attitude or state of mind (such as approval, or some other "pro-attitude"). Generally, of course, merely having certain attitudes toward an arrangement by itself grounds no new obligations and conveys to others no new rights. While we may, of course, and regularly do approve of arrangements to which we give our consent, such attitudes are in no way necessary to our successfully undertaking new obligations by our acts of consent. So because we are interested precisely in the connection between consent and certain kinds of obligations, we can leave behind such "subjective" accounts of consent.[3]

Why, though (beyond a societal historical fixation on consent), would we think of consent as privileged in this way to ground important obligations of political allegiance and obedience? First, of course, appealing to consent to explain such central obligations provides them with a clear and uncontroversial source: Voluntary undertakings such as promises and contracts are more readily acknowledged as grounding clear obligations than virtually anything else. And when it comes to moral justifications for interfering in another's life (as governments necessarily do to their citizens), the principle *volenti non fit injuria* (roughly, the willing person is not wronged) is equally widely accepted. Second, accepting consent as necessary for political obligation is the clearest possible rejection of the legitimacy of force, intimidation, and custom in structuring political relationships, and so constitutes the clearest possible rejection of the bloody and repressive past history of states. Instead, consent theory affirms the moral importance of individual autonomy or self-government, insisting that our important relationships be those that we choose, not those we are forced or born into. What we consent to (at least within the limiting conditions discussed below in section V) provides, the consent theorist tells us, the most reliable expression of our individual wills. So the consent theory of political obligation, far from being attractive only to those raised in a few odd public political cultures, should be attractive to anyone who regards individual freedom and self-determination as important goods or constraining rights.

II. History: From Social Contract to Individual Consent

The consent theory of political obligation, as we have described it in the previous section, is represented historically in texts as early as Plato's *Crito*. But the theory came to prominence as an offspring of the modern social contract tradition of thought in political philosophy. While it was certainly a natural offspring of that tradition, however, consent theory has not been an integral part of every social contractarian view. Indeed, neither the first generation of social contract theorists nor the most recent generation of them generally regard(ed) actual, personal consent as necessary for any individual's political obligations. Most of the theorists during the great modern emergence of contractarian thought—that is, most of the authors of the early Huguenot, Scottish Calvinist, and Puritan political treatises— took the contract that they thought bound contemporary persons to be either the originating, historical contract of each society or some more recent contract between the king (or government) and the "leading men" of the people (or the "lesser magistrates" representing the people). The *personal* consent of most of those said to be bound by the contract was in neither case necessary or expected, the relevant binding consent having supposedly been given on their behalf by their ancestors or representatives.

Similarly, in the Kantian "wing" of social contract thought—and most importantly in the extremely influential contemporary version of it developed by John Rawls and his many followers—the "consent" that grounds the political obligations (or duties) of contemporary persons is not their own actual consent. Rather, our political duties are derived from the conformity of institutional arrangements to the *hypothetical* choices of appropriately described rational choosers. It is thus on this view the hypothetical consent of nonactual persons (or, better, of the model-theoretic versions of persons[4]), not the actual, personal consent that we ourselves might give, that is thought to generate our political obligations/duties. Kant himself tested the legitimacy of laws by asking whether *actual* citizens *could* have given those laws to themselves, rather than, as in Rawls, by asking whether nonactual contractors *would* have chosen them (or chosen principles that permit them). But in neither case is the legitimacy of law determined by the actual consent of actual persons.

The rise of actual consent theory within the social contract tradition—most importantly through the influence of the political writings of George Buchanan and John Locke—can be seen in certain ways as an individualist "perfecting" of that tradition. This is evident when one considers the implications of the fact that the early modern social contractarian approach developed largely as a response to (what we can call) the "political naturalism" of the age. Political naturalism, deriving principally from Aristotle's *Politics* and from St. Paul's conservative doctrine on obedience to "the powers that be" (*Romans* 13:1–2), is the view that (most) persons are *naturally* subject to the political authority of others, that (at least within limits) simply by being born into a sociopolitical position of subjection to government we are bound to compliance with and support for that government. One standard contractarian response to the political naturalist was to argue that persons are all naturally equal—and so not naturally subject to anyone's authority (but God's and, temporarily, their parents')—and naturally free (to choose political subjection only on terms they find acceptable). Social contract theorists thus introduced accounts of the "state of nature" (a natural, apolitical condition of *nonsubjection*) and defended historical accounts of the origins of existing societies in historical contracts. (If existing political societies began in contracts, of course, then some nonpolitical condition of persons had to precede polities, so political subjection could hardly be man's natural condition.)

From our contemporary perspective, at least, it is surprising to find that many of the early social contract theorists defended the same kinds of absolutist political conclusions as did their naturalist rivals. Hobbes was far from alone among contractarians in defending absolute sovereignty. If people are free to choose their own terms of political subjection, the argument went, then they are free to choose subjection to a person or body that rules with unlimited rights. Such a choice was often (as in Hobbes) defended as a wise choice—and so the choice that persons *ought* to make—because of the necessity of absolute authority for concentrating the power of the state and thus keeping civil peace. But the choice of absolute government was often defended instead (or as well) as the choice that had *actually* been made by the historical representatives of contemporary persons, thus binding those contemporaries to absolute obedience. Kings/governments of the period, after all, frequently claimed (and/or ruled as if) they were entitled to absolute authority; and the (always hazy) ancient agreements that produced their authority—the "founding contracts" between kings and the peoples' leading men—were, after all, uncoerced contracts between relative equals in power, wealth, and education.[5] Understood in that way, absolute government appeared unsuspicious even in contractarian terms.

How, then, was social contract theory led from these origins to its more familiar (for us moderns) emphasis on individual consent and limited government? Historically, of course, the theoretical answer coincided with the gradual breakdown of the feudal hierarchy of political, social, and economic roles, with its associated complex network of expectations and obligations. The claims of history and peoples came to seem less authoritative, and "leading men" were less and less regarded as entitled to speak for and bind their social "inferiors" and descendants. Philosophically, these changes corresponded to a growing moral and political individualism. As the obscuring veil of custom and coercion was drawn back, persons could be seen not as bound by birth to economic and political roles, but as naturally free and equal, with social "inferiors" every bit as much the subject of an important life as were their "betters." Even more plainly, contemporary persons are seen as the moral equals of their ancestors; but as equals, they must be equally free to associate according to their own lights. As Locke famously put it, a person "cannot by any compact whatsoever bind his children or posterity."[6] The recognition of historical consent as binding on contemporary persons is inconsistent with the premise that persons of both ages are equally persons (and no more than that), born to the same rights and freedoms.

This emerging individualism thus naturally resulted in the famous Lockean insistence that only the actual, personal consent of those subject to government can legitimate its authority over them. But this new consent theory also brought with it certain new concerns about the binding power of individual consent (our subject in section V below). Once the consent of all (free, male) subjects (and not just society's "leading men") became the focus of political legitimation, obvious societal inequalities in power, wealth, and education raised concerns that the "consent" of the poor and powerless to unfavorable political arrangements might be secured through the use (by or on behalf of the powerful) of intimidation, misrepresentation, economic pressure, or simple duress. So the original, simple focus of social contract theory on "who had agreed to what" became a more complicated focus on the conditions under which agreements have been secured. Thus, Locke emphasized that no binding political (or other) consent could be thought to have been given where that consent was a product of duress or irresistible economic pressure: "a man can no more justly make use of another's necessity to force him to become his vassal . . . than he that has more strength can seize upon a weaker . . . [and] offer him death or slavery."[7]

Similarly, the egalitarianism of the new consent theory raised natural worries about whether uninformed consent or simply imprudent consent should be taken to bind the consenter. This emphasis on the limiting conditions of actual, personal consent's binding power, of course, led rapidly to the emergence of various doctrines of the *inalienability* of certain natural rights, doctrines that are best known from their roles in the great "rights manifestos" of the seventeenth and eighteenth centuries. Consent, the argument went, no matter how freely or sincerely given, simply cannot convey to others a range of basic rights over the consenter (such as the right to kill or to enslave the consenter). Justified *political* tyranny would have to involve a tyrant wielding rights over subjects that they could not have conveyed to the tyrant with their consent. So consent theory, once accompanied by a doctrine of inalienability, was taken to logically entail the conclusion that only suitably *limited* government could be justified or legitimate. The "rights retained by the people"— whether *necessarily* retained because inalienable, or simply *in fact* retained in the actual terms of the consent given—establish a permanent moral barrier to political tyranny.

III. Justification by Consent

Let us step back now from the history of the consent theory of political obligation and try to understand better its normative force, particularly the force of appeals to actual consent as these relate to other justificatory employments of the idea of consent. How, then, might we go about trying to justify or legitimate contemporary actions, policies, arrangements, or institutions (and so forth) by appeal specifically to *consent*? The most natural example, of course, involves justification by appeal to someone's actual, personal consent: I can justify or legitimate my driving away with your lawn mower in my pickup truck if you have given me your lawn mower, thus consenting to my taking it away. But as we have seen, some branches of contractarian thought have attempted justifications by appealing to historical consent, to consent by "representatives" or by "peoples," or to hypothetical consent. The idea that historical consent, given by our ancestors (or their representatives), could justify or bind persons to contemporary arrangements has, as we've seen, been (correctly) dismissed as inconsistent with our recognition of the natural equality and freedom of all persons. And, while our being bound by the consent of a representative (say, an attorney or a broker) is a perfectly familiar feature of our lives, the power of representatives to bind us with their consensual acts is normally[8] taken to require our own *prior* free consent to such representation. "Representative consent," then, is not typically a *free-standing* basis for justification or legitimation. And consent given by historical representatives (the "dead hand" of the past), of course, could not possibly bind us today, if being so bound requires our prior consent to representation. Our moral and political individualism has advanced sufficiently to produce a broad consensus on these points. Similarly, this individualism results in our generally taking consent given by the majority of the members of some *group* in which we are nonvoluntarily included (such as a racial or ethnic group, or a "people") to be insufficient to ground our personal obligations.

Appeals to nonactual (counterfactual), hypothetical consent, by contrast, do seem often to function as freestanding sources of justification (which explains, of course, the enduring popularity of Kantian contractarian thought). But they do not, of course, function in this way in any simple fashion. Sometimes simple appeals to what people "would have consented to" seem adequate to justify our conduct toward them, as when I am justified in carrying your unconscious, injured body to the emergency room for treatment, or in restraining your violently insane behavior—in both cases overcoming the usual prohibition on touching nonconsenting others because, we reason, this is what you would have consented to had you been able to give rational, binding consent to anything. Or we may reason (as legal courts sometimes do) that the best way to divide the property of one who cannot do so himself is to appeal to the division to which that person would have been most likely to consent. Sometimes, however, such appeals to what people "would have consented to" seem to have no justificatory force at all. The fact that you would have consented to marry me, had I proposed to you (which I did not), plainly does not legitimate my present demand that you treat me as your husband.

The obvious difference between these cases—that in the former cases it would have been impossible to obtain actual consent to the necessary actions while in the latter case actual consent could easily have been solicited (but was not)—suggests that this sort of appeal to hypothetical consent seems forceful primarily because the will of the person from whom consent was needed was temporarily or permanently inoperative or severely impaired. But these examples may suggest as well that even in the former cases it is not really *consent* that is being appealed to (to justify our actions) at all. Talk of what people "would have consented to" may, rather, just be a "suggestive" way of talking about what would be *best* for people, or what would best promote their interests. What justifies my carrying you to the emergency room seems to be simply that we think it best for all that people be left free to help others, at least where decisions must be made and where those others cannot decide for themselves. And, of course, talking about what is best for people seems quite different from talking about what they have agreed to, for we regularly give binding consent to arrangements that are demonstrably not (or that unexpectedly turn out not to be) best for us. Even where consenters are unimpaired moral agents and even where their consent is fully informed and fully free—so that the standard requirements for *binding* consent are satisfied—our consent can still be a product of bad reasoning or unhealthy preferences, thus resulting in consent to that which is not best for us.

This last fact—that real persons tend to be flawed (or "distinctive") in their desires and their reasoning—is an important source of skepticism about the moral importance of *actual* consent, and it thus serves as a push in the direction of trying to justify conduct or arrangements by appealing instead to hypothetical consent. Why should we take seriously, as either necessary or sufficient to justify restricting actions or arrangements, actual consent of persons that may flow from personal flaws? But the regular occurrence of "flawed" (but still free and informed) consent can push us toward greater justificatory reliance on hypothetical consent only if the sort of hypothetical consent appealed to is not similarly problematic. Notice that thus far our examples of reasoning from hypothetical consent have all involved appeals to *individualized* hypothetical consent—that is, we justify conduct by arguing that the *very individual in question* would have consented to that conduct (had she been asked or able). Further, the hypothetical consent at issue is *dispositional*, in that we determine what the individual in question would have consented to by asking ourselves what that individual was in fact disposed to consent to (though unable to consent to in the circumstances) in virtue of her existing desires and patterns of reasoning. But appealing in that way to "individual-dispositional" hypothetical consent involves the very same problem that is faced by appeals to actual consent—namely, that those existing desires and patterns of reasoning may be flawed or bizarre (without constituting disqualifying incapacities).

In light of this problem, it seems natural to suppose that the sort of hypothetical consent from others that could justify our policies or actions would be some more *idealized* form of consent. Thus, we might argue that we can justify our actions to you by appealing to "individual idealized" hypothetical consent, where we ask what you, the very individual in question, would have consented to had you been purged of your worst or most peculiar desires and patterns of reasoning. The "purged" version of you would still be recognizably you, and it would thus remain true that different persons often "would have consented to" different things. But in appealing to this "individual-idealized" hypothetical consent, we would no longer be trying to morally justify conduct by appealing to what flowed from your "worst" personal characteristics. We argue neither from what you actually did or did not consent to nor from what you, with all your oddities, would have consented to, but rather from what some cleaned-up, more respectable version of you would have agreed to. This at least appears to be how we are arguing when we try to justify our treatment of children or the insane (and so forth) by appealing to what they would have consented to. We guide our conduct neither by what they actually agree to (in childish or insane ways) nor by what their most childish or insane desires indicate they would have agreed to. But we are nonetheless inclined to take seriously in our reasoning about their hypothetical consent at least some of their less worrying distinctive traits or desires—such as taking seriously the fact that different restrictions might be justified for sensitive or artistic or athletic children.

If you have followed along this far, however, it is should be obvious that there is only one step more to the rationale for declining to appeal to *individualized* versions of consent—either actual or hypothetical—at all. If justifications seem more secure when the hypothetical consent at issue doesn't rest on individual flaws and peculiarities, why not simply eliminate appeal to distinctive individual characteristics altogether, justifying arrangements and conduct in terms of perfectly *generic* (idealized) hypothetical consent? Why not ask as our justifying question what a perfectly rational being with no unusual desires would have consented to? In one sense, of course, appealing in this way to perfectly generic hypothetical consent seems so distant from more familiar arguments utilizing actual consent that the justifications yielded may seem impossibly weak. I am not perfectly rational and I do have distinctive desires and interests. So why should the choices that would be made by beings so unlike me have any justificatory weight at all with respect to me? In another sense, however, such appeals to generic hypothetical consent may seem to yield the strongest possible justifications (with respect to *all* of us). The rational is that to which our actions toward others (and our enforced arrangements) ought to aspire, and their justifications ought not to be relative only to peculiar or distinctive interests. Institutions that rational, nonpeculiar persons would choose are, we might say, those institutions that are just or good or best.

Attempts to use this kind of idealized, generic hypothetical consent to explain our political obligations or duties are, as we saw in section II, central to the Kantian tradition in political philosophy, taking their most sophisticated form in the work of Rawls and his followers. We are bound to support and comply with our political institutions *not* if we have actually, personally consented to their authority over us, but rather if those institutions *would be* chosen by representative, rational parties, purged of bad reasoning and unhealthy desires.[9] Indeed, the hypothetical choices that matter here are the choices of "persons" with no distinguishing characteristics whatsoever. Rawls asks: What sort of basic institutional structure would be chosen by perfectly rational parties concerned only to advance their conceptions of the good, but with no knowledge of what their distinctive, individual ("thick") conceptions might be? The choosing parties are all "assigned" identical interests (according to a "thin" conception of "primary goods"). The hypothetical consent at issue in Rawls's account is thus perfectly general, perfectly nonindividualized hypothetical consent.

The motivation in such views to disregard *actual* consent (or its absence) in justifying political arrangements involves partly the difficulties involved in obtaining (unanimous) actual consent to arrangements at the level of national politics, partly the flawed nature of actual consenters (noted above), and partly the allegedly objectionable consequences of individually innocent-looking acts of actual consent (discussed below in section VII). While I believe that this Kantian approach to political obligation (or duty) is seriously misguided in several respects,[10] it is enough here to observe (again) that such appeals to hypothetical consent do not really seem to be much about *consent* per se. To say that subjection to certain political institutions would have been agreed to by perfectly rational, motivationally purged contractors seems to be simply to say that these institutions are *good* ones, whose virtues would be perceived and selected by ideal choosers. Making *that* point appears to have little in common with justificatory claims based on actual persons having actually agreed to be subject to certain political arrangements. The problem of *paternalism* (for instance) is a *problem* chiefly because of the basic tension between appeals to what people *actually choose* and appeals to what is *best* (or what is best *for them*). Hypothetical consent theories of political obligation thus seem in important ways not really to qualify as *consent* theories.

IV. Actual Consent

These conclusions about appeals to hypothetical consent naturally push us to think more about the force of appeals to actual, personal consent—that is, to appeals of the sort that are central to the consent theory of political obligation (as it was described in section I). Justifications in terms of actual, personal consent (far more than in terms of hypothetical, ancestral, or majority consent) are perfectly familiar from our everyday lives (and from our common-sense understanding of private law). Such consent is what typically distinguishes sexual intercourse from rape,[11] borrowing from theft, invasive medical treatment from battery, and so forth. In each case, our consent to others' actions conveys to them special rights to do what would otherwise be prohibited—thus justifying those actions—while generating for us a special obligation to permit or assist their actions.

The justificatory force of an appeal to actual, personal consent might seem to be as strong a justification for conduct (that affects another) as any we could hope to find. After all, where the person who is affected by our actions has consented to it, that person has given a clear, full indication of his willingness to be so affected. It is hard to see how he could then complain of any wrong to him on our part. On the other hand, when we remember that consent, even when given freely and with full information, may nonetheless rest on defective reasoning or "peculiar" desires, justifications by appeal to actual, personal consent may seem less obviously strong, at least in some cases. The wisdom or even justice of outcomes generated by actual, personal consent is far from guaranteed. Concerns about this fact are to some extent reflected in the legal doctrines of inalienability and unconscionability that we discuss in section V. For example, I typically cannot legally justify another's killing me or making me his slave simply by giving my consent to the arrangement. I cannot do this even if I act freely, with full information, and in so doing satisfy my strongest and most enduring desires.

Actual, personal consent, of course, can be given in a variety of ways. Contract law distinguishes *express* contracts (made in written or uttered words) from *implied* contracts (as well as contracts that are implied *in fact* [where the facts imply a contract without written or oral evidence] from those that are implied *in law* [so-called *quasi-contracts*][12]). Consent theorists have traditionally drawn a related distinction between *express* consent and *tacit* (implied, implicit, "virtual," "by inference") consent. In writing of express consent, political philosophers have mostly had in mind the kind of consent given by a direct, verbal oath of allegiance or some explicit agreement to become a citizen. But since consent can plainly be expressly given without the use of *words* (by, say, nodding, raising one's hand, and so forth), let us draw the distinction between express and tacit consent as follows. Express consent is consent given by acts (or omissions) whose default conventional point is precisely to give consent. Tacit consent is consent given by acts (or omissions) that acquire the significance of consent not by their default conventional points but rather by the special contexts in which they take place.

Thus, saying "I consent" is normally to consent expressly, since the standard-case linguistic point of such an utterance is precisely to give consent. Remaining silent, by contrast, lacks this standard-case conventional point, since we can remain silent without consenting to anything in a wide array of contexts. But remaining silent *can* be a way of tacitly consenting to something in virtue of the features of some special context in which it occurs—such as when it constitutes a free, deliberate response to a call for indications of *dissent.* Express consent binds us independent of special, nonstandard features of its context; it, as it were, creates its own context by positively invoking standing linguistic (or other) conventions for giving consent. The contexts in which acts or omissions constitute tacit consent, however, must exhibit a variety of special features that distinguish those acts or omissions from their nonconsensual analogues that could occur in other contexts. For instance, for silence to constitute tacit consent, the consenter typically must be awake, aware that silence will be taken to give consent, aware of the means available for indicating dissent, and so forth—that is, there must be a "clear choice situation" in which silence is a deliberate, significant response to a required choice.[13] Further, of course, those posing the choice must be entitled to do so (for example, your silence in response to my offer to you of a "clear choice" between killing yourself or by silence agreeing to be my slave would not constitute consent to slavery).

It has sometimes been suggested that tacit consent binds us (and conveys rights to others) less completely or for a shorter duration than does express consent.[14] On its face, this seems implausible, for consent is consent, regardless of the manner in which it is given. Even tacit consent must be free and deliberate (in order to bind), with the will as fully engaged as in cases of express consent. It would appear rather to be the specific nature of the consenter's acts (or of the context in which consent was given), not the mode of consent, that normally determines variations in the obligations (or the duration of obligation) generated by different acts of consent. Some, however, have thought of tacit consent as something to be simply inferred from inactivity or regularity of behavior, even in the absence of a clear choice situation. And on that weaker understanding of tacit consent, the ascription to it of weaker binding power perhaps makes sense, since there is no guarantee that the "consenter's" will is engaged at all. For instance, it is sometimes suggested that if we fail to resist or protest regular wrongs, we tacitly consent to them, or that if we regularly perform certain actions, we tacitly consent to continue performing them. While there is no denying that regularity of behavior can sometimes shade into or become a form of consent to continue (as when bridge players rely on each other to show up for their weekly game), and no denying that certain (in my view, morally questionable) legal doctrines of prescription might appear to accept such reasoning, there is also no denying that *mere* regularity of behavior, without strong contextual conditions, is insufficient to constitute consent, tacit or otherwise. I consent to nothing if I am regularly robbed (without resisting) of my lunch money by the class bully, nor did Kant consent to always take a daily morning walk just because the housewives of Konigsburg relied on his compulsive timeliness to set their clocks.

V. Limiting Conditions

Sometimes apparent acts of consent plainly do not bind us. Whether we say in such cases that real consent was given but that it was nonbinding or instead that there simply was no real consent matters little. What matters are the conditions under which the standard-case undertaking of obligation and conveyance of right do not occur. Most obvious among these conditions is when words or actions conventionally used to give consent are used with no intention of consenting—as when apparent consent is given by a speaker who does not understand the meaning of the words spoken or by someone who is only rehearsing her lines for a play. More generally (as we have seen), in order for our "consent" to bind us and to convey rights to others, we must *intend* for our actions to communicate (and must *succeed* in communicating) to others that we thereby undertake new obligations with respect to them and/or convey to them new rights. This is not to say, of course, that consent only binds us when we intend to *perform* as we have undertaken to do. Just as an insincere promise may nonetheless bind us to perform as promised, so consent that intentionally and successfully communicates our undertaking of obligation, even in the absence of any intention on our part to honor our consent, may (and typically does) still bind us.

A related requirement for binding consent concerns not so much the consenter's *intention* to alter the existing distribution of obligations and rights, but rather the consenter's *knowledge* and understanding of important nonmoral facts about and consequences of the act of consent (that is, binding consent must be adequately "informed"). In general, where the "consenter" does not adequately understand that to which he has "consented" (due to, say, incapacity or vagueness in the presentation of terms) or where the "consenter" has been wrongly induced to "consent" by, for example, others' fraud, nondisclosure, or misrepresentation, no genuine, binding consent has been given. While it does not seem possible to specify precisely (independent of specific contexts) which facts or consequences a consenter must understand in order to count as giving binding consent, the consenter's knowledge or understanding must at the very least suffice to make his action genuinely intentional.

Further (and relatedly), genuine, binding consent must be given *voluntarily* or *willingly*. The use of duress to secure another's consent obviously robs that "consent" of its moral force, as may various kinds of intimidation (and vast disparities in bargaining power) and the manipulation of circumstances in order to eliminate or to make excessively costly the available options to consenting.[15] While we may, of course, freely consent to an arrangement even where we have no viable options to doing so (just as a person whose exits have been secretly blocked may nonetheless freely choose to remain in her home for the evening), "consent" given only *because* of the absence of options—especially where others have removed those options precisely in order to compel consent—typically does not bind us. I will not attempt here to further clarify the fuzzy line between legitimate competition (as when another's playing "economic hardball" induces our consent) and the kinds of manipulation, exploitation, and compulsion that deprive "consent" of its justifying power.[16]

Many of these conditions, of course, determine the outlines of the legal concept of an *unconscionable* (hence, in certain respects, unenforceable) contract. *Procedurally* unconscionable contracts, which involve a "defective bargaining process," are those involving incapacity, lack of information, or involuntariness. The more controversial realm of *substantive* unconscionability is generally defined as covering contracts whose specific terms are such as to defeat the claim that a real "bargain" was made. Similarly, the perhaps more familiar legal doctrines of the *inalienability* of certain rights—for instance, we may not give legally binding consent to become another's slave or to allow another to murder us, thereby providing that other with a legal justification for his actions—seem to be based partly on the fact that certain types of agreements raise a virtually indefeasible presumption that one of the parties was *non compos mentis*. Further, of course, even where such presumptions are not inevitable, doctrines of inalienability could be rooted just as strongly in societal values that hold certain types of relationships to be inconsistent with civil or respectful social life.

There may, of course, be other limits on the binding power of consent—such as limits on the *duration* of consent's justifying capacity, which would motivate bans on consent in perpetuity.[17] If there are such limits, they will of course affect the binding power of acts of *political* consent, perhaps establishing requirements that genuine "government by consent" (the subject of our next section) involve occasions for regular reaffirmations of consent (or expressions of *dissent*). A few less obvious possible limits on consent will be considered in section VII.

VI. Government by Consent

If, as consent theorists believe, the political obligations of citizens in legitimate polities (and the political authority of their governments or states) rest on their actual consent, how might such "government by consent" actually manifest itself in real political life? Many social contractarians, of course, offered accounts of how the state might arise from a state of nature through the free consents of its members. Locke's is undoubtedly the most explicit description of the creation of a legitimate consensual "commonwealth," in which each individual freely consents to "membership" in a political society, thereby accepting (and undertaking an obligation to abide by) all of the terms necessary to the creation of a stable, enduring, peaceful society. Prominent among these terms are agreements to be governed by majority rule, to join one's land to the society (thus creating a unified national territory, under the jurisdiction of the society), and to assist in the enforcement of the society's rules and in its defense.[18]

Of course, few real political societies have had such clear or benign origins, typically arising and attaining their modern forms only through long and confusing periods involving much violence and assembled patch-works of complicated alliances. And, of course, few real persons are privileged to participate in the founding of a political society (through consent, violence, or otherwise), being mostly born within the territories of already existing states and, at their majorities, taking on (or being compelled to take on) the burdens of citizenship with little apparent choice in the matter. Are all such polities simply illegitimate according to consent theory, with their citizens, though subject to legal coercion, still free of political obligations?

It might, of course, be true that though a state was illegitimately founded, its subjects have since given to it their legitimating consent, freely undertaking their political obligations. And it is undoubtedly true that at least some citizens of modern polities have the look of consenters. This seems especially true of those who take express oaths of allegiance to their states. Oaths of political allegiance were once more common than they are today, with most of the clergy, teachers, and political officeholders of (for instance) Locke's England required to take such oaths. Even then, however, explicit oath takers constituted only a small minority of those subjected to the coercive powers of the state. In today's states, even the most obvious cases of oath

taking seem ill suited to serving as the foundation for a consensually legitimated polity. Naturalized citizens often freely take general oaths of allegiance,
though (in addition to being small in number) they equally often do so
somewhat less freely, having fled foreign oppression to the only state willing
to take them in. Political officeholders, members of the military, and voters
are frequently required to take such oaths, but the oaths tend to be either (at
least implicitly) limited in scope to the duration of the specific service in
question or administered under the threat of punishment for refusal (as in the
case of military conscripts). The oaths of allegiance taken by schoolchildren,
of course, are taken prior to the "age of consent" and are, in any event, too
much a matter of routine to be taken as the source of serious, long-term
obligations.

So while it might in principle be possible for a modern state's authority to
be legitimated by express consent, no actual state can lay claim to such a
pedigree. What seems more likely is that the masses of consenters required for
a modern state to be at least largely legitimated in its powers could have given
their consent in some less apparent, more tacit fashion. Locke (with Plato,
Hobbes, Rousseau, and others) suggested that tacit political consent is given
by continued residence within the established jurisdiction of the state—
indeed, by "the very being of anyone within the territories of" the state.[19]
Others have suggested that the consent in which we are interested is in some
way to be found in the processes through which the citizens of a democratic
society give voice to their collective will.

The first of these suggestions has been steadily criticized at least since
Hume's essay *Of the Original Contract*, primarily on the grounds that the
limiting conditions for binding consent emphasized in the previous section
are seldom satisfied in the cases of real citizens in real states. In Hume's attack
he argued that trying to understand continued residence as an act of consent
violates virtually *all* of those commonly accepted limiting conditions. First,
real citizens simply do not understand going about their ordinary lives as a
way of consenting to anything, thus violating the conditions (for binding
consent) of knowledge and intention. Further, we can add, no "clear choice"
is presented to them by anyone (that is, the choice between residence and
dissent is never clearly required), so silence or inactivity could not reasonably
be taken to indicate consent. Second, if such a clear choice *were* presented to
real citizens—say, a "love it or leave it" choice between emigrating and
"consenting by remaining"—Hume suggests that for many (especially the
poor) emigration is not really a viable option, so that the "choice" being
presented constitutes no genuine choice at all. This indicates that the voluntariness condition for binding consent cannot be satisfied for the case of

continued residence as an act of political consent. Even if consent is not exactly coerced by the state in requiring a choice between consent or emigration, it seems nonetheless true that in doing so the state counts as exploiting the vulnerability of those who find themselves within its claimed territories and thus rendering their choice insufficiently voluntary to count as binding.

It has been suggested that dramatic changes in the ways states operate might be able to address these worries.[20] But there seems to be a still larger difficulty with the idea that we might give binding political consent through our continued residence in some state: As noted previously (in section IV), in a "required choice" situation, the party requiring the choice must be clearly entitled to do so before choices made in that context can be thought to bind us. Are states clearly entitled to require us to either consent to their authority or leave "our" homes and land? Only, it would seem, if states have *prior moral title* to the land on which citizens live, such that states are entitled to remove citizens from that land for nonconsent. But the most plausible accounts of how states could acquire such moral dominion over geographical territories all make reference to the prior consent of those persons who live and work on the land in question. In short, states would already need the consent of their citizens to be in a moral position to require a choice between consent and emigration. And this, of course, just replicates, one level down, our original problem of finding evidence of political consent in the real lives of real citizens.

Such problems have led many to look for the "consent of the governed" in some other aspects of ordinary political behavior, the most popular candidate being the behavior of citizens involved in democratic political processes. In limiting our "discovery" of real political consent to this context, of course, we limit as well our account of consensual political obligations to the realm of democratic society, leaving the political obligations of citizens of nondemocratic societies either unexplained or dismissed. But at least voting in elections—or perhaps some more continuous democratic participation—unlike mere residing (and most else that real citizens do), *looks* like it involves consenting to something. And, of course, this would help to explain why we all think that there is something morally special about democracy.

The immediate obstacle to relying on such an identification of political consent, however, lies in the fact that many citizens in democracies choose not to vote in any elections, and even more citizens choose not to participate in any consistent fashion. Are those who fail to vote or to consistently participate thereby freed of political obligations? Worse, discrete acts of voting actually look far less like a way of consenting to the overarching authority of the state than they do like a way of consenting to the authority of some particular political officeholder (usually for a limited term of office). So we plainly need some better way to explain why democracy has some special connection to widespread (ideally, citizen-wide) consensual political obligations.

And it is easy to find apparent explanations in the familiar rhetoric of democratic political life. After all, we (mostly) vote and otherwise participate in democratic politics knowing that we are engaging in a process designed to produce elected legislative and executive bodies and knowing as well that we have a right to oust office holders we oppose. Further, we believe that contemporary democratic decision procedures (that is, "one-person, one-vote" plus majority rule) are fair to all. So when we decline to vote, we can reasonably be taken to agree to allow our fellow citizens to decide these matters; and when we vote for specific candidates, we can reasonably be taken to agree to the rules (and the outcomes) of the entire democratic system in which we participate—thence, the widespread citizen consent and authorization of governments that we seek.

Even if we accepted the premises of such arguments,[21] however, their desired conclusions (about the ubiquity of real political consent in democracies) simply would not follow. Democratic decision procedures are not self-justifying, applicable without condition to all and sundry. My students cannot cite the virtues of democracy in order to justify "out-voting" me concerning course requirements, nor can the United States simply extend voting rights to Peruvians and then out-vote them in matters concerning the governing of Peru. Democracy, however fine it may be, is still only legitimately applicable to those who are morally subject to a particular group's democratic procedures—for instance, to those who have previously *agreed* to be subject to it. And it was precisely *that* question—namely, the question of who is subject to and obligated to comply with which political authority—that we were trying to answer. We cannot appeal to the virtues of democracy to answer that question of who is legitimately subject to a particular state's democratic procedures. If we do, we simply beg the question to which we seek an answer.

VII. Objections to Consent Theory

We have now seen what should probably be taken to be the "classic objection" to consent theory[22]: that the political lives of real citizens in real contemporary states simply do not include sufficiently numerous cases of true, binding political consent to legitimate the activities of such states. It is easy to respond to this objection, however, by pointing out that, even if successful in its own terms, it actually does nothing to falsify consent theory itself. Actual, personal consent might still be the only possible ground of political obligation (and governmental authority). All that is falsified by the "classic objection" is a further, conservative claim, one that consent theorists have often, but by no means universally, wanted to defend (and one that is certainly not a necessary feature of consent theory): namely, that most of the citizens of at least decent contemporary states in fact *have* political obligations. Can the consent theorist regard his position as, though admittedly unconventional, at least safe from further objection, if he simply renounces such conservative ambitions?[23]

Many of consent theory's determined critics have taken its defects to go far beyond its mere failure to justify conservative assumptions about political obligations in contemporary states.[24] According to one of these more fundamental objections to consent theory, political consent, while perhaps sufficient to ground political obligations, is not necessary for these obligations. Some other, perhaps more fundamental, ground(s) of political obligation can be successfully defended. Such a claim constituted the second part of Hume's famous critique of Whig consent theory, where Hume argued that political obligations (or "obligations of allegiance") can be explained in terms that are both far more basic than consent and that apply far more widely than any principle of consent: namely, in terms of the *utility* of a stable, law-guided government. Many of us, of course, will reject the kind of rule-utilitarian analysis that guides Hume's account of the obligations associated with the virtue of allegiance (and with the other "artificial virtues"); but there are obviously many other candidate theories of political obligation from which to choose, from Hart's "mutuality of restrictions" account (utilizing what has come to be called the "principle of fairness") to associativist accounts to Kantian natural duty approaches.[25] Whether or not consent theory can defend its claim to identify the *sole* ground of political obligation will, of course, depend on how these alternative approaches to political obligation should be assessed. But each of the alternatives seems in principle consistent with acknowledging at least that consent to political membership (or to subjection to some political authority) can be *sufficient* for political obligation.

The most fundamental objections to consent theory reject even this sufficiency claim. The "classic objection" is sometimes taken to be (or to include) an "insufficiency" objection of this sort, since it can be read as claiming that our political consent can never be sufficiently voluntary to bind us, given the fundamentally nonvoluntary nature of birth and residence in our political communities. This, however, would be to misread or to overextend the classic objection, since even if birth and residence are largely nonvoluntary, there remain perfectly voluntary ways of giving our consent within that nonvoluntary context. A nonrequired, perfectly gratuitous oath of allegiance given in an utterly unintimidating and noncoercive context would seem adequate to ground political obligations, regardless of the nonvoluntariness of birth and residence. The classic objection, in short, should be taken as Hume first presented it—namely, as an attack only on the idea that *continued residence* can be taken to give consent to the powers that be.

How, then, could one argue that free, informed political consent is *not* sufficient for political obligation, especially recalling that it seems that consenters can hardly complain about others' conduct when those others act within the terms of the consent given (as the maxim *volenti non fit injuria* implies)? Perhaps it is not the consenters themselves, but rather *others*, who are entitled to complain if such consent is taken to be sufficient for obligation. Just as otherwise unobjectionable-looking consensual economic transactions between persons can have outcomes that seem unjust or indefensible with respect to those not involved in the transactions—as when they result in restrictive monopolies or the exclusion of already oppressed groups, or when many such transactions result in vast and debilitating economic inequalities— so, too, could otherwise unobjectionable-looking *political* consent result in the creation of political communities that are intolerant, uncharitable, and illiberal. Persons could unanimously give their perfectly free and informed consent to arrangements that excluded others on grounds of race, gender, ethnicity, religion, or sexual orientation, imposing all manner of distasteful restrictions on persons' basic liberties. If such communities are as a result illegitimate, then presumably their "citizens" would lack political obligations to obey and support them. If so, however, the free, informed consent that created those political arrangements was insufficient to ground political obligations.

One possible response to such concerns about the sufficiency of political consent is simply to confront them directly: Provided that people discharge their moral duties and obligations to others, one can argue, they are entitled to associate and enter into consensual transactions with others. The resulting arrangements are legitimate, and the consensually undertaken obligations binding, regardless of whether we find their choices distasteful. Then argument can proceed concerning precisely what moral duties and obligations we do in fact owe to others, with those independent moral requirements restricting what people can legitimately accomplish by consent. That, however, would not amount to rejecting the sufficiency of consent for political obligation, but would only (possibly) add others to the limiting conditions that already need to be satisfied for consent to be binding. The consent theorist must still allow, of course, that consent can create, sustain, and legitimate arrangements and associations that are admittedly ugly and distasteful—that are less good, that display fewer virtues than other possibilities—just as persons in their private lives can make unpleasant, but still binding, agreements with one another. The consent theorist can even concede that such arrangements are less well *justified*, morally, than would be others. The only point on which the consent theorist must insist is that authorities can be empowered over and genuine obligations undertaken between persons who freely and informedly consent to the arrangements while honoring their prior duties and obligations to others, no matter how unpleasant or illiberal those arrangements might be. And this, perhaps, is not too heavy a theoretical price to pay for affirming the otherwise inspiring ideal of legitimate government as deriving only from the consent of the governed.

VIII. Conclusions

As our discussion has indicated, there are a variety of possible conclusions that we might draw from the arguments considered in this chapter. If we were persuaded by the "classic objection" to consent theory, but not by any of the more "fundamental" objections, we could conclude that while consent theory is the correct theory of political obligation (that is, that it correctly identifies the necessary conditions for persons to have political obligations), persons in real political communities seldom have political obligations. This (my preferred option) would amount to defending a consent-based version of "philosophical anarchism," according to which real citizens generally lack political obligations and real states or governments generally lack the authority or legitimacy that correlates with those obligations.[26] And it would be to give up the "conservative claim" about political obligation that most political philosophers have intended to validate. Or, of course, we could try to defend the conservative claim by finding a more persuasive way to characterize the behavior of real citizens in decent states as in fact giving their binding political consent.

Alternatively, we might accept one of the arguments purporting to show that consent is neither necessary nor sufficient for political obligation, in which case we would need to defend either an alternative account of political obligation or an alternative version of philosophical anarchism (according to which real citizens still lack political obligations, but now according to the preferred alternative theory's criteria). An intermediate position would be to accept the limited claim that consent can be (and perhaps sometimes or often is in fact) sufficient for real political obligations, but that consent is not necessary for political obligation—that alternative grounds for such obligations are possible. In that case, we would be defending a multiprinciple, "pluralist" theory of political obligation. My own view is that it is extremely difficult to persuasively argue for any rejection of consent theory that is stronger than this intermediate, pluralist one. The ideal of government by consent is too powerful and plausible to permit the conclusion that the free, deliberate consent of rational persons *could not* justify political arrangements for those persons and ground obligations to support and comply with those arrangements.[27]

Notes

1. The right to govern (that is, governmental authority or legitimacy) is thus understood to be "assembled," right by right, from the rights to govern *them* that are transferred by individual citizens' acts of consent. If citizen consent is not unanimous, this raises the possibility that governments (or polities) may be "more or less" legitimate or authoritative, depending on the percentages of citizens who consent.

2. That is, one cannot consent without successfully communicating to another one's intention to consent. Consent is thus a *performative* notion.

3. On this point, and on consent more generally, see Joseph Raz, *The Morality of Freedom* (Oxford: Oxford University Press, 1986), 80–94.

4. In Rawls's "justice as fairness" (the name he gives to his "extension and generalization" of social contract thought), it is probably best not to think of the original position contractors as "persons" at all, given their lack of differentiating personal characteristics. The whole original position model simply constitutes an "intuitive" elaboration of the particular conception of fairness that Rawls wants to explicate.

5. Consider, for example, that the ancient agreement between the king and the leading men of England was largely forced *on* King John by them, not vice versa.

6. *Second Treatise*, section 116.

7. *First Treatise*, section 42.

8. "Normally" here refers to the case of "normal" adults—that is, those past the "age of consent" and unimpaired by conditions that (at least at the moment when choice is required) produce serious "defects of will" (for example, deep ignorance of fact, serious retardation, insanity, and so forth). Consent by representatives (or proxies) in non-normal conditions requires a different treatment.

9. The original position contractors of Rawls's thought experiment are perfectly rational (in the instrumental, means-ends sense of rationality) and have only one "desire"—namely, to maximize their shares of primary goods (that is, all-purpose goods that are important to advancing any meaningful life plan).

10. See my "Justification and Legitimacy" (essay 7 in my *Justification and Legitimacy* [Cambridge: Cambridge University Press, 2001]), *Is There a Duty to Obey the*

Law? For and Against (with C.H. Wellman) (Cambridge: Cambridge University Press, 2005), esp. chs. 7–8, and *Political Philosophy* (New York: Oxford University Press, 2008), esp. 58–62.

11. On consent in sexual relations, see David Archard, *Sexual Consent* (Boulder, CO: Westview Press, 1998), and Alan Wertheimer, *Consent to Sexual Relations* (New York: Cambridge University Press, 2003).

12. Consent and intention are irrelevant to the existence of quasi-contracts (the applicable obligations resting instead on considerations of equity and "natural justice"). We will thus ignore that legal doctrine here, where our concern is with consent proper, not with the acceptance and retention of benefits.

13. I discuss these (and other) conditions for silence giving consent in *Moral Principles and Political Obligations* (Princeton, NJ: Princeton University Press, 1979), 79–83.

14. Locke is generally taken to defend this view, at least with respect to *political* instances of tacit and express consent. I defend a different (and more charitable) reading of Locke in "'Denisons' and 'Aliens': Locke's Problem of Political Consent," in *Justification and Legitimacy*.

15. See Alan Wertheimer, *Coercion* (Princeton, NJ: Princeton University Press, 1987).

16. The conditions briefly summarized previously correspond to those characterized by John Horton as conditions of intention, knowledge, communication, and "appropriate background conditions of choice" (*Political Obligation* [Atlantic Highlands, NJ: Humanities Press, 1992], 30).

17. See, e.g., Raz, *The Morality of Freedom*, 90, and my "Consent Theory for Libertarians," *Social Philosophy & Policy* 22:1 (Winter 2005), 348–50.

18. *Second Treatise*, sections 95–99, 120.

19. Ibid., section 119.

20. Harry Beran, for example, argues that the voluntariness problem could be addressed by guaranteeing legal rights to emigrate and secede and by establishing a "dissenters' territory" to which those who decline to consent could move (*The Consent Theory of Political Obligation* [London: Croom Helm, 1987], 125). If we added to these requirements state assistance (financial or otherwise) to make emigration (to the dissenters' territory or to some other state) a realistic option for all and perhaps a wider range of citizenship levels or options, states would indeed come to more closely approximate the ideal of a voluntary society. But as the text below indicates, problems still remain for any version of consent theory that takes residence to give consent.

21. For reasons to worry further about the premises, see my *Political Philosophy*, 112–17.

22. Margaret Gilbert divides what I here call the "classic objection" into two distinct objections: "the no-agreement objection" (pointing to the absence of relevant acts of choosing) and "the no-obligation objection" (pointing to insufficiently free background conditions) (*A Theory of Political Obligation* [Oxford: Oxford University Press, 2006], 70–83). For another contemporary restatement of Hume's objection, see Ronald Dworkin, *Law's Empire* (Cambridge, MA: Harvard University Press, 1986), 192–93.

23. I have myself defended a version of "philosophical anarchism" based in this way on consent theory, arguing that existing modern states are in fact (though not *necessarily*) illegitimate and their citizens in fact largely free of political obligations. See, e.g., my *Moral Principles and Political Obligations,* esp. ch. VIII.

24. For a much more extended and systematic treatment of familiar and possible critiques of consent theory, see my "Consent Theory for Libertarians," 343–56.

25. I discuss the general character and principal weaknesses of all of these approaches—with special emphasis on natural duty accounts—in my portion of *Is There a Duty to Obey the Law?*

26. This would be an *a posteriori* form of philosophical anarchism, which leaves open the possibility that "government by consent" *could* exist. On the character and varieties of philosophical anarchism, see my "Philosophical Anarchism," in *Justification and Legitimacy.*

27. For a defense of this ideal from the perspective of left-libertarianism, see Michael Otsuka, *Libertarianism Without Inequality* (Oxford: Oxford University Press, 2003), ch. 5.

13

Advances in Informed Consent Research

Philip J. Candilis and Charles W. Lidz

Almost since the origins of the informed consent doctrine, physicians and researchers have been frustrated by the difficulty of attaining meaningful consents—consents that truly fulfilled the high ideals of the doctrine. This difficulty quickly led to a series of empirical studies showing that patients did not understand informed consent disclosures. Almost as quickly, critics pointed to methodological flaws in those studies.[1]

Recent years have seen empirical ethicists explore new directions in informed consent, both in the methods used to study consent and in innovative approaches for improving the consent process. Consequently some studies have clarified persistent problems while others have provided fodder for existing controversies. Research methodologies themselves have expanded substantially as investigators combine quantitative and qualitative methods to improve their recording of disclosures and testing of patient/subject understanding. Improved assessments of the quality of consent, of patient understanding and satisfaction, and of tools that enhance information sharing are all part of this new research. Of course, this work has not resolved all of the challenges of this complex social interaction, but there has been a substantial emphasis on the improvement of the informed consent process as a whole.

Our own starting point for this overview is that respect for persons is a foundational principle for informed consent and renders it a deontological commitment.[2] It is right and proper that physicians and researchers explain what they are proposing even if it does not alter behavioral outcomes. It is equally right that they expect changes in people's understanding and participation to flow from the consent process. For these reasons empirical research on informed consent is vital.

We will begin our overview with a description of the expanding research methodologies and consider some recent research findings. We will follow this by exploring some of the theoretical innovations that have resulted, describing certain problems that remain in consent, and considering the efforts being made to overcome them.

Methodological Developments

The earliest studies of informed consent consisted largely of physicians creating simple marketing-style questionnaires to assess what they thought a patient should understand. Usually the patient had already consented, and the questionnaires were administered months after the procedure itself. Investigators generally found that patients did not understand what they had consented to.

However, there were a number of problems with these early conclusions about patient understanding. First, investigators typically did not record their verbal disclosure or whether the patient had even read the consent form. Second, the consent forms were often obscurely written. Finally, the measures of understanding were often unsystematic and the questions themselves irrelevant to valid consent.

One solution was to use hypothetical research projects or treatment conditions. This has remained a common mechanism for ensuring that respondents use the same context or risk condition for their answers. With this approach, it was possible to fine-tune the analysis of consent studies since a large number of people could be asked the same questions.

However, questions were soon raised about this technique as well. What reason was there to believe that people would act the same way with a hypothetical scenario as they would in real life? After all, the personal relationship between clinician and patient—an influence critical to the consent process—would largely be removed from the hypothetical scenario.

The alternative for research consents was not simple. The difficulty in adding consent research to existing research projects (or "piggy-backing") is well known. It requires assurance to clinicians and families that their patients will not be discouraged from participating, that their consent procedures will not be judged inadequate, and that the burden on patients or staff will not be too great. Moreover, few clinical trials recruit enough subjects at one site to allow a single trial to form the basis for a piggy-back design. Thus, informed consent researchers were left with the choice of a hypothetical study that had limited external validity or a complex study using different consents to many different clinical trials. Nonetheless, some partial solutions would soon become apparent, from the use of semi-structured interviews to direct observation and video-taping.

Less Structured Interviews

Recent consent research is increasingly using semi-structured interviews to gather detailed reports from patients and research participants about their experiences of the consent process. Like a model consent discussion, this requires that interviewers be minimally leading in their questioning, use lay language rather than professional or academic terminology, and spend significant amounts of time listening. The text of the interview is then transcribed and coded for the relevant data. Although this can be complex and time consuming, there is more to this rich interplay of information, values, and choices than can be found in the discussion of a hypothetical scenario. This burgeoning ecological or contextual approach has the benefits both of quantitative research, in that it generates variables that can be analyzed statistically, and of qualitative research, in that it captures the subject's perspective relatively undistorted.[3,4]

One broadly applied—and somewhat more structured—approach is based on the MacArthur Competence Assessment Tools (or MacCATs). These instruments were designed to assess decision-making capacity, a psychological trait closely related to the legal concept of competence and empirically tested in consent to treatment, research, and choice of a health care proxy.[5-7] They require adaptation to the elements of a specific research protocol or treatment intervention, and assess four important domains of decision-making capacity: understanding, appreciation, reasoning, and choice.[8] MacCAT administration involves a structured disclosure of information about the study or treatment, followed by questions that assess the four domains. MacCAT interviews have been used to compare widely varied populations and to demonstrate three critical findings in informed consent: (1) medically ill, non-ill, and mentally ill research participants overlap considerably in their decision-making capacities; (2) part-by-part information disclosures are important to understanding; and (3) the decision-making capacity of subjects can improve with educative measures.[7,9-11] By removing the disclosure provided by the informed consent investigator, MacCAT-like instruments have been used widely to assess subjects' understanding of clinical and research disclosures.

Shorter tools for assessing capacity have been derived from the parent tool, including a 5-minute, 10-item screen for those needing less comprehensive assessment (that is, the University of California San Diego Brief Assessment of Capacity to Consent).[12] This short combination of open-ended and true-false questions is a welcome result of the approach found in the MacArthur model.

Other forms of semi-structured interviewing have played substantial roles in informed consent research. Swiss researchers used semi-structured conversations with almost 4,000 women to determine the best combination of written and oral consent for preoperative ob/gyn procedures.[13] Their finding that written material and illustrations were helpful to patients was not surprising, but served as an important reminder that consent forms do not have to interfere with consent discussions. The study also offered extensive data from in-depth interviews to demonstrate patients' strong interest in being active participants in the consent process.

Pediatric researchers Reynolds and Nelson[14] also used in-depth interviews to assess the affective influences on research participation of parents and adolescents. They described an intuitive and emotional response to the invitation to enter a research protocol. Thematic coding of this less structured approach led investigators to identify magnitude of risk, rather than probability, as the primary basis for their subjects' risk perceptions. Respondents made speedy decisions based on past experience, and—although some had past negative experiences with the procedures—most made decisions based in positive feelings of altruism.

Similar qualitative methods have also been useful in studying the motivation of participants to enter experimental protocols. In one study of parental reasons for enrolling their children with pneumonia, for example, researchers used open- and closed-ended questions to identify altruistic interests in increasing scientific knowledge.[15] Eighteen percent did cite benefit for their own child as their primary motivator, a potential signal of therapeutic misconception (that is, "the mistaken belief that decisions about one's treatment while a research subject would be made solely based on one's individual condition and needs").[16] The authors reported that parental decisions to enroll their children were best predicted by well-designed research that answered a clear clinical question.

More Structured Research

None of this should suggest that progress has not been achieved with more highly structured studies. Gurmankin et al.[17] used surveys and follow-up telephone interviews to describe some of the problems of providing patients with risk information. Of 108 women undergoing genetic counseling for breast cancer, a significant number showed higher-than-appropriate risk perceptions and resistance to the information itself. The investigators worried that information disclosure itself could lead to poor medical decisions. However, Upadhyay et al.[18] used four vignettes with varying risk and benefit to explore the interest of 210 patients in participating in medical decisions and research studies. They found that 85% of respondents showed *significant* interest in participating in even "trivial risk" protocols and similarly strong interests in participating in decisions for common, low-risk treatments. Few patients expressed interest in forgoing consent procedures even for more mundane interventions or treatments.

In Scotland, a structured interview was used as a tool to increase the effect of standard consent disclosures in surgical patients.[19] One hundred and thirty-eight patients in two groups received either a standard consent (and form) or the structured interview. The enhanced methodology resulted in better awareness of risk and of postoperative pain and a higher percentage of patients that actually read the consent form.

Observational Studies of Disclosure

The study of interactions between health care professionals and patients is also allowing new insight into the dynamics of consent interactions.

Kodish et al.[20] conducted a large multisite study of the informed consent communication process for randomized clinical trials (RCTs) of childhood leukemia. Informed consent conferences were observed and audio-taped on inpatient pediatric oncology wards at six major U.S. academic children's hospitals. The information obtained was coded and analyzed; parents were interviewed shortly after the conference to ascertain their understanding. The investigators found that randomization was explained by physicians in only 83% of cases, although a consent document containing the term was presented during 95% of the conferences. Interviews after the consent conference demonstrated that 50% of parents did not understand randomization.

This is consistent with an earlier study in Great Britain that audio-taped 82 RCT discussions. Jenkins et al.[21] demonstrated significant variation in the practice of oncologists who frequently omitted the term "randomization" or neglected to provide information leaflets specifically describing the clinical trial.

Ness et al.[22] have recently adopted an alternative approach to the study of consent interactions. Using linguistic techniques, they have analyzed tapes of interactions between researchers and potential research subjects. One finding is that there are marked differences in turn-taking processes in more and less successful consent interactions. Researchers in more successful interactions, for example, left genuine openings for subject turn-taking. These are easily identifiable in transcripts of the discussions. Likewise, these researchers have been able to show how, in some situations, the therapeutic misconception is built into the *frame* of the interaction between researcher and subjects. They underscore the difficulty of even well-intentioned researchers in transforming that frame. However, this technique is still in its early stages: There has been no large-scale effort to apply this linguistic approach to a systematic sample of interviews.

Although direct observation and videotape show promise by providing a more rigorous approach to the interaction patterns of researcher and subject, their use in studying how the consent process occurs is limited. This is because the analysis suffers from the difficulty of observing or taping consent interactions that are often fleeting and informal. Classic work in informed consent indicates that consent discussions can begin as early as the patient introduction and the unobserved walk to the office door.[23]

Neuroethics

Recent advances in functional neuroimaging and related technologies have led to the development of neuroethics, a controversially named field that explores the ethical and policy implications of our newest brain-related interventions and technologies.[24–26] Government interest in improving the wakefulness and attention of its soldiers and academic enthusiasm for scientific reductionism have led to great strides in this neuroscientific frontier.[27] With them comes the claim that neuroscientific findings raise important philosophical issues for research and clinical ethics.

For example, is it empirically possible to trace thoughts, behaviors, and motivations to their neuronal origins? Could we, for example, trace the neurological patterns of adequate or inadequate consent? Brain images of patients with serious mental illnesses like schizophrenia differ, in aggregate, from non-ill brains, although normal images may also show "abnormalities."[26] What conclusions, then, can ethics draw from these images? The application of general findings to specific cases is a core controversy in this kind of clinical and research thinking.[28,29] Yet, some companies now offer brain scans as lie detectors—although there is considerable doubt that they can truly tell when someone is lying.

Physician-ethicist Georg Northoff[30] has proposed an empirical framework for identifying the neuropsychological functions required for informed consent. Specific brain changes in Alzheimer's disease, depression, and schizophrenia, he argues, lead directly to the emotional and cognitive deficits that undermine consent. Using tools assessing emotional and cognitive elements of decision making together (that is, a MacCAT tool in addition to a test such as the Iowa Gambling Task) would allow consent researchers access to the exact neuronal deficits undermining consent. Working memory, executive function, and their related brain regions could then be targeted specifically to treat and improve consent discussions.

This approach is not dissimilar to the work already being conducted by empirical researchers who identify specific deficits among participants in their consent studies and seek to remediate them. Working memory, executive dysfunction, and cognitive impairment have been identified as factors influencing consent for years.[6,31–33] Moreover, there is some evidence that remediation is possible with enhanced consent processes.

So, are the challenges of informed consent reducible to neuronal substrates, or do personal values, decision-making heuristics, and social context require individual cognitive rather than neuronal assessment? It will take both philosophical analysis and a robust empiricism indeed to answer such questions.

Current Findings in Informed Consent

Despite new and heterogeneous methodologies, recent empirical work underscores a number of persistent problems in the practice of informed consent. For example, surrogate consents seem more problematic than might be expected. After all, surrogate decision makers are expected to know and support the values of their principal decision makers. But physicians in one study were willing to override patient wishes at the request of surrogates,[34] and another study showed that proxies were unable to describe accurately a patient's wishes about ophthalmologic surgery.[35]

Among professionals, differences in approaches to consent persist as well. A British team coded thematic information from interviews to show how a group of nurses differed from a group of general practitioners in their preparation of patients for cervical (or Pap) smears.[36] The physicians varied their presentations depending on the reason for the smear, while nurses followed a set protocol more closely. Both groups missed important areas of consent, from the sensitivity and specificity of the test, to the possibility of an abnormal finding, to what follow-up might be required. The interviews seemed to uncover a correlation to the clinicians' enthusiasm for the national screening program.

Communication between physicians and patients or research participants also remains problematic. In a study of lung and colon cancer patients entering experimental protocols, Sorensen et al.[37] found that physicians underestimated patient competence and satisfaction with consent information. This discrepancy underscored the difficulty physicians often have in determining the amount and kind of information their patients want, and emphasizes the need for early and frequent values discussions.

This kind of communication difficulty is evident in the persistent finding that many professionals view informed consent simply as part of routine clinical explanations.[38,39] These routine discussions are often paternalistic monologues rather than collaborative decision-making processes. For many, consent discussions are still not an ongoing exchange of information and values, but a method for ensuring a desired outcome.

There continues to be research showing that patient understanding of consent forms and procedures is less than ideal.[39–42] Akkad et al.'s survey[43] of over 700 patients demonstrates that many patients view informed consent merely as a protection for physicians and hospitals. The same research group's earlier surveys showed that consent forms themselves were perceived as "ritualistic and bureaucratic hurdles."[42,44,45] In the 700-patient survey, the investigators found that 68% of patients thought the consent form permitted physicians to take control of decision-making.

In surgical outpatients, too, although there was good understanding of consent materials among 141 individuals undergoing gastroscopy, few received full disclosure of risks, benefits, and consequences of declining the intervention.[41] Joffe et al.[46] have also described the deficits in informed consent among cancer patients in early-phase research. Of 207 patients enrolled in clinical trials, many had difficulty understanding the risks and benefits, and could not distinguish standard from nonstandard treatment. King et al.'s[47] look at consent forms in gene transfer research highlights the role of consent form language itself in contributing to the therapeutic misconception. Taken together, these findings seriously undermine informed consent doctrine, for, as Nixon et al.'s[19] use of the structured consent aid noted, it is having enough information to make decisions that builds trust in one's physician.

These consent problems may be even stronger when patients perceive themselves as desperate enough to take any risk for even the least possibility of relief. Elements of desperation and strong trust in their caregivers have long been found to be important in patients who enter research, including among HIV patients, persons with cancer or cardiovascular disease, and those with debilitating disorders such as arthritis.[48–50]

Patient interviews conducted during the groundbreaking Advisory Committee on Human Radiation Experiments (ACHRE) investigation indicated specifically that subjects trust their physicians to guide them through research decisions.[51] Misplaced trust in the researcher—that is, overconfidence in the protection, goodwill, and treatment competence of the researcher—is considered so significant that commentators are now suggesting it is as detrimental to research consents as the therapeutic misconception itself.[52]

Some research suggests that money can be a problematic inducement, especially in recruiting vulnerable research participants.[53–55] For example, money was the most important motivator among 136 healthy volunteers entering phase I studies, particularly those who were less educated or less well off financially.[56] In-depth interviews of cocaine abusers in economically disadvantaged neighborhoods point to research inducements as part of *daily* economic choices among poor participants.[57]

Conceptual Changes Driven by Research

One of the most interesting results of research into informed consent has been its interplay with ethical theory and policy. This is a complex area that we can only touch on here, but we will consider a few examples.

Ethicist Kenneth Kipnis has explored the concept of "vulnerability" of research participants that is so prominent in the regulation of research with human subjects. Kipnis found that vulnerability is not merely a matter of "subpopulations" such as prisoners or pregnant women, but of criteria that can describe any individual regardless of class membership.[58] Kipnis identifies a group of easily recognizable vulnerabilities that can be found in any number of research participants, including being subject to the authority of others, being undervalued by society at large, and being deprived of important goods and services.

A South African case study puts this construct into stark relief. Public health ethicist Lyn Horn explored the vulnerability of mine workers, often infected with tuberculosis or HIV, who are pressed into service as research participants.[59] The mining industry's economically driven commitment to research that might improve the health of its employees creates a unique vulnerability among workers: They become willing to undertake research risks in order to preserve their livelihoods. These are vulnerabilities that have been well established in other socioeconomically disadvantaged people and those under the influence of debilitating illnesses.

Research has also played a major role in the development and modification of the construct of the therapeutic misconception. This concept was first coined in 1982 as a result of a research project designed to improve informed consent.[16] Therapeutic misconception has generally been understood as research subjects' belief that their individual needs will determine treatment, or that the likelihood of benefit is greater than is actually the case.[60] Empirical studies dating to ACHRE have established its extensive presence among research participants.[51] Recent studies have identified it among cancer patients, in pediatrics and psychiatry studies, and among those participating in randomized clinical trials.[46,61,62] Sixty-two percent of participants in one seminal study—drawn from 44 treatment studies ranging from heart disease and cancer to asthma and depression—were thought to exhibit one form of misconception or the other.[63]

These results have led to much discussion about the meaning of therapeutic misconception. Some have noted the difficulty of connecting actual decisions to the presence of the misconception,[64] while others have attempted to parse out the overestimation of benefit as a separate construct (therapeutic *misestimation*).[65] Others have suggested that the core concept is simply a misunderstanding of the purpose of research.[66] Further research may further refine the construct, but its presence as a barrier to informed consent remains an important conceptualization backed by empirical evidence.

Attempts to Improve Informed Consent

Research findings about the understanding of consent disclosures, then, have not been entirely encouraging. Pervasive therapeutic misconception in research consents[63] and limited understanding of clinical and research interventions have led to efforts to improve the process through both enhanced education and the use of technological assistance.

Carpenter et al.[6] used educational assistance from the research staff, including formal 30-minute sessions, question-answer periods, flip-charts, and computer aids, to improve understanding among subjects diagnosed with schizophrenia (arguably the most devastating of mental disorders). Others have used multimedia or computer-aided educational interventions to raise performances of patients with schizophrenia to the level of comparison groups.[33,67] Eyler et al.[68] used interactive questioning with schizophrenia patients to offer corrective feedback and improve the consent process. An alternative consent process using a structured interview in surgery patients[19] improved awareness of risks and outcomes. Combs et al.[69] like Eyler, have also used cuing and verbal recognition of prompts to ensure improved comprehension of consent information.

Because consent forms do not encourage the active collaboration of discloser and disclosee, Sorenson et al.[70] emphasized the educational component of their own decision aid. In this study of 139 women considering genetic testing, participants identified personal reasons for enrolling so that the consent process was directly relevant to them. This value-based assistance in assessing the consequences of participating appears to be superior to the usual risk-benefit focus of generic consent discussions.

In one small study, a structured decision aid specifically mined patient values and developed a personal worksheet to facilitate decisions on intubation and ventilation.[71] This was an intervention not simply to improve understanding but to apply personal values to a specific decision. This approach has proven useful among chronic lung patients as well.[72,73]

In order to assess the quality of the informed consent process, investigators at the Berman Institute of Bioethics at Johns Hopkins developed a brief instrument called the BICEP, or Brief Informed Consent Evaluation Protocol.[74] This 8- to 9-minute telephone survey assessed patients' satisfaction with a recently completed consent process as well as elements of informed consent, including therapeutic misconception. Poor scores on the therapeutic misconception scale demonstrated some decision-making weaknesses among participants, but the study confirmed the ease of use of this kind of instrument.

Taking a similar approach with over 800 participants who had just completed a research consent process, the same lead investigators attempted to enhance the informed consent process itself.[75] Used as a quality assurance process, however, the cumulative exposure to the informed consent questionnaire did not appear to improve understanding by participants. There were still significant elements of therapeutic misconception, and understanding of risks and voluntariness was less than ideal. The authors suggested that more in-depth interviews and less heterogeneous populations could well show the expected effect.

Although these efforts, and others, appear to have produced improved understanding and participation, there has been considerable criticism of the process of assessing informed consent in such studies.[76] Because the educational interventions are so closely tied to the tools for measuring outcomes, improved understanding may actually be an artifact of the assessment process. Thus, improved scores may only reflect memorization of the correct answers rather than true understanding. Likewise, although Carpenter's[6] lengthy interactions between research staff and subjects may well be an ideal approach, it is hard to imagine this as a routine feature of either research or clinical care in the current health care system.

Lessons Learned

Empirical research is clearly making advances in our understanding of the informed consent process, although admittedly the progress may be limited. Through the direct analysis of the experiences of patients, subjects, clinicians, and researchers, new methods have expanded the boundaries of research, identified continued areas for improvement, and led to new empirically grounded conceptualizations.

We leave the topic of informed consent research with exhortations from the Informed Consent Project researchers, a group committed specifically to the study and improvement of this critical social interaction:[3,4]

1. The combination of qualitative and quantitative methods remains critical for the advancement of consent research.
2. The difficulties in enrolling consent subjects must be overcome by contact with and education of researchers about the importance of the research.
3. Policies must be developed to identify appropriate interventions when the consent being observed is inadequate.
4. Policies must also be developed for how consent research itself will be used to improve institutional standards without exposing researchers who have agreed to being observed to punitive sanctions.

References

1. Meisel, A., and L. Roth. 1983. Toward an informed discussion of informed consent: A review and critique of the empirical studies. *Arizona Law Review* 25(2):265–346.
2. Ethical principles and guidelines for the protection of human subjects. 1979. In *The Belmont Report.* Washington DC, National Commission for the Protection of Human Subjects of Biomedical and Behavioral Research.
3. Hougham, G., G. Sachs, D. Danner, J Mintz, M. Patterson, L. Siminoff, L. Roberts, et al. 2003. Empirical research on informed consent with the cognitively impaired. *IRB: Ethics and Human Research* 25(5):S26–S32.
4. Sachs, G., G. Hougham, J. Sugarman, P. Agre, M. Broome, G. Geller, N. Kass, et al. 2003. Conducting empirical research on informed consent: Challenges and questions. *IRB: Ethics and Human Research* 25(5):S4–S10.
5. Appelbaum, P., T. Grisso, and C. Hill-Fotouhi. 1997. The MacCAT-T: A clinical tool to assess patients' capacity to make treatment decisions. *Psychiatric Services* 48(11):1415–19.

6. Carpenter, W., J. Gold, A. Lahti, C. Queern, R. Conley, J. Bartko, J. Kovnick, and P. Appelbaum. 2000. Decisional capacity for informed consent in schizophrenia research. *Archives of General Psychiatry,* 57(6):540–42.

7. Candilis, P., K. Fletcher, C. Geppert, C. Lidz, and P. Appelbaum. 2008. A direct comparison of research decision-making: mentally ill, medically ill, and non-ill subjects. *Schizophrenia Research* 99:350–58.

8. Appelbaum, P., and T. Grisso. 2001. *MacCAT-CR: MacArthur Competence Assessment Tool for Clinical Research.* Sarasota, FL: Professional Resource Press.

9. Dunn, L., P. Candilis, and L. Roberts. 2006. Emerging empirical evidence on the ethics of schizophrenia research. *Schizophrenia Bulletin* 32(1):47–68.

10. Moser, D., S. Schultz, S. Arndt, M. Benjamin, F. Fleming, C. Brems, J. Paulsen, P. Appelbaum, and N. Andreasen. 2002. Capacity to provide informed consent for participation in schizophrenia and HIV research. *American Journal of Psychiatry* 159:1201–7.

11. Jeste, D., C. Depp, and B. Palmer. 2006. Magnitude of impairment in decisional capacity in people with schizophrenia compared to normal subjects: An overview. *Schizophrenia Bulletin* 32(1):121–28.

12. Jeste, D., B. Palmer, D. Jeste, B. Palmer, P. Appelbaum, S. Golshan, D. Glorioso, et al. 2007. A new brief instrument for assessing decisional capacity for clinical research. *Archives of General Psychiatry* 64(8):966–74.

13. Ghulam, A., M. Kessler, L. Bachmann, U. Haller, T. Kessler. 2006. Patients' satisfaction with the preoperative informed consent procedure: A multicenter questionnaire survey in Switzerland. *Mayo Clinic Proceedings* 81(3):307–12.

14. Reynolds, W., and R. Nelson. 2007. Risk perception and decision processes underlying informed consent to research participation. *Social Science and Medicine* 65:2105–15.

15. Sammons, H., M. Atkinson, I. Choonara, and T. Stephenson. 2007. What motivates British parents to consent for research? A questionnaire study. *BMC Pediatrics* 7:12–18.

16. Appelbaum, P., L. Roth, and C. Lidz. 1982. The therapeutic misconception: Informed consent in psychiatric research. *International Journal of Law and Psychiatry* 5:319–29.

17. Gurmankin, A., S. Domchek, J. Stopfer, C. Fels, and K. Armstrong. 2005. Patients' resistance to risk information in genetic counseling for BRCA1/2. *Archives of Internal Medicine* 165(5):523–29.

18. Upadhyay, S., A. Beck, A. Rishi, Y. Amoateng-Adjepong, and C. Manthous. 2008. Patients' predilections regarding informed consent for hospital treatments. *Journal of Hospital Medicine* 3:6–11.

19. Nixon, I., N. Balaji, O. Hilmy, B. Fu, and C. Brown. 2005. A prospective study comparing conventional methods against a structured method of gaining

patients' informed consent for tonsillectomy. *Clinical Otolaryngology* 30(5):414–17.

20. Kodish, E., M. Eder, R. Noll, K. Ruccione, B. Lange, A. Angiolillo, R. Pentz et al. 2004. Communication of randomization in childhood leukemia trials. *Journal of the American Medical Association* 291(4):470–75.

21. Jenkins, V., L. Fallowfield, A. Souhami, and M. Sawtell. 1999. How do doctors explain randomized clinical trials to their patients? *European Journal of Cancer* 35(8):1187–93.

22. Ness, D., S. Kiseling, and C. Lidz. Why does informed consent fail? A discourse analytic approach. *Journal of the American Academy of Law and Psychiatry* forthcoming.

23. Lidz, C., L. Fisher, and R. Arnold. 1992. *The erosion of autonomy in long-term care.* New York: Oxford University Press.

24. Fins, J., and Z. Shapiro. 2007. Neuroimaging and neuroethics: Clinical and policy considerations. *Current Opinion in Neurology* 20(6):650–54.

25. Annas, G. 2007. Foreword: Imaging of neuroimaging, neuroethics, and neurolaw. *American Journal of Law and Medicine* 32(2–3):163–70.

26. Greely, H., and J. Illes. 2007. Neuroscience-based lie-detection: The urgent need for regulation. *American Journal of Law and Medicine* 33(2–3):377–431.

27. Moreno, J. 2006. *Mind wars: Brain research and national defense.* Washington, DC: Dana Press.

28. Beresford, E. 1991. Uncertainty and the shaping of medical decisions. *Hastings Center Report* 24(4):6–11.

29. Brett, A. 1984. Ethical issues in risk factor intervention. *American Journal of Medicine* 78(4):557–61.

30. Northoff, G. 2006. Neuroscience of decision making and informed consent: An investigation in neuroethics. *Journal of Medical Ethics* 32:70–76.

31. Holzer, J., D. Gansler, N. Moczynski, and M. Folstein. 1997. Cognitive functions in the informed consent evaluation process: A pilot study. *Journal of the American Academy of Psychiatry and the Law* 25(4):531–40.

32. Basso, M., P. Candilis, J. Johnson, C. Ghormley, D. Combs, and T. Ward. Capacity to make treatment decisions in multiple sclerosis: A potentially remediable deficit. *Journal of Clinical and Experimental Neuropsychology* Under review.

33. Jeste, D., B. Palmer, S. Golshan, L. Eyler, L. Dunn, T. Meeks, D. Glorioso, I. Fellows, H. Kraemer, and P. Appelbaum. Jan 31, 2008. Multi media consent for research in people with schizophrenia and normal subjects: A randomized controlled trial. *Schizophrenia Bulletin [Epub ahead of print].*

34. Sypher, B., R. Hall, and G. Rosencrance. 2005. Autonomy, informed consent and advance directives: A study of physician attitudes. *West Virginia Medical Journal* 101(3):131–33.

35. Mantravadi, A., B. Sheth, R. Gonnering, and D. Covert. 2007. Accuracy of surrogate decision-making in elective surgery. *Journal of Cataract and Refractive Surgery* 33(12):2091–97.

36. Chew-Graham, C., E. Mole, L. Evans, and A. Rogers. 2006. Informed consent? How do primary care professionals prepare women for cervical smears: A qualitative study. *Patient Education and Counseling* 61:381–88.

37. Sorensen, J., P. Rossel, and S. Holm. 2004. Patient-physician communication concerning participation in cancer chemotherapy trials. *British Journal of Cancer* 90:328–32.

38. Delany, C. 2007. In private practice, informed consent is interpreted as providing explanations rather than offering choices: a qualitative study. *Australian Journal of Physiotherapy* 53(3):171–77.

39. Yousuf, R., and A. Fouzi. 2007. Awareness, knowledge, and attitude toward informed consent among doctors in two different cultures in Asia: A cross-sectional comparative study in Malaysia and Kashmir, India. *Singapore Medical Journal* 48(6):559–65.

40. Fisher, C., C. Cea, P. Davidson, and A. Fried. 2006. Capacity of persons with mental retardation to consent to participate in randomized clinical trials. *American Journal of Psychiatry* 163(10):1813–20.

41. Woodrow, S., and A. Jenkins. 2006. How thorough is the process of informed consent prior to outpatient gastroscopy? *Digestion* 73:189–97.

42. Paris, A., C. Cornu, P. Auquier, P. Maison, A. Radauceanu, C. Brandt, M. Salvat-Melis, M. Hommel, and J. Cracowski. 2006. French adaptation and preliminary validation of a questionnaire to evaluate understanding of informed consent documents in phase 1 biomedical research. *Fundamental and Clinical Pharmacology* 20:97–104.

43. Akkad, A., C. Jackson, S. Kenyon, M. Dixon-Woods, N. Taub, and M. Habiba. 2006. Patients' perceptions of written consent: Questionnaire study. *British Medical Journal* 333(7567):528–30.

44. Akkad, A., C. Jackson, S. Kenyon, M. Dixon-Woods, N. Taub, and M. Habiba. 2004. Informed consent for elective and emergency surgery in obstetrics and gynecology: A questionnaire study. *BJOG: An International Journal of Obstetrics and Gynecology* 11:1133–38.

45. Habiba, M., C. Jackson, A. Akkad, S. Kenyon, and M. Dixon-Woods. 2004. Women's accounts of consent to surgery: A qualitative study. *Quality and Safety in Health Care* 13:422–27.

46. Joffe, S., E. Cook, P. Cleary, J. Clark, and J. Weeks. 2001. Quality of informed consent in cancer clinical trials: A cross-sectional survey. *Lancet* 358:1772–77.

47. King, N., G. Henderson, L. Churchill, A. Davis, H.S. Chandros, D. Nelson, P. Parham-Vetter, et al. 2005. Consent forms and the therapeutic

misconception: The example of gene transfer research. *IRB: Ethics and Human Research* 27(1):1–8.

48. Logue, G., and S. Wear. 1995. A desperate solution: Individual autonomy and the double-blind controlled experiment. *Journal of Medicine and Philosophy* 20(1):57–64.

49. Minogue, B., G. Palmer-Fernandez, L. Udell, and B Waller. 1995. Individual autonomy and the double-blind controlled experiment: The case of desperate volunteers. *Journa Medicine and Philosophy* 20(1):43–55.

50. Fureman, I., K. Meyers, A. McLellan, D. Metzger, and G. Woody. 1997. Evaluation of a video supplement to informed consent: Injection drug users and preventive HIV vaccine efficacy trials. *AIDS Education and Prevention* 9(4):330–41.

51. *Advisory Committee on Human Radiation Experiments Final Report.* 1995. Washington, DC: U.S. Government Printing Office.

52. de Melo-Martin, I., and A. Ho. 2008. Beyond informed consent: The therapeutic misconception and trust. *Journal of Medical Ethics* 34(3):202–05.

53. Dickert, N., and C. Grady. 1999. What's the price of a research subject? Approaches to payment for research participation. *New England Journal of Medicine* 341(3):198–203.

54. Tishler, C., and S. Bartholomae. 2003. Repeat participation among normal healthy research volunteers: Professional guinea pigs in clinical trials? *Perspectives in Biology and Medicine* 46(4):508–20.

55. Russell, M., D. Moralejo, and E. Burgess. 2000. Paying research subjects: Participants' perspectives. *Journal of Medical Ethics* 16(4):353–66.

56. Almeida, L., B. Azevedo, T. Nunes, M. Vaz-da-Silva, and P. Soares-da-Silva. 2007. Why healthy subjects volunteer for phase 1 studies and how they perceive their participation? *European Journal of Clinical Pharmacology* 63:1085–94.

57. Slomka, J., S. McCurdy, E. Ratliff, S. Timpson, and W. Williams. 2007. Perceptions of financial payment for research participation among African-American drug users in HIV studies. *Journal of General Internal Medicine* 22(10):1403–09.

58. Kipnis, K. 2003. Seven vulnerabilities in the pediatric research subject. *Theoretical Medicine and Bioethics* 24(2):107–20.

59. Horn, L. 2007. Research vulnerability: an illustrative case study from the South African mining industry. *Developing World Bioethics* 7(3):119–27.

60. Appelbaum, P., and C. Lidz. 2008. The therapeutic misconception. In *The Oxford textbook of clinical research ethics*, Emanuel E, C. Grady, R. Crouch, R Lie, F. Miller, D. Wendler eds. New York: Oxford University Press.

61. Snowden, C., J. Garcia, and D. Elbourne. 1997. Understanding randomization: Parental responses to the allocation of alternative treatments in a clinical trial

involving their critically ill newborn babies. *Social Science and Medicine* 45:1337–55.

62. Daugherty, C. 1999. Impact of therapeutic research on informed consent and the ethics of clinical trials: A medical oncology perspective. *Journal of Clinical Oncology* 17:1601–17.

63. Appelbaum, P.S., C. Lidz, and T. Grisso. 2004. Therapeutic misconception in clinical research: Frequency and risk factors. *IRB: Ethics and Human Research* 26(2):1–8.

64. Kimmelman, J. 2007. The therapeutic misconception at 25: Treatment, research, and confusion. *Hastings Center Report* 37(6):36–42.

65. Horng, S., and C. Grady. 2003. Misunderstanding in clinical research: Distinguishing therapeutic misconception, therapeutic misestimation and therapeutic optimism. *IRB: Ethics and Human Research* 25(1):11–16.

66. Henderson, G., L. Churchill, A. Davis, M. Easter, and C. Grady. 2007. Clinical trials and medical care: Defining the therapeutic misconception. *PLoS Medicine* 4(11):e324.

67. Dunn, L., L. Lindamer, B. Palmer, S. Golshan, L. Schneiderman, D. Jeste. 2002. Improving understanding of research consent in middle-aged and elderly patients with psychotic disorders. *American Journal of Geriatric Psychiatry* 10(2):142–50.

68. Eyler, L., H. Mirzakhanian, and D. Jeste. 2004. A preliminary study of interactive questioning methods to assess and improve understanding of informed consent among patients with schizophrenia. *Schizophrenia Research* 75:193–98.

69. Combs, D., S. Adams, T. Woods, M. Basso, and W. Gouvier. 2005. Informed consent in schizophrenia: The use of cues in the assessment of understanding. *Schizophrenia Research* 77(1):59–63.

70. Sorenson, J., C. Lakon, T. Spinney, and T. Jennings-Grant. 2004. Assessment of a decision aid to assist genetic testing research participants in the informed consent process. *Genetic Testing* 8(3):336–46.

71. Wilson, K., S. Aaron, K. Vandemheen, P. Hebert, D. McKim, V. Fiset, I. Graham et al. 2005. Evaluation of a decision aid for making choices about intubation and mechanical ventilation in chronic obstructive pulmonary disease. *Patient Education and Counseling* 57(1):88–95.

72. Dales, R., A. O'Connor, P. Hebert, K. Sullivan, D. McKim, and H. Llewellyn-Thomas. 1999. Intubation and mechanical ventilation for COPD: Development of an instrument to elicit patient preferences. *Chest* 116(3):792–800.

73. Graham, I., J. Logan, C. Bennett, J. Presseau, A. O'Connor, S. Mitchell, J. Tetroe et al.. 2007. Physicians' intentions and use of three patient decision aids. *BMC Medical Informatics and Decision Making* 7:20–29.

74. Sugarman, J., P. Lavori, M. Boeger, C. Cain, R. Edsond, V. Morrison, and S. Yeh. 2005. Evaluating the quality of informed consent. *Clinical Trials* 2(1):34–41.

75. Lavori, P., T. Wilt, and J. Sugarman. 2007. Quality assurance questionnaire for professionals fails to improve the quality of informed consent. *Clinical Trials* 4(6):638–49.

76. Flory, J., and E. Emanuel. 2004. Interventions to improve research participants' understanding in informed consent for research: A systematic review. *Journal of the American Medical Association* 292(13):1593–1601.

14

Consent to Medical Care: The Importance of Fiduciary Context

Steven Joffe and Robert D. Truog

An eminent bioethicist visited his dermatologist to discuss the management of a lump on his back. The lesion had recently been diagnosed by biopsy as a basal cell carcinoma, a benign skin cancer that is easily treatable by surgical removal. After stating, "Here's what we are going to do," the dermatologist drew a picture of the proposed minor surgical procedure and mentioned sutures and the probable appearance of the scar. The physician then asked the bioethicist if he had any questions, and finally gave him a generic consent form for subsequent perusal and signature. At no time did the physician mention any risks of or alternatives to the proposed surgery.

As a bioethicist, the patient recognized that what transpired during this visit was minimally informed acquiescence rather than true informed consent. Nevertheless, he denied feeling any substantive offense at the nature of the interaction. As he later noted, "If I didn't happen to be a bioethicist, and hadn't gone into it with an eye to observing how the doctor handled the process, the encounter would probably have seemed perfectly appropriate and unremarkable."

Introduction

According to the standard conception of medical ethics, informed consent is fundamental to ethical practice because it is the mechanism by which patients autonomously authorize medical interventions or courses of treatment.[1] This prerogative to control one's medical destiny, which functions as a constraint on physicians' power and a curb to their paternalistic instincts, is elemental.[2] As the President's Commission for the Study of Ethical Problems in Medicine and Biomedical and Behavioral Research stated, "Informed consent is rooted in the fundamental recognition—reflected in the legal presumption of competency—that adults are entitled to accept or reject health care interventions on the basis of their own personal values and in furtherance of their own personal goals."[3] Or, as Justice Cardozo famously declared almost a century ago in *Schloendorff v. Society of New York Hospitals,* "Every human being of adult years and sound mind has a right to determine what shall be done with his own body."[4]

The case of the bioethicist with the basal cell carcinoma illustrates a basic problem for the standard conception of informed consent for treatment. Physicians often do not live up to their obligation to facilitate autonomous authorization. More important, patients often do not demand the robust decision-making responsibility that the concept of autonomous authorization presupposes, and in fact frequently prefer a lesser decision-making role.[5] Should ethics and policy seek to educate and exhort patients to assume, and physicians to encourage, greater patient responsibility for medical decisions? Or, taking into account the psychological realities of illness and the nature of the physician–patient relationship, is current practice normatively defensible? In light of the magnitude and persistence of the gap between the theory and practice of informed consent, answering this question constitutes a critical challenge for contemporary bioethics.

The Fundamentals of Informed Consent

When is a patient's consent to a course of medical treatment valid? Ethical and legal commentators have identified five elements that together establish the conditions for valid consent.[6] First, the patient must be situated so as to be able to make a *voluntary* decision. A decision that is substantially coerced is incompatible with valid informed consent. Second, the patient must be *competent* to make the decision. Significantly diminished consciousness or cognitive ability, among other impairments, invalidates a patient's apparent consent. Third, the patient must receive sufficient *disclosure* of the relevant facts, typically from the physician or another member of the medical team, to be able to reach a considered decision (note, however, that informed consent can occasionally be valid in the absence of disclosure, such as in the case of the physician-patient who is already an expert on his or her condition[1]). Elements to be disclosed include the nature and purpose of the procedure or intervention, its risks and potential benefits, and the available alternatives to the proposed course of action.[7] Fourth, the patient must achieve an adequate degree of *understanding* of the disclosed facts, as well as of the nature of consent as authorization, to form the basis of his or her decision.[1] Finally, the patient must *authorize* (informed consent) or *decline* (informed refusal) the proposed course of treatment.

Because most patients must rely on their physicians' assistance to gather and interpret the relevant facts, the process of autonomous authorization almost always requires professional input. How, then, should patients and clinicians work together to achieve the goal of informed consent? The President's Commission, Jay Katz, and many others have advocated a process of *shared decision making*.[2,3,8–11] Wide agreement on this label, however, masks deep uncertainties about its precise meaning. The term is often used without definition or further explanation, and likely means different things to different authors. On one view, shared decision making has three features: (1) information flow is two-way, (2) both the patient and the physician (as well as perhaps others) participate in deliberations about the decision, and (3) the patient and physician share the final decision.[12] On another view, shared decision making involves a division of labor: Physicians present and contextualize the facts that are material to the decision, whereas patients integrate those facts with their own values and preferences to make a final decision.[7,10,13,14] This division of labor is too sharp. Especially in the Internet age, patients often contribute material facts to medical discussions. In addition, physicians have a duty, based on their own values and status as moral agents, to respectfully challenge their patients when they perceive patients' choices to be contrary to their own interests.[8,11,13] Nevertheless, the concept of a division of labor captures an essential, if partial, truth about the distinct roles of patients and clinicians, as well as about the power differential and lack of symmetry between these parties, in the decision-making process.[2]

Emanuel and Emanuel provide further insight into the range of conceptual models that can reside under the heading of shared decision making.[11] They articulate four models of the physician–patient relationship; with the exception of their paternalistic model, all of these are consistent with the notion of shared decision making. In the informative model, physicians serve as competent technical experts, whose duty is to provide relevant factual information and implement the selected intervention even as patients retain control over choices about medical care. In the interpretive model, physicians serve as counselors or advisers, who perform all the functions of the informative physician while also helping to elucidate and interpret patients' health-related values. In the deliberative model, which the authors favor for most medical relationships and interactions, the physician is expected to step further onto the terrain of values, articulating and advocating for important health-related ends.

Although the dominant ethical conception of informed consent in medical care is one of autonomous authorization, it is important to identify at least two other senses in which the term *informed consent* is commonly used. First, it may describe a set of legal and institutional norms and practices that govern interactions in the health care setting. A patient's informed consent in this sense may provide legally or institutionally *effective* authorization for clinicians to proceed along a particular course, but does not guarantee that the authorization will be autonomous or otherwise ethically valid according to the criteria described previously.[1,7] Second, informed consent may denote a mechanism for the acceptance or assumption of risk by the patient. Under this conception, when a patient gives her informed consent, she accepts the possibility of certain adverse outcomes, especially those that the physician has disclosed to her. By doing so—presuming no negligence in execution on the physician's part—she absolves the physician of liability should a disclosed risk come to pass.[1,15] Although informed consent in these two senses is necessary to the smooth functioning of the health care system, and we later return briefly to the question of how ethical and legal conceptions of informed consent might align or diverge, our focus is on the ethical norm of informed consent as autonomous authorization for medical care.

Controversies Surrounding Informed Consent

Despite the volumes that have been written about informed consent in medical care, conceptual controversies as well as empirical evidence of gaps between theory and practice remain. On the conceptual side, defining what level of understanding is sufficient to serve as the basis for valid consent has proved elusive. Faden and Beauchamp, in their classic treatment of the subject, reject the view that informed consent requires "full" understanding. (The misconception that informed consent implies full understanding often leads to cynicism about informed consent and about ethics in general, as exemplified by the view of some physicians that informed consent is a mere formality—"if we took it seriously all patients would have to go to medical school before consenting to any procedure.") Instead, Faden and Beauchamp advocate a standard of "substantial" understanding, by which they mean (*1*) understanding that one is in fact authorizing some action, and (*2*) understanding of those aspects of the situation that are material to the action that one is authorizing.[1] Without minimizing the importance of their acknowledgment that valid consent does not require "full" understanding, the standard they articulate leaves unanswered many questions at the level of implementation about the threshold for adequate understanding. Furthermore, although the *patient* may require substantial understanding of the relevant facts to provide autonomous authorization, the basis of the *physician's* presumptive obligation to ensure the patient's understanding is obscure. Indeed, in most other consent contexts, A has no affirmative duty to ensure B's understanding prior to accepting B's consent.[15,16] Second, as noted previously, questions persist about the best way to interpret the claim that patients and physicians should "share" in decision making. Third, there is debate about whether informed consent is appropriately considered to be a right or an obligation for patients.[1,5,7] Finally, and perhaps most important for our present purpose, considerable empirical evidence suggests that, although the desire to receive medical information is generally strong, many patients—even physician-patients—frequently prefer to delegate medical decisions to their physicians rather than assuming responsibility for those decisions.[5,17–26]

Beyond the controversies highlighted previously, all of which have received considerable attention in the bioethics literature, the concept of informed consent calls out for further development in at least two other areas. First, although Katz and Brody have separately explored the relational context of informed consent,[2,8] there has been no systematic analysis of the ways in which the *fiduciary* character of the physician–patient relationship should influence conceptions of informed consent for medical care.[27] Second, although Faden and Beauchamp do acknowledge that "many decisions about routine and low-risk aspects of the patient's medical treatment [should] remain the exclusive province of the physician,"[1] the question of whether and how expectations for informed consent should be sensitive to the *nature* of the specific decision has largely escaped notice. In what follows, we contend that filling in these two gaps—which, as it turns out, intersect in interesting and important ways—helps to resolve the conundrums that continue to bedevil the theory and practice of informed consent.

Informed Consent and the Fiduciary Character of the Physician–Patient Relationship

The claim that the physician–patient relationship is fiduciary in nature, or at least that the fiduciary metaphor aptly characterizes the relationship in its essential aspects, is widely accepted.[1,27-30] According to Rodwin:

> The law defines a fiduciary as a person entrusted with power or property to be used for the benefit of another and legally held to the highest standard of conduct. Fiduciaries advise and represent others and manage their affairs. Usually they have specialized knowledge or expertise. Their work requires judgment and discretion. Often the party that the fiduciary serves cannot effectively monitor the fiduciary's performance. The fiduciary relationship is based on dependence, reliance, and trust.[27]

Trust in physicians as professionals, and a corresponding duty of loyalty that binds physicians to their patients, are at the heart of the fiduciary relationship between them. As Sokolowski writes, "The client trusts the professional and entrusts himself or herself . . . to the professional . . . . There is an elegant anonymity to professional trustworthiness; if I get sick away from home and must go to the emergency room of a hospital, I can in principle trust doctors and nurses I have never met before. I enter into a fiduciary relationship with them because they are presented as members of the medical *profession*" (italics in the original).[30]

How does the fiduciary nature of the physician–patient relationship affect physicians' obligations to obtain informed consent to medical procedures or courses of action? Is a robust obligation to obtain informed consent for each medical procedure truly necessary in light of patients' reliance on physicians' specialized knowledge and expertise, their expectations that physicians will exercise judgment and discretion on their behalf, and their acceptance that their relationships with physicians are based on dependence and trust? Might assumptions by patients about the duty of physicians to promote patients' best interests, rooted in patients' expectations about the fiduciary nature of the relationship, help explain why so many are so ready to delegate responsibility for medical decisions to their physicians? Or, conversely, does the fiduciary nature of the physician–patient relationship buttress, rather than weaken, physicians' obligations to seek autonomous authorization for medical interventions?

Answering these questions requires a precisely specified conception of the way in which the physician–patient relationship is a fiduciary one. Although there is no single model to guide us, Shepherd has identified three broad classes of fiduciary relationships recognized in the law: the fiduciary as property holder, the fiduciary as agent or representative, and the fiduciary as adviser.[31] The first of these has no direct bearing on the physician–patient relationship. The second and third, however, are potentially relevant to the medical setting. Their implications for informed consent merit close examination.

The Fiduciary as Agent

In the agency or representative model, the fiduciary acts on the client's behalf and in service of the client's welfare in the relevant domain. In the typical case, there is no need for the agent-fiduciary to seek authorization for each action; rather, the overarching authorization that the client grants to the fiduciary upon entering into the relationship—to represent the client and to act as an agent for his welfare—entails the license to act on the client's behalf. For example, in the political sphere, within the confines of her mandate and the limits of the law, there is no requirement that an elected official seek the voters' assent for each decision that she makes. Similarly, in the business arena, directors need not poll shareholders before making important decisions that affect the prospects of the company.[31] Rather, they must use their best judgment to select the course of action that optimally serves shareholders' interests. As applied to the medical setting, the agency model is most consistent with the paternalistic model articulated by Emanuel and Emanuel, predicated on the patient's authorization to enter into the relationship in the first place.[11]

If the agency model best describes the physician–patient relationship, then the requirement for informed consent for particular interventions is overblown. Of course, physicians must understand the broad objectives that they serve in assuming responsibility to care for each patient. However, consistent with those broad goals, physicians have the discretion to determine which course of action to select. As agents for patients, physicians must integrate their medical knowledge, practical experience, and technical expertise with their conception of individual patients' preferences and goals to select the course of action that best serves patients' medical needs.

The agency model of fiduciary relationships is unsatisfactory as a general account of the physician–patient interaction, at least when the patient is a competent adult, for at least two reasons. First, agency relationships are most appropriate when a robust, real-time decision-making role for the client is either not possible, as in the examples of director-shareholder and elected official-citizen relationships cited previously, or has been explicitly delegated. Second, physicians cannot be expected to know or anticipate their patients' values and preferences in sufficient detail to make important medical choices on the latters behalf, in part because those values and preferences likely evolve as patients' medical and other life circumstances present new challenges. Nevertheless, as we discuss further below, it is impossible to deny the elements of truth in the agency model of the physician–patient relationship.

The Fiduciary as Adviser

If the agency model paints an inadequate, or at least substantially incomplete, picture of the physician–patient relationship, perhaps the adviser-fiduciary model is a better fit. Indeed, Shepherd's only mention of doctors comes in the section of his book devoted to the adviser model, and on this basis Morreim claims that the concept of an adviser best captures the physician's role.[29,31] Other types of advisers, according to Shepherd, include attorneys, real estate agents, and financial planners. Advisers differ from agents in that the main role of the former is to provide information and guidance to their clients, whereas the main role of the latter is to represent their clients in decision-making situations. Although duties of fidelity and loyalty govern the fiduciary's advice-giving role, the adviser-fiduciary lacks authorization to act on the client's behalf without the client's explicit consent. Depending on how broadly one conceives the scope of the physician's duty to advise, this model may be consistent with the informative, interpretive, or deliberative models of the physician–patient relationship.[11]

If Morreim is correct that physicians are advisers to their patients, the fiduciary nature of the physician–patient relationship supports a robust requirement for informed consent. Physicians must provide their patients with information about their medical conditions, the available treatment options, and the risks and benefits of each, but have no license to act unless and until patients specifically authorize them to do so. Furthermore, under the more demanding interpretive and deliberative models,[11] the physician must go beyond providing information to help the patient clarify her values, or even to help shape and direct those values. Fulfilling these obligations will require respectful conversation, as envisioned by Katz and by Brody,[2,8] in the service of what Fried has called "the life plans of . . . patients."[32]

The adviser model of the fiduciary relationship between physicians and patients helps to explain one of the central problems identified previously with the standard conception of informed consent. Although the parties to a consent interaction frequently have positive obligations to disclose information, it is uncommon for one party to have an affirmative obligation to ensure the other party's understanding prior to accepting his or her consent.[15,16] However, viewed as an adviser-fiduciary, the physician has a duty not simply to act as an agent for the patient's welfare, but rather to help the patient make choices that cohere with and advance his individual life plan. In order to satisfy this demanding duty, the physician must do more than merely provide information that can serve as the basis for the patient's decision; she must take affirmative steps to ensure that the patient has a sufficient understanding of that information to make a decision that promotes his life plan.

Despite the undeniable appeal of the adviser model as a normative description of the physician–patient relationship, it is at best incomplete. In some circumstances, as with the patient who, having agreed to undergo a surgical procedure, is now under general anesthesia, physicians must make decisions without the possibility of securing input from the patient. Perhaps more important, during the course of complex medical care, physicians must inevitably make many choices about lesser issues on the basis of an implicit grant of authority from the patient rather than on the basis of explicit consent for each choice. Although these choices may relate to the "routine and low-risk aspects of the patient's medical treatment" noted by Faden and Beauchamp,[1] it nevertheless seems evident that when making such choices physicians unavoidably step out of their advisory roles.

We contend that every interaction involving a physician and a competent adult patient inevitably straddles the agency and adviser models of fiduciary relationships. Furthermore, different physician–patient dyads occupy different points on the continuum between these two archetypal relationships, and individual dyads move back and forth across the continuum as medical and other circumstances change. Finally, except when the patient is temporarily incapacitated as during general anesthesia, there is no natural or objectively correct place on this continuum for any particular relationship at any particular point in time. Rather, the specific blend of adviser and agent roles is the product of an ongoing negotiation between patient and physician, and is therefore always characterized by dynamic tension.

What considerations militate in favor of the adviser model of the physician–patient relationship, and what considerations militate in favor of the agency model? As noted previously, the major distinction between these two models is which party retains presumptive power to authorize actions. If we adopt the agency model in a particular circumstance, we will view some prior higher-order consent, up to and including the patient's general agreement to enter into the relationship with the physician in the first place, as entailing that authority, and for practical purposes will therefore vest authority for the particular decision in the physician. Conversely, if we adopt the adviser model, we will expect the physician to use his or her medical knowledge to make diagnostic or treatment recommendations, and perhaps to deliberate with the patient about the best course of action, but in each case will retain for the patient the authority to make the decision. Deciding which approach to decisions fits best, and therefore which fiduciary model to invoke, requires close attention to the features of the decision at hand. It is to this task that we now turn.

Ends, Means, and Presumptions About Authority in Medical Decisions

Let us review the ground we have covered so far. We have pointed to the frequent gap between the strong view of informed consent as autonomous authorization on the one hand, and the degree to which patients commonly prefer to delegate responsibility for many medical decisions on the other, as a reason to question the former's pragmatic if not its normative force. We have further argued that the superficial consensus surrounding the notion of shared decision making masks deep uncertainties about the appropriate allocation of responsibility for decisions between patients and physicians. We have also explored the various conceptions of the fiduciary physician–patient relationship, recognizing that the literature to date has failed to consider informed consent in this particular relational context. In doing so, we have shown that the agency and adviser models each captures essential elements of the fiduciary physician–patient interaction, but point in opposite directions with regard to the role of informed consent and autonomous authorization in the medical encounter. In light of the various tensions and uncertainties surrounding decision-making roles in the physician–patient relationship, how should we allocate responsibility for particular medical decisions between patients and physicians?

One potential approach to this problem is to consider a division of medical decisions into choices about ends or choices about means. Ends and means, of course, are interdependent.[33] Nevertheless, the distinction between ends and means is useful because it offers a first step toward identifying the appropriate roles of patients' values and of physicians' expertise in medical decisions. To oversimplify (temporarily) the issue: Patients' values inform decisions about ends, whereas once patients and physicians reach agreement about ends, technical considerations that lie within the domain of medical expertise inform decisions about means.

The literature on informed consent in lawyer–client relationships offers an instructive parallel to our proposal for assigning responsibility for decisions according to a distinction between ends and means. Spiegel notes the traditional view that the "subject-matter/procedure rule" governs the allocation of decision-making authority between lawyer and client. According to this rule, "the attorney has implied authority to do everything necessary and proper in the conduct of a case, provided his actions affect the remedy and not the cause of action."[34] So, for example, responsibility for deciding whether to settle a suit or to contest it at trial belongs with the client, whereas responsibility for deciding whether or not to call a particular witness, or to strike a particular juror, rests with the lawyer. Spiegel also points to the American Bar Association's (ABA) Code of Professional Responsibility[a] (EC 7-7), which states, "In certain areas of legal representation *not affecting the merits of the cause or substantially prejudicing the rights of a client*, a lawyer is entitled to make decisions on his own. But otherwise the authority to make decisions is exclusively that of the client . . . ." (italics added).[35] The subject-matter/procedure rule and the ABA code bear obvious similarities to the proposal articulated previously for allocating medical decision-making authority according to a distinction between ends and means.

There is, of course, a problem with allocating decision-making authority between patients and physicians (or between clients and lawyers) on the basis of a distinction between ends and means. Deciding whether a particular decision is primarily about ends or primarily about means is rarely straightforward. At the extremes, of course, we have no difficulty determining which is at stake. For example, consider George Zimmer, a professor of English who wrote of his decision to participate in several phase I anticancer trials: "We who are struggling to escape cancer do not, obviously, want to die of it. We do prefer death in the struggle to life under cancer's untender rule."[36] Professor Zimmer's preference for continued struggle undeniably reflects a choice about the ends of medical interventions at that particular point in his life. In contrast, the selection of 3-0 versus 4-0 sutures during the surgical removal of the bioethicist's basal cell carcinoma patently involves a decision about means, not ends.

In most decisions between alternative treatments, however, the distinction between means and ends is less clear-cut. Different choices may have different positive and negative consequences, and deciding which set of potential consequences to prefer may require selecting among ends. Consider the classic decision whether to undergo mastectomy (removal of the whole breast) or lumpectomy (local excision with breast preservation) plus radiation therapy for localized breast cancer. Although it is possible to view the choice between these two surgical approaches as merely a decision about which means will best minimize the chance of death from breast cancer, such a view misrepresents the situation. Instead, the choice between these procedures necessarily involves important decisions about ends, such as the psychological and social meaning to the patient of losing a breast and the acceptability of living with an increased possibility of local recurrence. As this example shows, the choice of medical means intended to address an overarching end frequently entails consideration of other, logically subsidiary but no less consequential ends.

A picture thus emerges of a taxonomy of decisions, characterized by the extent to which the decision is best described as a choice between ends or a choice between means. Decisions regarding the overall objectives of a course of therapy occupy one end of this spectrum, and technical choices about which no reasonable patient could have a preference lie at the other. Decisions that, although ostensibly about means, entail choices between more or less important subsidiary ends occupy various intermediate points along this spectrum. For instance, as discussed previously, the decision whether to undergo lumpectomy or mastectomy undeniably involves important choices about ends. The decision about which drug to use first to treat a patient's hypertension is closer to a choice among means, although it may nevertheless raise considerations of ends such as cost or the acceptability of the various potential toxicity profiles (the logically prior decision about whether or not to initiate drug therapy for hypertension, in contrast, plainly involves consideration of ends). What defines the place that a particular decision occupies on this spectrum, then, is the degree to which it can reasonably be viewed as entailing choices among ends. And this, in turn, depends on the extent to which important patient values are plausibly at stake in the outcome of the decision at hand.

Again, consideration of the lawyer–client analogy is instructive. Spiegel, who writes about informed consent between lawyers and clients, rightly rejects the subject-matter/procedure rule, at least in its simplest form, as a guide to whether or not informed consent is required. His primary criticism of the rule is that, although many decisions appear at first blush to be about means or procedures, upon deeper inspection they often involve important considerations of clients' values. As he writes, "The basic problem is that the division between subject matter and procedure is inevitably artificial. It is based on a false view of an ends/means dichotomy."[34] For example, the decision about whether or not a plaintiff should testify at trial turns not only on tactical decisions about whether testifying is most likely to lead to a favorable verdict, but also on questions such as the value the plaintiff places on telling his story in court. Spiegel therefore advocates replacing, or at least extending, the subject-matter/procedure rule: "a lawyer should be affirmatively required to obtain informed consent when *client values* or lawyer conflicts of interest are involved" (italics added).[34]

As an aside, it is worth noting that the examples chosen to illustrate the theoretical literature on informed consent have largely been drawn from among those decisions, such as the choice between mastectomy and lumpectomy, that clearly implicate important subsidiary ends and patient values. This class of decisions has thus become the paradigm for normative discussions of informed consent. For example, the first case that Katz discusses at length in his classic *Silent World of Doctor and Patient* involves "Iphigenia," a young woman with breast cancer faced with this very decision.[8] Because of the surgeon's belief that mastectomy was the best option for Iphigenia, he had at first obtained her "consent" for the procedure without telling her about the option of an alternative, more limited operation. However, as the surgery approached, he had doubts about not having disclosed the alternatives to her, and therefore initiated a second conversation about the available options that ultimately led Iphigenia to opt for lumpectomy. Eddy illustrates his article on the "Anatomy of a Decision" with the case of a 55-year-old asymptomatic woman who is considering whether or not to undergo mammography screening for breast cancer, a decision that trades a possible reduction in risk of dying from breast cancer against the possibility of a false-positive result, the risks associated with the radiation used in mammography, and the discomforts and anxiety of the exam itself.[10] If the normatively defensible approach to informed consent varies according to the nature of the particular decision, as we have argued, then biases in the literature that derive from its focus on a specific class of decisions may limit the generalizability of insights drawn from those examples to other classes of medical decisions.

Even if we are roughly correct in arraying decisions along a spectrum of ends to means, with patient values increasingly implicated to the degree that ends are at stake, what, if any, are the consequences for informed consent? After all, if a necessary justification for a medical intervention involving a competent patient is his or her autonomous authorization, then all decisions about medical interventions, even those that unarguably involve choices among means to a settled end, require the patient's explicit, voluntary informed consent. There are at least two problems with this position. First, as discussed above, compelling evidence indicates that many patients prefer to delegate decisions, or aspects of decisions, to their physicians. Second, most medical interventions or courses of action are not unitary, but rather reflect packages of elements that are at least logically distinguishable from one another. Furthermore, the elements of the package are frequently not fixed, and choices must be made about precisely which elements will be included as well as about how they will relate to one another. For example, once a patient has agreed to proceed with resection of an early-stage lung cancer, must the surgeon engage the patient in discussion and decision making about each particular element of that complex surgical package? Although an extreme view of informed consent might insist that patients explicitly authorize each element of the package, such an arrangement would be both fatally inefficient and seriously inconsistent with the wishes of the vast majority of patients. Physicians must therefore regularly decide when to proceed as though a patient's higher-order consent to an intervention entailed his or her agreement to all its elements versus when to draw the patient's attention to a particular aspect of the intervention and seek additional, explicit consent. In other words, physicians must constantly make judgments about what constitutes the "smallest decision unit." How can they know where to draw the line?

It is now time to refine and restate our earlier crude hypothesis that patients are responsible for decisions about the ends of medical care, whereas physicians are responsible for decisions about the means to the agreed-upon ends. A more precise formulation of this position, which acknowledges the frequent inextricability of ends and means, is:

1. Patients are always responsible for medical decisions about the ultimate ends or goals of therapy, which necessarily involve weighing of values.
2. Patients are presumptively responsible for decisions about the means to those ends, to the extent that such decisions entail value-laden choices among subsidiary ends.
3. Physicians may assume presumptive responsibility for those decisions about means that are unlikely to entail value-laden choices between subsidiary ends.

A corollary to this position is that, when a decision can plausibly be viewed as involving a choice among ends, the physician has an obligation first to frame the decision for the patient in a way that assists the patient to appreciate the values and ends at stake, and then to offer the patient the opportunity to choose among the available alternatives.

Under the formulation we have proposed, physicians may proceed with interventions without explicit consent, or with only (in the words of our eminent bioethicist) "minimally informed acquiescence," in certain precisely delimited circumstances. Specifically, such implicit or *de minimus* consent is permissible when—after appropriate consideration of patient values—the patient and physician have agreed on all the important ends, and the intervention or procedure in question may reasonably be characterized as merely a means to the agreed-upon ends. Three questions, however, immediately arise. First, is there an objectively determinable normative threshold in the hierarchy of decisions beneath which important ends are no longer at stake, or does this threshold vary from one case to the next? Second, if the threshold varies among cases, who has the ultimate authority to determine whether or not ends are at stake in a particular decision? Finally, is explicit agreement on ends always required, or are there circumstances in which physicians may identify and pursue means on the basis of implicit agreement with patients about ends?

The variation among patients in attitudes toward the assumption versus delegation of responsibility for medical decisions lends support to the contention that there is no objective threshold beneath which all observers can agree that ends are no longer at stake. Rather, precisely when all the important ends, and the values that inform them, have been accounted for in a particular chain of decisions is open to negotiation among the parties. Some patients may decide that the ends and values that are important to them have been accounted for at a relatively high level of decision making, whereas other patients may decide that ends and values require exploration at a much more granular level of decisions. To take an example that we have already cited, one patient may be comfortable that his informed decision to initiate pharmacotherapy for hypertension adequately addresses all his important ends and values, and therefore leave the choice of agents to his physician. In contrast, another patient might decide that the differing toxicity profiles of the various pharmacological options require her active participation in, and ultimately her consent to, the selection of the first-line drug.

The forgoing discussion suggests that, in general, determining the point at which there is sufficient agreement on ends to justify treating subsequent decisions as touching only on means is the prerogative of the patient rather than of the physician. This leads to a conundrum: If a physician elects to treat a particular decision as touching only on means, how can the patient know whether or not ends or values that are important to him are at stake? Although the determination of whether or not ends are at stake may be the patient's prerogative, without guidance from the physician he may not know enough about the decision—indeed, he may not even be aware that the particular decision awaits—to be able to determine whether or not additional discussion about ends is required. If this is correct, then perhaps we are back to requiring autonomous authorization on the basis of substantial understanding, or explicit delegation of decision-making authority, in every case.[1]

Although there is no perfect solution to this conundrum, we can at least make pragmatic headway by recognizing that both physicians and patients bear responsibility for identifying when medical choices implicate values or ends. Physicians, in their roles as adviser-fiduciaries, must always strive to evaluate each decision from the patient's point of view and to consider whether any important values or ends might reasonably be at stake. In doing so, they must take into account both their general norms about what sorts of information are likely to be material to patients (in the sense of relevant to their values or ends) as well as their knowledge of the particular patient before them. Patients, for their part, must assume responsibility for asserting themselves whenever questions arise about the impact of medical choices on ends of importance to them. It would, after all, be paradoxical to claim simultaneously that patients are adults who are responsible for their own medical decisions and that their position in the patient–physician relationship is so weak that they cannot reasonably be asked to assert themselves. It is essential, however, to recognize and accept that no workable system for deciding whether important ends or values are at stake will lead to satisfactory outcomes in every case. Despite the best efforts of patients and physicians, physicians will at times unnecessarily highlight minor decisions, whereas at other times they will fail in good faith to engage patients in decisions that the latter would view as implicating important ends.

The complexity of this dynamic is illustrated, albeit in the context of surrogate rather than autonomous decision making, by the case of a young man admitted to the intensive care unit with severe meningitis and septic shock. Despite efforts at resuscitation, his condition deteriorated, and eventually his physician suspected that he may have progressed to the state of brain death (at which point he would legally be dead). In order to diagnose brain death, it was necessary to perform a radioisotope test to determine if blood was still flowing to the brain. The boy's father was an Orthodox Jewish rabbi, who, unknown to the physician, belonged to a group that does not accept that patients diagnosed as brain dead are actually dead. Following usual procedure, the physician ordered the test without seeking the consent of the father. When the father learned from the nurse that the test was about to be done, and that a likely outcome of the test would be that his son would be pronounced legally dead, he refused permission for the test to be performed.

In this case, the physician regarded the blood flow study as a means to providing appropriate medical care. The physician was unaware, however, that the results of the study would impact significant values and ends for the patient's father. Ideally, the physician might have anticipated the religious implications of the test and discussed them with the father before ordering the test, but in this case it was not until the father learned about the test on his own and objected that it became clear the test was more about ends than about means.

Even if patients, as a rule, retain the prerogative to determine whether or not a decision touches on ends, there are circumstances in which this presumption may not hold. Consider the patient who seeks to "micromanage" care, for example, by dictating choices, such as size of suture, settings of mechanical ventilation, or selection of tests ordered for the evaluation of severe chest pain, that most physicians would consider to be within their toolkit of means. Although physicians may not legally or ethically be permitted to impose unwanted interventions on competent patients, they nevertheless are entitled to challenge such micromanagement or even, outside of emergency situations, to decline to care for patients who unreasonably constrain their choices of means. Similar issues arise in the lawyer–client relationship; in arguing for broader obligations of informed consent than had previously been accepted, Spiegel nevertheless concedes that excessive client control over the means and methods of legal work risks compromising various interests of the lawyer, including an interest in professional autonomy and "craft interests in not being forced to do substandard work."[34] In the medical setting, excessive patient control over the means and methods of doctoring would place the analogous interests of physicians as professionals at risk.

Finally, we contend that it may sometimes be ethically acceptable for physicians to proceed with tests or treatment, either without specific authorization or with minimally informed acquiescence, on the basis of implicit agreement with patients about ends. Consider the young, healthy adult who presents to the emergency room with classic early appendicitis. What is required of the surgeon who proposes to move expeditiously toward the operating room to remove the inflamed appendix? Must she secure explicit agreement on the goal of removing the appendix before the risk of serious complications becomes substantial, and then engage in a detailed conversation about the various theoretical options for management, including immediate resection and watchful waiting, before insisting that the patient select from among the options on offer? Alternately, may she presume agreement on the goal of removing the appendix and preventing complications, briefly describe the proposed procedure and the main attendant risks, and accept the patient's often-perfunctory agreement to proceed? Or consider the dermatologist caring for our bioethicist. Plausibly, the bioethicist's lack of serious objection to the superficial nature of the dermatologist's consent conversation stemmed from the implicit agreement between the physician and patient on the goal of removing the skin cancer to prevent local spread or recurrence, combined with the patient's sense that the choice of means to achieve this goal implicated no important ends or values. If so, then under the framework we have advanced, the dermatologist cannot be charged with failing to fulfill his professional obligation to secure the bioethicist's informed consent.

Although the subject of consent to research participation is addressed elsewhere in this volume, a few brief words of contrast between the medical and research settings are in order. We have argued that physicians may assume presumptive responsibility for decisions to the extent that those decisions can reasonably be seen as having implications only for means. Such assumption of responsibility is permissible only because of the fiduciary character of the physician–patient relationship, and the duty of loyalty that the physician owes to the patient. It follows, then, that given the nonfiduciary character of the researcher–participant relationship, in which the researcher does not owe the participant an undivided duty of loyalty,[29] the investigator's ability to assume responsibility for decisions about means is more limited than that of the physician. This fundamental difference in the natures of the physician–patient and researcher–participant relationships suggests that the obligations of investigators to obtain informed consent are more demanding and less easily set aside than are those of physicians.

The framework we have articulated here for allocating decision-making responsibility between patients and physicians on the basis of the nature of the decision at hand, and in particular on the extent to which it implicates important patient ends or values, helps explain empirical observations of the gap between the theory and practice of informed consent. Braddock et al., in a much-cited medical journal article describing findings from a large study involving audiotapes of consultations between patients and primary care physicians or surgeons, concluded that "surgeons and primary care physicians in office practice infrequently had complete discussions of clinical decisions with their patients . . . . [T]he ethical model of informed decision making is not routinely applied in office practice."[37] The investigators divided decisions into three levels of complexity, and applied a sliding scale to determine whether or not discussions preceding those decisions were complete (see the Table 1). They found that, by their definition, discussions were complete for only 17% of "basic" decisions and for less than 1% of the "intermediate" and "complex" decisions. Even more striking, when intermediate and complex decisions were scored according to the minimal criteria for completeness developed for basic decisions, only 20% of intermediate and 38% of complex decisions were judged complete.

These apparent flaws in the implementation of informed consent norms become more comprehensible when considered in light of the framework we

Table 1: Criteria for completeness of basic, intermediate, and complex decisions according to Braddock et al.[37]

Criterion	Required for Decisions to Be Judged Complete?		
	Basic Decision[*]	Intermediate Decision[†]	Complex Decision[‡]
1. Discussion of patient's role in decision	Yes (1 or 7)	Yes (1 or 7)	Yes
2. Discussion of the clinical issue or nature of the decision	Yes	Yes	Yes
3. Discussion of alternatives	No	Yes	Yes
4. Discussion of pros and cons of alternatives	No	No	Yes
5. Discussion of uncertainties associated with decision	No	Yes	Yes
6. Assessment of patient's understanding	No	Yes	Yes
7. Exploration of patient preferences	Yes (1 or 7)	Yes (1 or 7)	Yes

[*] Basic decisions are defined as those that have minimal effect on the patient, are supported by medical consensus, and have clear, singular outcomes. An example of a basic decision is thyroid function testing to evaluate the cause of fatigue.

[†] Intermediate decisions are defined as those that have moderate effect on the patient, have wide medical support but not medical consensus, and have moderately uncertain outcomes. An example of an intermediate decision is changing the dose of an existing medication, versus adding a new medication, to obtain better control of blood pressure.

[‡] Complex decisions are defined as those that have extensive effects on patients, are medically controversial, and have uncertain, multiple outcomes. An example of a complex decision is screening for prostate cancer.

have developed here. Agreement, whether implicit or explicit, on the goal of seeking to identify a cause for fatigue may be sufficient to justify the physician's obtaining a blood test to assess thyroid function (a basic decision) without much additional discussion or explicit consent. Although the rare patient may disagree, it is reasonable for the physician to conclude that the decision to test thyroid function is a decision about means, not ends, and that it is unlikely to implicate important patient values. At the other extreme of complex decisions, the decision to screen a man for prostate cancer undoubtedly implicates ends: In the face of uncertainty, some men prefer aggressive measures to minimize cancer risk, whereas others are reluctant to accept screening and its consequences (for example, the potential need to decide about undergoing morbid procedures such as prostatectomy or prostate radiation) in the absence of clear evidence and consensus that screening reduces the likelihood of death from prostate cancer.[38] Finally, in the middle, some patients might reasonably prefer to treat decisions about whether to increase their current blood pressure medication or to add a second agent as decisions about means, in which case relatively limited discussion followed by passive acquiescence might be acceptable. In contrast, other patients might view this decision as touching on important values and ends, and might wish a robust discussion about the advantages and disadvantages of the various options, together with the opportunity to select the alternative that best coheres with their personal life plans.

One final point is in order before concluding our discussion of ends and means in medical decision making. The heuristic we have articulated here should not be confused with the familiar idea, advanced by others, that shared decision making involves a division of labor between patients, who supply values, and physicians, who supply facts.[10,13,14] Whatever the merits of their position, those who write of a division of labor between facts and values address the structure of *individual decisions*. They view patients and physicians as jointly responsible for each decision, and seek to allocate responsibility for the components of each decision between patients and physicians. The framework we have developed aims instead to distinguish various types of decisions from one another, and on the basis of this typology to allocate presumptive responsibility for those decisions between patients and physicians.

Objections to Allocating Responsibility for Decisions According to the Degree to Which Patients' Ends and Values Are at Stake

We will briefly review two major objections to our proposal for allocating decision-making responsibility. First, critics of our argument might object that all decisions are in some greater or lesser way about ends, and that the class of decisions that exclusively implicate means is so narrow as to be of little theoretical importance. If so, then at best our argument reduces to a footnote to theoretical discussions of informed consent. There are several reasons, however, why this cannot be right. First, as we have noted, the degree to which decisions implicate patients' ends and values represents a continuum. At one end of the continuum, where decisions unarguably implicate critical ends, all patients should be encouraged or even required to understand their choices and to take responsibility for decisions. However, below a certain threshold on that continuum—the precise specification of which undoubt-edly varies among patients and among circumstances, and is subject to negotiation within the dynamic patient–physician interaction—virtually all patients would cease to see that any important ends or values are at stake. Indeed, we hypothesize that when patients delegate decisions to physicians, they typically view those decisions as touching primarily on means, and therefore as best informed by physicians' medical expertise. Second, most decisions can be decomposed into a package of component choices. At a certain point in that process of decomposition (that is, the point at which the "smallest decision unit" is reached), it becomes neither practical nor consis-tent with patients' preferences to insist dogmatically that all component choices implicate ends and therefore require full patient engagement. Finally, the claim that all decisions require consideration of ends, and there-fore require robust informed consent, runs into arguments from efficiency. The resources required to undertake robust informed consent—mainly patient and physician time—are not unlimited, and it seems unlikely that patients or society at large would be willing to pay for time spent on decisions that have few implications for patients' important ends or values.[15]

A second, related objection is that, even if we accept that some decisions are only about means, respect for patients' autonomy means that they should be offered the opportunity to make them. At a certain level of abstraction, this objection is correct—for example, physicians may not impose interventions, whether or not they can be characterized as pure means to an agreed-upon end, over the explicit refusal of a competent patient. But as a practical guide this claim fails for the same reasons as the argument that all decisions implicate ends: It is inconsistent with patients' preferences, ignores the notion of the "smallest decision unit," and has unacceptable implications for the efficient deployment of medical resources. Finally, the claim that explicit informed consent is required even for choices that are unarguably about means constitutes an open invitation to micromanaging, with all the implications for professional autonomy and physicians' craft interest in the practice of medicine that micromanaging entails.

The Relationship Between Legal and Ethical Norms of Informed Consent

We suggested above that, in addition to its use as shorthand for autonomous authorization, the term *informed consent* has a distinct institutional and legal meaning. In this latter sense, informed consent denotes a set of procedures that permit physicians to obtain effective authorization from patients to proceed with medical interventions, and that allows patients to accept the possibility of and assume responsibility for certain disclosed risks.[15] Is it possible to reconcile these legal and institutional norms with the ethical model of informed consent as patient responsibility for decisions that entail choices between important ends? And if so, can a single set of practices support both the legal and ethical objectives of informed consent? Or, alternately, must we concede that the legal and ethical purposes of informed consent are sufficiently distinct that they should part company in either theory or practice?

It is important not to overstate the gap between the legal and ethical senses of informed consent. Both ethics and the law seek to establish and protect patients' rights to be informed about the important consequences of medical choices, and to select the choice that is most consistent with their values and goals. Furthermore, in some respects, the ethical model we have advocated here is reflected in the current institutional practices surrounding legal authorization for treatment of hospitalized patients. On admission to the hospital, all patients or their surrogates must sign a document to indicate their general consent for treatment. This consent typically covers a wide range of diagnostic and therapeutic interventions, including laboratory and radiology studies, prescription of medications, and nursing care. For certain procedures, however, additional specific consent is required. These include surgeries and anesthetics, as well as risky treatment regimens such as chemotherapy protocols.

This distinction between general and specific consent broadly mirrors the distinction we have drawn between the agent- and adviser-fiduciary models and between decision making about means and ends. On admission, patients provide their consent for procedures consistent with the implicit goal of diagnosing and treating their medical conditions; clinicians implement these procedures, with varying degrees of discussion and patient involvement in decisions, as agent-fiduciaries under the global grant of authority conveyed by the general consent to treatment. Once decisions begin to implicate ends, or when a certain level of risk is exceeded, however, current practice requires physicians to assume the role of an adviser-fiduciary and to engage the patient in a discussion about ends with regard to the procedures under question.

If this conceptual bridge between our theory and current practice is correct, then it points to at least one way in which current practice could be improved. Some surgical procedures (for example, a punch biopsy of the skin) entail no more than minimal risk, and therefore should not require more than the general consent for treatment. Requiring the same level of informed consent for such a procedure as is required for major surgery leads many physicians to become cynical about the paperwork and administrative hurdles that they must overcome, a development that risks undermining their commitment to ethical practice overall. Conversely, some diagnostic or therapeutic procedures currently performed under the general consent for treatment (for example, use of anticoagulants in situations where the risk of thrombosis must be balanced against the risk of hemorrhage) probably deserve a more deliberate and thorough consent process then they currently receive. Efforts to better align the legal requirements in hospitals with the ethical "first principles" described here could lead to more effective patient involvement in decision making as well as improved support from clinicians for the ethical requirements themselves.

Notwithstanding these areas of compatibility between the ethical framework we have advanced and contemporary legal and institutional practices, it is difficult to square informed consent as a mechanism whereby patients accept and assume responsibility for risk with informed consent as a model for facilitating patients' decisions about which choices best serve important ends. Howard Brody brings this distinction into sharp focus in considering whether or not valid informed consent obligates physicians to disclose remote risks of serious adverse outcomes (he uses the example of a 1 in 40,000 risk of death associated with contrast injection for intravenous pyelography, a procedure used historically to image the urinary tract).[2] According to the legalistic approach to informed consent, such a risk should probably be disclosed, if for no other reason than that the physician who opts not to disclose it might reasonably fear legal jeopardy in the unlikely event that the patient dies due to a contrast reaction. Conversely, according to the ethical model we have advocated here, disclosure of the remote risk is necessary only if it is likely to help the patient decide among the available choices in light of their likely impact on his important ends, or if the patient conveys a desire for such information. Viewed from this perspective, the duty to disclose the remote risk of death is less clear. Thus, it may not be possible to map a legal regime of informed consent onto the ethical conception we have outlined here. In some situations, such as the expectation of full disclosure about and written consent to a risky procedure that is nevertheless the only reasonable means to a certain set of agreed-upon ends, the legal requirements of informed consent are more demanding than are its ethical mandates. In contrast, in others, such as the choice of a patient with advanced cancer to opt for best supportive care rather than aggressive, low-benefit anticancer interventions, the physician's ethical obligation to support deliberative decision making about ends is considerably more robust than is his legal obligation to obtain informed consent. More broadly, the ethical framework we have advanced emphasizes discussions about ends, whereas the legal mandate to obtain informed consent emphasizes discussions about means. Ultimately, recognizing the substantial differences between the legal and ethical goals of informed consent, the only coherent path may be to abandon the fiction that a single set of consent practices can adequately serve both its legal and ethical purposes.

Conclusion

We set out to address three of the central challenges in the literature on informed consent to medical treatment. First, how does the nature of the physician–patient relationship, which establishes the context in which medical decisions are made, influence norms of informed consent for medical care? Second, how do the characteristics of the particular decision at hand affect expectations for informed consent? Finally, how can we bridge the persistent gap between the theory and practice of informed consent, and in particular between the robust decision-making rights accorded to patients and the often limited extent to which patients claim decision-making responsibility for themselves? We have argued that progress in resolving these three questions is possible if we take seriously two features of medical relationships and decisions that to date have been neglected in conceptual discussions about informed consent: the complex fiduciary nature of the physician–patient relationship and the notion that some medical decisions involve choices among, or at least substantially impact upon, important ends, whereas others are best understood as choices among means to a settled end.

The relationship between these two strains of our argument should now be evident. The sense in which the physician–patient relationship is a fiduciary one hinges on the nature of the decision to be made. When considering decisions about ends—or decisions about means that necessarily entail important choices among ends—physicians function as adviser-fiduciaries to their patients. Their role is to provide patients with information, and to guide patients in interpreting that information, so as to maximize the likelihood that patients will make choices among ends that are consistent with their priorities and values. Indeed, viewing physicians as adviser-fiduciaries helps explain their affirmative duty to ensure that patients understand the facts that are material to a decision, an obligation that at first blush appears anomalous compared with other contexts of informed consent.[15] In contrast, when considering decisions about means to settled ends, physicians may legitimately function as agent-fiduciaries to their patients. As agents, physicians must use their expertise and experience to determine which course of action is most likely to achieve patients' desired ends. Of course, the boundaries between decisions that do or do not entail important choices among ends, and therefore between these two senses of the fiduciary physician–patient relationship, are often less than clear-cut. As a result, physicians will sometimes find themselves wondering which of the two fiduciary roles they should play. It is precisely at such times that reflective physicians should step back from substantive consideration of the choices at hand to engage patients in conversation about the decision-making process itself.

Note

a. The Model Code of Professional Responsibility was created in 1969. At the time Spiegel wrote, the Code was used by Bar Associations in all 50 states. However, in 1983, the Code was largely replaced by the ABA's Model Rules of Professional Conduct. At present, only New York State still uses the Model Code.

References

1. Faden, R.R., and T.L. Beauchamp. 1986. *A history and theory of informed consent.* New York: Oxford University Press.
2. Brody, H. 1992. *The healer's power.* New Haven, CT: Yale University Press.
3. President's Commission for the Study of Ethical Problems in Medicine and Biomedical and Behavioral Research. 1982. *Making health care decisions: The ethical and legal implications of informed consent in the patient-practitioner relationship.* Washington, DC: U.S. Government Printing Office.
4. *Schloendorff* v. *Society of New York Hospitals.* 211 N.Y. 125 (1914).
5. Schneider, C.E. 1998. *The practice of autonomy.* New York: Oxford University Press.
6. Meisel, A., L.H. Roth, and C.W. Lidz. 1977. Toward a model of the legal doctrine of informed consent. *American Journal of Psychiatry* 134(3):285–89.
7. Berg, J.W., P.S. Appelbaum, C.W. Lidz, and L.S. Parker. 2001. *Informed consent: Legal theory and clinical practice.* 2nd ed. Oxford: Oxford University Press.
8. Katz, J. 1984. *The silent world of doctor and patient.* New York: The Free Press.
9. Charles, C., A. Gafni, and T. Whelan. 1997. Shared decision-making in the medical encounter: what does it mean? (or it takes at least two to tango). *Social Science and Medicine* 44(5):681–92.
10. Eddy, D.M. 1990. Anatomy of a decision. *Journal of the American Medical Association* 263(3):441–43.

11. Emanuel, E.J., and L.L. Emanuel. 1992. Four models of the physician-patient relationship. *Journal of the American Medical Association* 267(16):2221–26.

12. Charles, C., A. Gafni, and T. Whelan. 1999. Decision-making in the physician-patient encounter: revisiting the shared treatment decision-making model. *Social Science and Medicine* 49(5):651–61.

13. Brock, D.W. 1991. Facts and values in the physician-patient relationship. In *Ethics, trust and the professions: Philosophical and cultural aspects,* ed. E.D. Pellegrino, R.M. Veatch, and J.P. Langan, 113–38. Washington, DC: Georgetown University Press.

14. Donagan, A. 1977. Informed consent in therapy and experimentation. *Journal of Medicine and Philosophy* 2(4):307–29.

15. Schuck, P.H. 1994. Rethinking informed consent. *Yale Law Journal* 103(4):899–959.

16. Wertheimer, A. 2003. *Consent to sexual relations.* Cambridge, UK: Cambridge University Press.

17. Strull, W.M., B. Lo, and G. Charles. 1984. Do patients want to participate in medical decision making? *Journal of the American Medical Association* 252(21):2990–94.

18. Ende, J., L. Kazis, A. Ash, and M.A. Moskowitz. 1989. Measuring patients' desire for autonomy: Decision making and information-seeking preferences among medical patients. *Journal of General Internal Medicine* 4(1):23–30.

19. Ende, J., L. Kazis, and M.A. Moskowitz. 1990. Preferences for autonomy when patients are physicians. *Journal of General Internal Medicine* 5(6):506–09.

20. Guadagnoli, E., and P. Ward. 1998. Patient participation in decision-making. *Social Science and Medicine* 47(3):329–39.

21. Arora, N.K., and C.A. McHorney. 2000. Patient preferences for medical decision making: who really wants to participate? *Medical Care* 38(3):335–41.

22. Sutherland, H.J., H.A. Llewellyn-Thomas, G.A. Lockwood, D.L. Tritchler, and J.E. Till. 1989. Cancer patients: Their desire for information and participation in treatment decisions. *Journal of the Royal Society of Medicine* 82(5):260–63.

23. Cassileth, B.R., R.V. Zupkis, K. Sutton-Smith, and V. March. 1980. Information and participation preferences among cancer patients. *Annals of Internal Medicine* 92(6):832–36.

24. Deber, R.B., N. Kraetschmer, and J. Irvine. 1996. What role do patients wish to play in treatment decision making? *Archives of Internal Medicine* 156(13):1414–20.

25. Degner, L.F., L.J. Kristjanson, D. Bowman, et al. 1997. Information needs and decisional preferences in women with breast cancer. *Journal of the American Medical Association* 277(18):1485–92.

26. Ingelfinger, F.J. 1980. Arrogance. *New England Journal of Medicine* 303(26):1507–11.

27. Rodwin, M.A. 1995. Strains in the fiduciary metaphor: Divided physician loyalties and obligations in a changing health care system. *American Journal of Law and Medicine* 21(2–3):241–57.

28. Buchanan, A. 1988. Principal/agent theory and decision making in health care. *Bioethics* 2(4):317–33.

29. Morreim, E.H. 2005. The clinical investigator as fiduciary: Discarding a misguided idea. *Journal of Law, Medicine and Ethics* 33(3):586–98.

30. Sokolowski, R. 1991. The fiduciary relationship and the nature of professions. In *Ethics, trust and the professions: Philosophical and cultural aspects,* ed. E.D. Pellegrino, R.M. Veatch, and J.P. Langan, 23–43. Washington, DC: Georgetown University Press.

31. Shepherd, J.C. 1981. *The law of fiduciaries.* Toronto: The Carswell Company.

32. Fried, C. 1974. *Medical experimentation: Personal integrity and social policy.* New York: American Elsevier Publishing Co., Inc.

33. Kant, I. 1996. Groundwork of the metaphysics of morals. In *Practical Philosophy,* Ed. M.J. Gregor, 49–108. Cambridge: Cambridge University Press.

34. Spiegel, M. 1979. Lawyering and client decisionmaking: Informed consent and the legal profession. *University of Pennsylvania Law Review* 128:41–140.

35. American Bar Association. 1983. Model Code of Professional Responsibility. Available at http://www.law.cornell.edu/ethics/aba/mcpr/MCPR.HTM. Accessibility verified July 27, 2009.

36. Daugherty, C.K., M. Siegler, M.J. Ratain, and G. Zimmer. 1997. Learning from our patients: One participant's impact on clinical trial research and informed consent. *Annals of Internal Medicine* 126(11):892–97.

37. Braddock, C.H., K.A. Edwards, N.M. Hasenberg, T.L. Laidley, and W. Levinson. 1999. Informed decision making in outpatient practice: Time to get back to basics. *Journal of the American Medical Association* 282(24):2313–20.

38. Barry, M.J. 2006. The PSA conundrum. *Archives of Internal Medicine* 166(1):7–8.

15

Consent to Clinical Research

Franklin G. Miller

Consent to clinical research—biomedical research involving human subjects—is a vast topic, worthy of book-length treatment. In this chapter, I introduce the topic; present a famous historical case with enduring implications; briefly discuss the key normative concept of personal sovereignty, which consent serves and respects; and examine in depth two issues: the therapeutic misconception and the justifiability of research without consent.

Background

Informed consent is considered a fundamental norm governing clinical research. The Nuremberg Code of 1946, promulgated in the wake of the Nazi concentration camp experiments, declares that "The voluntary consent of the human subject is absolutely essential."[1] The normative significance of consent in this domain can be seen by contrasting animal experimentation with human research. There is no consent for animal experimentation, not only because animals are not capable of consent—human infants are not capable of consent either—but because we presume that researchers are entitled to exercise control over the use of animals for experimentation, subject only to regulations relating to their care and the imposition of painful procedures. Central to the normative foundation of consent to research is *personal sovereignty*—that persons are entitled to control their lives and others are not free to exercise control over them.[2] Hence, as a rule, consent is ethically necessary for research participation. The Nazi concentration camp experiments are notable for treating human beings as laboratory animals.[3] They took place within a regime of total control of a captive population, in which the inmates could be used as their captors saw fit, including exploiting them in brutal and often fatal experiments.

Outside of regimes of total control, clinical research has been grounded, as a matter of fact, on some element of consent, though often falling far short of informed consent to research participation. With respect to research involving healthy persons living outside institutions, researchers have had no means of access to them without soliciting consent. They need to be invited and agree to participate. Even within the coercive environment of prisons, often used in the past as a site for access to healthy subjects, consent was solicited. Whether prison research has involved (sufficiently) voluntary or informed consent is another issue. To be sure, although some form of consent was necessary for research involving noninstitutionalized subjects, it could be grossly defective, as in the Tuskegee Syphilis study. Poor African American men with late-stage syphilis were recruited for a "natural history" research experiment under the ruse of receiving treatment for "bad blood."[4]

Historically, the situation was different with respect to research involving hospitalized patients. Being available to physician-investigators, hospitalized patients were frequently used for experimentation without any specific consent for research participation. Still, underlying practices that we now see as abusive and exploitative, there was some form of consent to treatment. In some cases there was an element of consent to research, without any detailed disclosure about the nature of the research or its risks. For example, in the famous randomized trials evaluating internal mammary artery ligation for treatment of angina in the late 1950s, patients consented to surgery and were informed that there would be an "evaluation" of the procedure.[5] However, they were not informed about randomization to the real procedure or to a sham operation involving a chest incision without ligation of the artery. Physician-investigators saw themselves as licensed to experiment on hospitalized patients who had consented to treatment without obtaining informed consent for research. In a telling comment in 1962, Walter Modell, a distinguished investigator, remarked, "I think that when a patient goes to a modern physician for treatment, regardless of whether he consciously consents to it, he is also unconsciously presenting himself for the purpose of experimentation."[6]

Historical Case Study: Jewish Chronic Disease
Hospital Experiment

A justly famous watershed case of clinical research experimentation without informed consent occurred in July 1963 at the Jewish Chronic Disease Hospital in New York City.[7] The publicity generated by this case played an important role in stimulating the U.S. government to promulgate guidelines for biomedical research funded by the National Institutes of Health, requiring independent prior review concerning the protection of research subjects and written informed consent.[8] This case was also described in Henry Beecher's path-breaking medical journal article exposing the existence of unethical research conducted by leading academic medical institutions.[9] Unlike the Tuskegee Syphilis study, this experiment was based on sound science and the research subjects arguably were not exposed to risks of harm as a result of participation. It retains enduring interest in highlighting key issues of informed consent to research that remain relevant, in more subtle ways, to the current practice of clinical research.

The research, funded in part by the National Cancer Institute, was planned and overseen by Chester Southam, a leading physician-investigator affiliated with Sloan-Kettering Institute for Cancer Research. Since 1954, Southam had been interested in an immunological approach to understanding cancer, particularly in the differential ability of the human body to reject "cancer cell homografts"—injections of live cancer cells drawn from cell lines. In previous research, he had found that advanced cancer patients reject these injected cancer cells at a considerably slower rate than healthy volunteers. These findings posed the question whether the delayed rejection was due to the pathophysiology of cancer or to the debilitated state of patients with advanced disease. In order to address this question, he arranged a joint research venture with physicians at the Jewish Chronic Disease Hospital, to measure the rate of rejection of live cancer cells in chronically ill patients without diagnoses of cancer. The research procedures involved two hypodermic injections to the thigh of patients at the facility, frequent monitoring of the nodules produced by the injections, and periodic blood draws. With respect to the risks of the research, Southam commented in a letter to the medical director of the facility, "It is, of course, inconsequential whether these [injected cells] are cancer cells or not, since they are foreign to the recipient and hence are rejected."[10]

Consent was solicited from the patients, but it clearly was not informed consent to research participation. Oral consent for a "skin test" was obtained by the medical director for the facility in the first two subjects and by a staff medical resident for the next 20. There is dispute in the records of the subsequent investigation of this case by the New York State Board of Regents about whether the patients involved were mentally capable of giving informed consent. But I will presume for the sake of the argument that they were capacitated decision makers. The disclosure to the patients was described by the resident as follows:

> The patient was told that an injection of a cell suspension was planned as a skin test for immunity or resistance. The patient was also told that a lump would form within a few days which would last several weeks and gradually disappear. The patient was not told that the injection would contain cancer cells. The reason for this is that we did not wish to stir up any unnecessary anxieties, disturbances or phobias in our patients.[11]

Southam explained the rationale for not mentioning the injection of cancer cells in more technical language:

> Since the initial neoplastic source of the test material employed was not germane to the reaction being studied and not, in my opinion, a cause of increased risk to the patient, I believe that such revelation is generally contraindicated in the best consideration of the patient's welfare and therefore to withhold such emotionally disturbing details (unless requested by the patient) is in the best tradition of responsible clinical practice.[12]

These two descriptions of the consent process are noteworthy in conflating research experimentation and routine clinical care. The consent was obtained by clinicians employed at the hospital who were familiar to the patients. By being presented as a skin test, without any mention of research, it would be natural for patients to presume that this was a routine procedure being done in their medical interests. Given this context, not only did the consent disclosure withhold information that research was being conducted and that live cancer cells were being injected, but it was also deceptive in presenting research procedures in the guise of routine clinical care. Southam's rationale for not disclosing the nature of the cell suspension displays the lack of any understanding of the ethically significant differences between medical care, oriented to the medical best interests of particular patients, and clinical research, aimed at developing knowledge for the purpose of improving the medical care of future patients.

The ethical abuse evident in this research is radically different from the Nazi concentration camp experiments. In the latter there was not even the semblance of consent and subjects were treated brutally. To be sure, the potential for harm from this experiment may not have been entirely absent, as Southam insisted. The record contains testimony challenging the harmless nature of the experiment; however, there is no solid evidence that any of the research subjects were harmed. It was difficult at the time for clinical investigators to see that consent for research involves ethical considerations other than protecting patients from risks of harm that they are not prepared to assume. One expert medical witness testifying on behalf of Southam stated, "The reason I say that I believe that informed consent was obtained was because I don't think there was any risk involved here."[13] Missing from this attitude toward consent is sensitivity to how considerations of human dignity, respect, and autonomy ground the stance that participation in scientific experimentation should be based on the informed choice of the research subject. These patients, though not harmed, were used merely as a means to scientific investigation. They provided informed consent to a skin test, ostensibly for their benefit, but not to an experiment involving injection of live cancer cells that could be of no benefit to them.

Two key related points are underscored by the Jewish Chronic Disease Hospital case. First, informed consent to medical care does not itself encompass valid consent to research experimentation associated with medical care. Second, in order to obtain informed consent to clinical research, prospective patient-subjects need a fair opportunity to understand how research participation will differ from standard medical care. In discussing below "the therapeutic misconception," it will become apparent that a fully adequate disclosure about the nature of a research study and the research procedures may not be sufficient for valid consent. In any case, it is clear that the patients enrolled in Southam's experiment had no fair opportunity for comprehending what research participation involved. Though not coerced, they were deceptively enrolled in research without valid consent. It is inconceivable that any reputable investigators today would endorse the consent process that was considered routine and satisfactory in 1963. Yet the idea that consent is primarily a matter of protection from risk and the conflation of clinical research and medical care remain pertinent to the ethics of research consent. Part of what makes this case of more than merely historical interest is its illustrating that the purpose of soliciting consent to research is not limited to protecting patient-subjects from harm.

Personal Sovereignty

Other chapters in this volume address in depth the nature of consent and the values that it serves. Here I will tread lightly in this territory by outlining the concept of personal sovereignty and indicating its relevance to research participation. The idea of personal sovereignty—an inviolable zone of personal conduct and enjoyment of property free from invasion by others—has deep roots in liberal moral and political thought. In the introductory chapter to *On Liberty* Mill declares that "Over himself, over his own body and mind, the individual is sovereign."[14] Despite deep philosophical differences, Mill's appeal to individual sovereignty overlaps substantially with Kant's principle of humanity: "the human being . . . *exists* as an end in itself, *not merely as a means to be used by this or that will at its discretion*."[15] The legitimacy of the way that competent adults treat each other depends on it being consistent with their autonomy (literally, self-rule).

Personal sovereignty involves both protective and facilitative dimensions. Recognizing personal sovereignty in the law and common mores protects individuals from unwanted intrusions on their freedom and property. It also demarcates a zone of interpersonal conduct in which individuals should have the opportunity to cooperate with others free from external interference, provided that they do not harm third parties or violate their rights. The requirement to obtain consent protects persons from invasions of their personal sovereignty, thus respecting their freedom to be left alone. It also facilitates permissible interaction with others, thus respecting freedom of cooperative activity. In other words, consent and personal sovereignty go hand in hand: A zone of personal inviolability and control is manifested in respect for the ability to give and withhold consent.

Although the morality of consent is a ubiquitous feature of ordinary life, typically there is no requirement of soliciting *informed* consent in the sense that in order for A to validly consent to doing X in cooperation with B, B must prospectively provide pertinent information to A. This holds for purchasing most commodities, taking a job, playing competitive games, sexual interaction, and so forth. To be sure, we presume that consent is valid only when the consenter is sufficiently informed about what he or she is consenting to. However, we typically do not recognize an affirmative obligation of the party receiving consent to provide an information disclosure to the other. Indeed, valid consent in ordinary life is often implicit or tacit. We presume that competent adults will know what they are consenting to when they offer a token of unforced consent, absent deception, based on either common-sense understanding of how the world works or an expectation that it is up to them to undertake inquiry about whether what they consent to is in their interest.

Why, then, do we require investigators to obtain informed consent before enrolling individuals in their research? Research, especially human experimentation in clinical research, is characterized by a significant imbalance in knowledge and power between the investigator and the subject. This imbalance has several dimensions. First, the investigator typically has professional status and often represents an esteemed academic institution; second, the investigator has superior knowledge relating to disease and treatment; third, the investigator has an expert understanding of the nature of the research and risks to subjects that it poses; fourth, the physician-investigator has the authority to prescribe treatments; and finally, in the case of clinical trials, the investigator has access to experimental interventions not available in clinical practice. We cannot expect subjects of clinical research to have adequate knowledge of what research participation involves—its risks and likely benefits (if any). Furthermore, patient-subjects may be strongly motivated to volunteer to obtain medical benefits that are not otherwise available to them. If they are to be adequately informed so as to give valid consent for research participation, then the investigator must provide the information needed to make an autonomous choice.

The ethics of consent to research, grounded in personal sovereignty, has traditionally been understood as antithetical to paternalism. Yet the requirement for *informed* consent can be seen as based on an element of soft paternalism.[16] Given the imbalances in knowledge and power between investigators and subjects adumbrated above, individuals are considered to have decisional defects that make it impossible to protect their interests by virtue of the kind of informal consent that characterizes much of ordinary life. Consequently, investigators have an affirmative obligation to supply the information that individuals need to validly authorize their research participation. Moreover, according to prevailing ethical and regulatory standards, individuals are not invited to participate in research unless an independent research ethics committee has reviewed and approved the study, based on a set of criteria including risk-benefit assessment. This all the more so reflects a context of soft paternalism underlying research ethics—a thesis developed and defended elsewhere.[17]

The Therapeutic Misconception and Consent to Randomized Trials

In the Jewish Chronic Disease Hospital case, the lack of valid consent derived from the failure to inform prospective subjects that they were being invited to participate in an experiment not for their benefit, which involved injection of live cancer cells believed on scientific grounds not to pose any risk of harm to them. The fact that these patients were long-term residents of a hospital does not obviate their personal sovereignty with respect to medical and research decisions. Indeed, a careful process of informed consent is all the more important when research involves enrollment of patient-subjects who are vulnerable to undue influence in contexts in which it is easy to confuse research participation with medical care. Their consent may be compromised if they are unable to understand how research participation differs from standard medical care.

Paul Appelbaum et al. coined the term "therapeutic misconception" to describe the tendency of individuals enrolled in randomized clinical trials to confuse the scientific orientation of their research participation with the therapeutic orientation of medical care.[18] In clinical trials, methodological considerations govern such factors as the choice and delivery of treatment interventions, whereas in medical care, physicians are expected to recommend and adapt treatment based on judgments about what is best for the particular patient. The notion of the therapeutic misconception has become the dominant lens through which bioethicists view questions about informed consent to clinical research.[19] It is therefore surprising that there has been little systematic analysis of how the existence of a therapeutic misconception among patient-subjects matters ethically, or of the resulting policy implications. How does the therapeutic misconception impair informed consent? Is an understanding of clinical trial participation that is free from any therapeutic misconception a necessary condition of valid informed consent? Is such an understanding more important for some trials than for others? What steps should investigators take to counteract therapeutic misconceptions among prospective subjects?

In what follows I examine critically the way in which Appelbaum et al. characterize the therapeutic misconception. An important ambiguity about the nature and scope of the disadvantages that stem from randomized trial participation has hindered the quest for clarity regarding the significance of the therapeutic misconception. One plausible interpretation of their understanding of the therapeutic misconception is that clinical trial participation necessarily disadvantages subjects by exposing them to predictably inferior outcomes as compared with receiving standard medical care. Clarifying the nature of disadvantages that may result from clinical trial participation paves the way for a cogent account of the therapeutic misconception's ethical significance and for discussion of the appropriate policy response.

Characterizing the Therapeutic Misconception

In each of their articles on the topic from 1982 to the present, Appelbaum et al. have explicated the therapeutic misconception against the background of Charles Fried's distinction between the scientific orientation of randomized controlled trials, designed to answer questions about the efficacy of treatments, and the therapeutic, patient-centered orientation of standard medical practice.[20] Physicians practicing clinical medicine aim at providing individualized treatment for particular patients according to the principle of "personal care," which involves tailoring treatment to the clinical features and individual situations of particular patients. In contrast, physician-investigators conducting clinical trials adopt scientific methods to produce valid data, derived from groups of patient-subjects, with the aim of improving medical care for future patients. These methods, including randomization, double-blind administration of treatment, and protocol-defined restrictions on treatment flexibility, necessarily depart from the principle of personal care.

Based on empirical research on the informed consent process in psychiatric randomized trials, Appelbaum et al. observed that patient-subjects frequently failed to understand or appreciate how their trial participation involved departure from the therapeutic orientation of medical care.[21] For example, despite being informed about randomization and other key aspects of study design, interviewed subjects frequently stated that their treatment in the trial would be selected based on what the responsible physicians judged best for them, thus manifesting therapeutic misconceptions about research participation.

Recently, in the first systematic effort to determine the prevalence of the therapeutic misconception, this research group reported results of interviews with 225 research participants in 44 clinical trials across a wide range of conditions.[22] Based on their operational definitions, they found that 62% of the participants manifested therapeutic misconceptions.

The Consequences of Research Participation

Why does the therapeutic misconception matter? In their classic 1987 article, Appelbaum et al. stated, "To maintain a therapeutic misconception is to deny the possibility that there may be major disadvantages to participating in clinical research that stem from the nature of the research process itself."[23] According to this perspective, since the scientific requirements of clinical trial design potentially disadvantage participants as compared with standard medical care, prospective subjects cannot give informed consent to enroll in a clinical trial unless they understand how participation constrains their treatment.

What are the "major disadvantages" that might arise as a result of trial participation? In elucidating what is at stake ethically in the therapeutic misconception, it is important to distinguish between *potential* disadvantages to subjects owing to the scientific methods employed by all clinical trials—the chance that subjects may fare worse than they would if they received standard medical care—and *predictable* disadvantages stemming from the actual design of particular trials. In many trials, potential disadvantages associated with scientific design may or may not materialize; furthermore, these may be justified or outweighed by potential benefits from trial participation, such as more frequent attention from expert clinicians or access to effective new interventions. Though patient-subjects may experience worse outcomes than they would if they received standard medical care, their outcomes might also be similar or even better. In contrast, a subset of trials presents subjects with predictable disadvantages. These include trials employing placebo control groups that withhold proven effective treatment, as well as trials that administer burdensome or risky procedures that are necessary for research but lack the prospect of direct benefits for participants.

When stated explicitly, the distinction between potential and predictable disadvantages of trial participation seems obvious. Nevertheless, Appelbaum et al. blur the distinction between theoretical disadvantages deriving from scientific design and actual disadvantages likely to be experienced by all or some patient-subjects in particular trials. The previous quote refers to the possibility of disadvantage. However, they also state that "... reliance on randomization represents an inevitable compromise of personal care in the service of attaining valid research results."[24] Unless personal care is viewed as a purely intrinsic good, "inevitable compromise" invokes what might be called *the disadvantage thesis* that participants in randomized trials are likely to experience worse outcomes as compared with standard medical care. The purpose of clinical medicine, governed by the principle of personal care, is to do what is best for patients. Randomization deviates from individualized treatment selection according to the principle of personal care. Whether or not this deviation leads to worse outcomes, however, is an empirical issue, which is examined below.

Appelbaum et al. further assert that "The use of a study protocol to regulate the course of treatment—essential to careful clinical research—also impedes the delivery of personal care."[25] They do not define, however, whether "impeding the delivery of personal care" means merely departing from the treatment flexibility characteristic of medical care, or whether it implies a predictably worse outcome. The authors also raise the question, "Are these disadvantages so important that they should routinely be called to the attention of research subjects?"[26] The lack of qualification of these disadvantages as "potential" suggests the inference that trial participants are likely to experience worse outcomes or greater burdens as compared with standard medical care.

Finally, the following observation by Appelbaum et al. again implies the disadvantage thesis: "Our findings suggest that research subjects systematically misinterpret the risk/benefit ratio of participating in research because they fail to understand the underlying scientific methodology."[27] One plausible reading of this quote is that research subjects who harbor therapeutic misconceptions routinely overestimate benefits or underestimate risks of trial participation compared with standard medical care. Such subjects certainly fail to see how trial participation differs in its orientation from medical care. But this difference in orientation, by itself, entails nothing about whether the risk-benefit ratio for participants is more or less favorable than treatment in standard medical practice.

To be sure, certain randomized trials are designed in a way that an unfavorable risk-benefit ratio compared with standard medical care, at least for some participants, is predictable. For example, randomized trials that involve placebo controls when proven effective treatment exists offer a less favorable risk-benefit ratio than standard medically indicated treatment, at least for those participants who receive placebo. Since many of the trials that Appelbaum et al. studied in their original and recent research are in this category, the predictable disadvantage to subjects as a result of participation in these placebo-controlled trials may have influenced their characterization of what is at stake globally in the therapeutic misconception. Patients enrolled in such trials who evidence therapeutic misconceptions fail to understand how the chance of receiving a placebo predictably disadvantages them as compared with standard medical care. Nevertheless, the statements quoted above, and other similar statements about the ways in which clinical trial participation differs from medical care, are not limited to trials that predictably disadvantage participants as compared with receipt of standard medical care.[28] This ambiguity about the scope of the disadvantage that results from randomized trial participation colors views about the nature and significance of the therapeutic misconception.

Assessing the Disadvantage Thesis

The disadvantage thesis has intuitive plausibility. Physicians recommend treatment and adjust their recommendations with the aim of producing optimal medical outcomes for their patients. Investigators in randomized trials do not determine which treatment under investigation particular participants receive, and accept reduced treatment flexibility according to the scientific design of study protocols. It is thus natural to presume that patients are likely to do better medically under a personal care orientation than in randomized trials. But is this true? Are patient-subjects, as a matter of fact, disadvantaged in clinical outcomes by virtue of participating in clinical trials?

Existing evidence does not support the assumption that, as a group, participants in randomized controlled trials have inferior outcomes as compared with standard clinical practice. Stiller, studying oncology trials, argued that "Inclusion in a clinical trial . . . is often linked with a higher survival rate for the cancers which have been studied,"[29] and Braunholtz et al. suggested on the basis of their systematic review that "[Randomized controlled trials] are more likely to be beneficial than harmful."[30] Peppercorn et al. noted that of 26 trial versus nontrial comparisons in oncology, "no studies recorded worse outcomes in trial-enrolled patients than in non-trial controls."[31] Finally, Vist et al. concluded in a systematic review of relevant research across all medical specialties that "Participating in a trial is likely to result in similar outcomes to patients who receive the same or similar treatment outside a trial."[32] As many of the studies comparing the outcomes of clinical trial participation and ordinary medical care have focused on oncology trials, more research is needed to assess relative outcomes in other settings. Nevertheless, these data indicate that, as a rule, we cannot assume that patients will experience worse outcomes as a result of clinical trial participation. Accordingly, these studies raise questions about the ethical significance of the therapeutic misconception. If a given clinical trial offers eligible patients a personal risk-benefit ratio no less favorable than standard medical care, why should we have any ethical concerns about the therapeutic misconception?

The evidence challenging the disadvantage thesis as a general proposition about randomized trials thus may lead to the conclusion that the therapeutic misconception lacks ethical traction. This conclusion, however, would be erroneous. As noted above, the design of some randomized trials predictably disadvantages patient-subjects as compared with standard medical care. Hence, although the disadvantage thesis as a general rule is not supported by available evidence, it is true about a subset of these trials, especially those that include placebo controls despite proven effective treatment—for example, placebo-controlled trials of new treatments for depression, anxiety, allergies, headaches, low back pain, irritable bowel syndrome, and so forth.[33] Research participants also are disadvantaged by trials that include risky or burdensome procedures, such as lumbar punctures or biopsies, to measure study outcomes. Such research procedures offer no compensating prospect of direct benefit to subjects. If trial participants harbor therapeutic misconceptions such that they think that everything that is done to them in a clinical trial is for their personal benefit, then with respect to particular trials they will fail to recognize that they are forgoing potentially effective treatment or undergoing procedures involving burden or discomfort without any prospect of benefit to them. Moreover, the therapeutic misconception merits attention and concern even when participants are not placed at a predictable disadvantage as compared with standard medical care.

Why the Therapeutic Misconception Matters

To develop an accurate account of the ethical significance of the therapeutic misconception, it is essential to assess it in light of an analysis of the principles or values underlying informed consent to clinical trials. As argued above, the requirement of informed consent flows from the normative commitment to personal sovereignty, coupled with recognition of the imbalances in knowledge and power between investigators and research subjects. The Nuremberg Code, in explicating its first principle stipulating the necessity of "voluntary consent" to human experimentation, states that the prospective subject "should have sufficient knowledge and comprehension of the elements of the subject matter involved as to enable him to make an understanding and enlightened decision."[34] The norm of informed consent to clinical research is generally thought to include the idea that people should understand the purpose and the nature of the activity to which they are being invited to participate. Accordingly, to enroll in a clinical trial under the misunderstanding that this is a form of personal medical care is to be confused about what one is doing. It is not a fully understanding and enlightened decision. Thus, there is reason to be concerned about the adequacy of informed consent insofar as patient-subjects fail to comprehend how trial participation differs from medical care, especially because the purpose of the activity is not to provide personal benefit for participants but to generate knowledge that can improve medical care for the benefit of future patients. When participants who harbor therapeutic misconceptions enroll in research, there remains a legitimate doubt about whether they would have volunteered were they clear about the purpose and design of clinical trials.

Yet, if participation in a particular randomized trial does not predictably disadvantage subjects, why would a reasonable person care to avoid therapeutic misconceptions in making decisions about research participation?

Although the risk-benefit ratio of trial participation will often be just as favorable as that of standard medical care based on current knowledge, randomized trials, as a rule, have greater uncertainty of risks and benefits, especially when experimental treatments are evaluated. Participants harboring therapeutic misconceptions may fail to understand that they are taking part in a scientific experiment to evaluate treatment, which may produce more or less favorable results than they would receive in standard medical care. Moreover, treatment decision making differs in these two activities. In medical care, either patients and their doctors choose together what is the best treatment or patients decide to defer to their doctors to choose *for them* what is considered best. This personalized decision-making process is precisely what is forgone in volunteering for a randomized trial. While many competent patients under-going medical care may not be interested in choosing treatment for them-selves, it is reasonable to presume that they will be interested in having their doctors select what is considered to be the best treatment for them. Therefore, the validity of informed consent to clinical trial participation is open to question for those patients who fail to understand that clinical management decisions are not guided by individualized medical judgment. Trial partici-pants manifesting therapeutic misconceptions fail to understand or appreciate this key difference in treatment decision making.

These considerations imply that the understanding component of informed consent is not a matter solely of comprehending risks and benefits of trial participation, thus underscoring the point made previously with respect to the Jewish Chronic Disease Hospital case that consent is not merely a tool to protect subjects from risks they are not prepared to assume. In the context of randomized trials, comprehending the personal meaning of trial participation as *distinct from* being a patient receiving standard medical care is relevant to informed consent. For many clinical trials, the invitation to participate presents eligible patients with a choice between two alternative ways of addressing the condition from which they are suffering. They can receive standard medical treatment provided by their doctor according to the personal care orientation, or they can receive treatment provided by clinical investigators within the context of a scientific experiment designed to evaluate treatment. Patients under the influence of a therapeutic misconception, who view clinical trial participation as essentially a form of medical care, fail to understand the meaning of the choice they are making in consenting to enroll in a trial. They fail to see that the purpose and design of the trial is to generate scientific knowledge, not to provide individualized therapy for them. Their comprehension of what they are doing by consenting to trial participation is defective, even when they are not exposed to any predictable clinical dis-advantage as compared with standard medical care.

Recognizing how treatment selection differs in randomized trials compared with medical care will have more or less personal importance depending on the nature of the treatments under investigation and the associated research procedures. For example, consider a randomized trial comparing two treatments that differ substantially in invasiveness (for example, surgery versus pharmacological treatment) or expected toxicity. As part of informed consent, prospective subjects should understand that whether or not they receive the more invasive or toxic, but potentially more beneficial, treatment is based not on an expert judgment of what is best for them but rather on a process of random selection. In addition, they should be aware at the time of enrollment that the prospective benefits of the experimental treatment are unproven, and may or may not ultimately justify its incremental risks and burdens.

Finally, a reasonable person considering trial participation would want to avoid the therapeutic misconception because, in most trials, benefits to society must be invoked to a greater or lesser degree to justify at least some risks and burdens of the trial. For example, prospective subjects considering a trial that involves research-specific procedures should be aware that those procedures, even if they involve limited risks and burdens, are being undertaken for reasons unrelated to their own direct benefit. Prospective subjects should have the opportunity to consider whether or not they wish to participate in an activity that is justified in part by benefits that do not accrue directly to themselves. By negating or circumventing the need to consider this question, the therapeutic misconception interferes with decision making about research participation.

To be sure, these concerns must be tempered by recognition that the therapeutic misconception is a matter of degree. Participants may be more or less confused about what trial participation involves; elements of accurate understanding may coexist with elements of confusion. Furthermore, the presence of a therapeutic misconception does not mean that a given participant would have declined to enroll had she been clear about the distinctions between trial participation and medical care. Patient-subjects who harbor therapeutic misconceptions fail to give *fully* informed consent. Nevertheless, as Sreenivasan has argued, we should not confuse "an ethical aspiration with a minimum ethical standard."[35] Valid consent does not require perfect understanding. Ideally, all trial participants would be free of therapeutic misconceptions, but it is not clear that each and every manifestation of a therapeutic misconception invalidates consent.

In sum, when evaluating the ethical significance of the therapeutic misconception, we must avoid two errors. On the one hand, the presumption or implication that randomized trials necessarily involve "major disadvantages" with respect to clinical outcomes exaggerates the import of the therapeutic misconception. On the other hand, the claim that there is no reason to be concerned about the therapeutic misconception in the case of randomized trials that offer patient-subjects a risk-benefit ratio no less favorable than standard medical care understates the import of this phenomenon. The therapeutic misconception always warrants attention with respect to the quality of informed consent, but the degree to which it matters ethically and the policy implications of this phenomenon depend on the contextual details of particular clinical trials.

Policy Implications

How should investigators and research ethics committees address the problem of the therapeutic misconception? Therapeutic misconceptions by research participants raise concerns about informed consent even when trial participation offers a risk-benefit ratio no less favorable than that of standard medical care. This implies that general efforts by investigators to dispel the therapeutic misconception are imperative. These include affirmative efforts both to inform prospective subjects about how the scientific purpose of clinical trials makes participation different from the therapeutic orientation of medical care and to avoid reinforcing therapeutic misconceptions by careful attention to the language used in informed consent documents and conversations.[36] As an example of the latter, consent documents that describe placebos as one of the treatments that participants may receive or the investigator as "your doctor" blur relevant differences between research and medical care. In their early research, Appelbaum et al. found that a "preconsent discussion" relating to methodological characteristics of research that depart from the therapeutic orientation of medical care, led by a neutral professional unassociated with the research team, produced substantial improvement in prospective subjects' understanding of key elements of trial design.[37] A recent review by Flory and Emanuel of experiments designed to enhance informed consent in clinical trials lends support to this observation.[38] Such educational efforts to improve the understanding of prospective clinical trial participants should focus on explaining scientific design issues such as the underlying purpose of clinical trials, randomization, double blinding, the use of placebo controls, and restrictions on treatment flexibility.

While efforts to dispel the therapeutic misconception as described previously may be helpful in enhancing informed consent, they are unlikely to eliminate this problem. Do investigators have a further obligation to detect whether prospective subjects manifest therapeutic misconceptions and to exclude those whose defects in understanding persist despite attempts at correction? The answer to this question depends not only on the ethical significance of therapeutic misconceptions in any given circumstance, but also on whether there are valid reasons—especially participant-centered reasons—to avoid imposing such a requirement. These include the time and burden that such a mandate would require of prospective subjects, the risk of paternalistically imposing an idealized rational decision-making process on individuals who prefer to make decisions in other ways, and the potential for harm and insult that would result from excluding individuals from trial participation owing to inadequate comprehension.

As noted previously, the ethical importance of the therapeutic misconception varies depending on the design of particular clinical trials, the types of treatments under investigation, and the interventions administered to measure trial outcomes or gather other research data. Concern with identifying and correcting therapeutic misconceptions among particular prospective subjects also should vary in light of these contextual factors. A differential standard for the extent to which investigators are obligated to ensure adequate comprehension free of therapeutic misconceptions depending on the personal consequences of clinical trial participation is reasonable in view of the ethical purpose of informed consent. In determining when investigators are subject to the more stringent set of obligations relating to informed consent, a useful rule of thumb is that therapeutic misconceptions are unacceptable when there is a significant likelihood that the individual would have made a different decision in the absence of such misconceptions.

Consider the case of a prospective participant with adequate decision-making capacity who chooses to enroll in a randomized trial comparing a promising experimental agent with a standard medication, but is confused about how research participation differs from routine medical care. Suppose that this trial involves no burdensome procedures undertaken solely for research purposes. There is no reason to think that this individual will be disadvantaged as compared with treatment in clinical practice. Assuming that she is seeking optimal medical care, treatment within the trial is likely to serve her purpose and values even though she misunderstands features of trial design. Although it is desirable to be free of therapeutic misconceptions, in this case neither well-being nor self-determination is markedly impaired by trial participation. Thus, adequate disclosure and voluntary choice should be sufficient to satisfy the investigator's obligations with respect to informed consent. Provided that the informed consent process clarifies the pertinent differences between trial participation and routine medical care, informal practices of assessing comprehension, as a rule, should be sufficient when clinical trials offer eligible patients a risk-benefit profile commensurate with that of standard medical care. By disclosing pertinent information about trial participation in this type of research, investigators give participants a fair opportunity to decide whether or not to participate. The fact that in this context patient-subjects remain unclear about how research participation differs from routine medical care does not invalidate their consent. However, heightened scrutiny is necessary when treatments under investigation are substantially more invasive, toxic, or burdensome than standard treatment.

As what is at stake for prospective participants in choosing between treatment in routine medical care and research participation increases, assurance of adequate understanding takes on greater ethical significance. Because there is a substantial likelihood that the decision about trial entry might be affected, trials that place subjects at a significant and predictable disadvantage compared with standard medical care deserve extra precautions to ensure that participants do not harbor strong therapeutic misconceptions. Placebo-controlled trials that withhold proven effective treatment are an important example. Although controversial, these trials are common and use of placebo controls has been defended by some commentators as necessary to promote scientific validity and acceptable as long as they do not pose undue risks of harm from withholding treatment.[39] Studies involving research-related procedures that impose substantial risks or burdens without the prospect of compensating direct benefit to subjects are another example. For trials in these categories, formal tests of comprehension should be instituted to address understanding of factors such as randomization, the meaning and use of placebo controls, the scientific rather than therapeutic purpose of burdensome or risky research procedures, and the alternative of medically indicated treatment in standard practice.[40] Subjects who fail to demonstrate minimally adequate comprehension should be offered further education relating to points of the misunderstanding, and should be excluded from participation if failure of understanding persists.

In sum, informed consent to clinical trials requires that investigators provide prospective research subjects with pertinent information about research participation, including the purpose of the study, the risks and benefits of the study procedures, and available treatment alternatives. In light of the pervasiveness of the therapeutic misconception, informed consent disclosures should explain salient differences between trial participation and standard medical care. Nevertheless, the extent to which research subjects must comprehend this information in order for consent to be valid is an unsettled issue of research ethics. Given that the therapeutic misconception involves the mental state of patient-subjects, there can be no obligation on the part of investigators to *guarantee* that they are free of elements of therapeutic misconception. Efforts to dispel the therapeutic misconception in service of personal sovereignty should be a routine part of the informed consent process and should vary in intensity depending on the risk-benefit profile of particular clinical trials. We have come a long way from the Jewish Chronic Disease Hospital case, in which the consent process systematically produced total therapeutic misconceptions by virtue of failing to solicit consent for research participation. Yet much work remains to be done to secure informed consent to clinical research enrolling sick patients seeking treatment in the context of clinical trials.

Research Without Consent

In view of the strong moral grounds for informed consent, based on personal sovereignty, it might seem impossible to justify human research without consent. However, a substantial range of research is routinely conducted entirely without consent for research participation, either from the subjects themselves or from surrogate decision makers for those subjects who lack the capacity to consent. This includes epidemiological and health services research using medical records, quality improvement research in medical settings, cluster randomized trials in which the unit of randomization is not individual subjects but entire hospital units or community-based health programs, and emergency research under conditions in which subjects are incapacitated and surrogate consent is not available. The fact that these research practices occur without consent does not entail that the absence of consent is justifiable. On the other hand, the moral importance of consent does not entail that there are no valid exceptions to a requirement of obtaining consent in order to undertake human research. Here I examine one area of research without consent—observational research using medical records. This is perhaps the easiest form of research without consent to justify. However, the justification is of philosophical interest by virtue of the need to investigate the scope and limits of personal sovereignty.

Research drawn from data contained in medical records is a common and immensely important means of scientific investigation in epidemiology and health services research. It provides valuable knowledge regarding risk factors for disease, the safety of pharmaceuticals and medical procedures, and the quality of medical care.[41] Electronic information technology has greatly enhanced the capability of conducting research using medical records, but has also generated increasing concern about invasions of privacy. Both practical and scientific considerations militate against soliciting consent for population-based observational research. Retrospective review of existing medical records, especially with large samples, poses insuperable barriers to locating human subjects to obtain their informed consent.[42] When efforts are made to obtain informed consent for prospective research drawn from disease and treatment registries, mounting evidence has accumulated that substantial selection biases are introduced into the data, as those who consent are not necessarily representative of the population of relevant patients.[43] Can it be ethical for researchers to obtain access to private personal medical information without informed consent?

Two separate but converging ethical norms call into question the common practice of medical records research without informed consent. First, there is the principle that clinical research involving competent adults ethically requires their informed authorization. Second, persons have a right to control access to private information about them, especially sensitive medical information obtained in the course of standard medical care. Investigators who obtain access to medical records for the purposes of observational research without the consent of human subjects appear to violate both of these norms. Given that research ethics demands respect for the rights of research subjects, how can this practice be justified?

When faced with an ethical conundrum, a reasonable initial response is to search for a convenient way to make the problem go away. If researchers are restricted to anonymized or de-identified data, it might seem that the ethical difficulty vanishes. Medical records research is merely observational, without any interaction between investigators and human subjects. When researchers lack access to personally identifiable data, how can there be any objection to the absence of consent for valuable records research? Yet if we think of medical records as belonging to individual patients, or at least as their having control over access to them, and if individuals have a right to consent to or refuse research participation, then it is not clear that de-identification makes the ethical problem go away. The individuals whose data are being accessed for research are still being used for research without their authorization. Moreover, some individuals whose data are used might object to the purpose of the research.

In any case, de-identification cannot solve the problem. Much important observational research, especially studies that link different sets of medical records and databases or track health outcomes over time, would be impossible or unfeasible to conduct without researchers having access to identifiable data. It is necessary, therefore, to examine more closely the two norms that appear to preclude access to medical records without consent to see if, indeed, a reasonable interpretation of their scope would rule out access to private, identifiable information without informed consent.

The Right to Control Participation in Research

As discussed previously, the recognition of an ethical requirement for informed consent to clinical research emerged out of concern over abusive medical experimentation. Medical experimentation typically involves more or less invasive bodily intervention on human subjects or planned manipulation of their medical treatment for the purpose of generating scientific knowledge. Personal sovereignty—interests in bodily integrity and personal autonomy relating to control over the way one is treated by, or interacts with, others—is strongly implicated in medical experimentation with human subjects.

Observational research drawn from medical records does not involve experimentation with human subjects or even any interaction between researchers and human subjects. Hence, the ethical prohibition of experimentation without informed consent does not apply to this type of research. Moreover, as nothing is being done to or with the persons whose records are accessed, it is not clear that merely observational research is unethical without consent. It might be objected that individuals are being used merely as a means to scientific investigation and the interests of society when information about them is accessed without their consent. Their personal information is being used as a means, but there is no interference with their freedom or the course of their lives, especially if the confidentiality of the data is protected. These considerations call into question any claim that categorically prohibits research involving competent adults without consent, regardless of the nature of the research. There is no ethical requirement to obtain consent for purely observational research in a public place—for example, field research by a social scientist on the behavior of people in a public park. If consent is required for medical records research, this would seem to be due to the expectation and right of privacy associated with medical records, rather than the mere fact that research involving human subjects is being conducted.

The Right to Privacy

Persons have a strong interest in the privacy of their medical information, to control access so that it is not used adversely against them by others. As Beauchamp and Childress observe, "The principle of respect for autonomy, therefore, includes the right to decide as far as possible what will happen to one's person—to one's body, to information about one's life, to one's secrets, and the like."[44] Yet invasions of privacy, depending on their consequences, provoke more or less ethical concern. When researchers have access to medical records (without consent) under rigorous procedures to protect confidentiality, the intrusion on privacy is minimal, especially when balanced against the public interest in research with the potential to improve medical care or promote public health. Gostin and Hodge assert that "Finding a balance between individual choice and public goods requires an assessment of consequences and, therefore, is frankly utilitarian."[45] They go on to argue that "Where the potential for public benefit is high and the risk of harm to individuals is low, public entities should have discretion to use data for important public purposes (e.g., cost-effective health care, public health, and research). In such cases, public entities should be able to acquire and use the data regardless of individual informed consent or other privacy protections."[46]

The standard objection to such a utilitarian perspective, however, is that it has the potential to run roughshod over the rights of individuals, sacrificing their legitimate claims to the welfare of society. To be sure, Gostin and Hodge affirm a set of reasonable safeguards for the use of private data for research without consent, including demonstrating an important public purpose for the research, de-identifying the data when possible, and mandating strict standards for protecting the private data from unwarranted use that can be harmful to individuals. But if individuals have a *right* to control access to their private information, then the utilitarian balancing advocated by Gostin and Hodge (and many other commentators) is ethically suspect. In setting up their argument, they note that "Rather than seeing autonomy as a 'trump card' that always prevails, our framework values both privacy and common goods, without a priori favoring either."[47] Gostin and Hodges are certainly correct that the value of privacy should not necessarily trump the common good. However, appeal to the common good will illegitimately trump valid claims of autonomy if rights are not respected. Indeed, the very ethical point of positing rights is to protect a zone of personal sovereignty free from the intrusion of others, including the state or other institutions acting in pursuit of the common good. In explicating the concept of personal sovereignty, Feinberg notes that "Sovereignty is an all or nothing concept; one is entitled to absolute control of whatever is within one's domain however trivial it may be."[48] Although it is questionable that personal sovereignty involves *absolute* control, a valid claim that the conduct of others intrudes on personal sovereignty or infringes rights carries strong moral force. What, then, are the boundaries of personal sovereignty in the domain of control over access to private information in medical records?

To determine whether personal sovereignty includes control over access to medical records for research, we need to inquire into the scope of the right to privacy. The issue of control over access to private information is often considered as a matter of ownership. Although medical records are not physically in the possession of patients, we view the personal information they contain as belonging to them. It is up to them to decide who gets access, which means that others are not entitled to access without their consent. Hence, unauthorized access to private information is akin to trespass on a person's property. There may be no palpable harm done by the trespass, but it violates the rights of the owner, thus making it wrongful.

Whether the right to privacy of medical information should be understood as a property right is an interesting theoretical question. Starr accuses strong advocates of privacy rights as "confusing the concept of a privacy and a property right."[49] He proceeds to assert (without argument) that "The essential interest in privacy is not control, but dignity—the protection of the individual from offensive and embarrassing disclosures." This begs the question. It is not clear why the interest in privacy does not include control as well as dignity. We are concerned not only about loss of dignity resulting from others obtaining and misusing private information but also with the fact that they have access to information that they have "no business" seeing because access has not been authorized. Indeed, Starr is not consistent about distinguishing the right to privacy from property rights, as he writes about data security measures that may "minimize the highly publicized cases of individual trespass and misuse of data that have raised public concern about the security of health information."[50] Trespass is a matter of unauthorized access to property, thus violating a property right, whereas misuse concerns inappropriate use of private information, which violates dignity or causes other harms to personal interests. A detailed analysis of the connection between privacy and property rights is outside the scope of this chapter. Here it will be presumed that at least the analogy to property rights is appropriate in explicating the scope of the right to privacy.

It is important to recognize that ownership rights, though central to personal liberty and autonomy, are distinctly limited in scope for a variety of reasons. People are not entitled to use their homes and their land in a way that is a nuisance to their neighbors. Hence, laws properly restrict noise and keeping of certain types of animals. Building codes further restrict the use of real estate. Some jurisdictions prohibit land owners from erecting billboards on their property. Under "eminent domain," the state is entitled to take private property for public use with fair monetary compensation to the owner. Property owners are obliged to pay real estate taxes. Additionally, ownership of income is subject to taxation. Instead of asking us to donate our money to contribute to public purposes, the state levies property and income taxes. It has the legitimate power to enforce payment. Accordingly, we generally acknowledge limitations on property rights both to prevent harm to others and to promote the common good.

Within the tradition of liberal political thought, the legitimacy of compulsory state action is brought into line with personal sovereignty via the idea of the consent of the governed (see Chapter 12). Yet whatever might be meant by "the consent of the governed," in representative governments, it is not individual consent that authorizes state action. The legitimacy of taxation does not depend on the individual consent of the taxpayer; nor does the taxpayer consent to the uses to which his or her money is put.

Reasonable restrictions on the ownership of physical property and income suggest that there may be comparable restrictions on personal control of private information. Limitations on privacy for the sake of public health are universally recognized. Physicians are required to report the infectious disease status of their patients to public health authorities. Likewise, professionals are subject to reporting requirements relating to child abuse and neglect. In both cases, the confidentiality of private information is limited to prevent harm to others. Some research drawn from medical records can lead to preventing harm to patients, as in research on the safety of medical treatments, and other research can contribute to improving medical care or preventing disease. Owing to the public purposes served by medical records research, and the potential to conduct this research with minimal intrusion on individual privacy, it is reasonable to restrict the scope of the right of privacy such that consent is not necessarily required for this research.

Access to medical records for the sake of research aimed at improving population health is supported by the fact that for the most part medical records are connected with coverage of health care through insurance or a national health service. The community is involved in funding health care according to evidence-based standards, making medical records a public resource for generating evidence relating to improving health care and promoting health. Because these records contain sensitive personal information, stringent privacy protections are ethically necessary in the conduct of research. Making access to medical records for research dependent on consent, however, fails to do justice to the legitimate interest of the public in developing important knowledge relating to health—knowledge that may be impossible to obtain if consent is required.

The case for permitting medical records research without consent is further bolstered by expanding on the analogy with taxation and restriction on ownership rights to income. Not only do we regard compulsory taxation as legitimately limiting the right to control the use of personal income, but also we regard individuals as having a moral obligation to pay taxes. Having derived benefit from the multitude of public goods financed by taxation, including public security and the rule of law that make it possible to enjoy the personal benefits of property and income, individual citizens are ethically bound to do their fair share in supporting the common good via paying the taxes they owe. Rawls articulates "the principle of fairness" at stake here as follows:

> The main idea is that when a number of persons engage in a
> mutually advantageous cooperative venture according to rules, and
> thus restrict their liberty in ways necessary to yield advantages for all,
> those who have submitted to these restrictions have a right to a
> similar acquiescence on the part of those who have benefited from
> their submission. We are not to gain from the cooperative labors of
> others without doing our fair share.[51]

The quality of medical care depends on the accumulation and dissemination of scientific evidence. Patients receiving evidence-based medical care benefit from the research conducted on medical records in the past. They do their fair share in maintaining the benefits of this sort of research by means of having their personal data available for research.

To make participation in medical records research depend on consent makes it likely that some will refuse. Yet those who refuse participation are positioned, when in need of medical care, to receive the benefits that flow from such research, as well as those who consent. It seems unfair for some to refuse to make their private data available for research, thus free-riding on the participation of those who consent. The principle of fairness might be understood as simply grounding an obligation to consent when asked to contribute data to research. Can a stronger position supporting a waiver of consent be justified? If we see this as a violation of personal sovereignty, then we will insist on consent and tolerate the free-rider problem, though rightfully encouraging (but not compelling) research participation. Arguably, this is how we should approach consent to medical experimentation in the case of randomized clinical trials, which also can be brought under the principle of fairness given the importance of clinical trials for guiding evidence-based medicine.[52] However, if we see access to medical records for research as an appropriate exercise of power in pursuit of the common good, which does not violate individual rights, then medical records research without consent can be justified. Mill, in the introductory chapter of *On Liberty*, remarked that "There are also many positive acts for the benefit of others, which he may rightfully be compelled to perform; such as to give evidence in a court of justice; to bear his fair share in the common defence; or in any other joint work necessary to the interest of the society of which he enjoys the protection."[53]

I contend that in view of these considerations, medical records research involving access to personally identifiable data is justifiable without consent under the following conditions: (1) the proposed research is socially valuable; (2) there are severe practical impediments to soliciting consent or requiring consent would be likely to compromise the scientific validity, and consequently the value, of research; and (3) adequate safeguards for access by researchers are implemented to minimize the intrusion on privacy. Because it is reasonable to make taxation compulsory, rather than condition financial contribution to the common good on consent of the taxpayer, it would seem all the more reasonable to adopt a public policy of permitting medical records research without consent under these conditions. Taxation involves a much more consequential restriction of the domain of personal sovereignty than research access to medical records. Provided that adequate procedures are in place to protect the security of the data and preserve confidentiality, individuals are not required to make any sacrifice to support medical records research without consent. Because inherently there is no infringement of rights or diminishment of personal well-being associated with a sound public policy supporting medical records research without consent, no one has any reasonable grounds for objecting to its adoption. In sum, personal sovereignty does not encompass control over medical records research when the appropriate justificatory conditions are satisfied.

Conclusion

Although informed consent from research participants is a basic norm governing clinical research, it is not necessary for ethical research for at least two reasons. First (and outside the scope of this chapter), valuable research can be justified that enrolls research subjects who are not capable of giving informed consent—children and incompetent adults. In this situation we look to informed authorization by parents and surrogate decision makers, usually family members, to serve the same values of personal well-being and autonomy that underlie the consent of decisionally capacitated research participants. Second, some types of research, including observational research using medical records, can be justified without consent. More controversially, deviation from informed consent *may* be justifiable in behavioral research that employs deception to promote scientific validity. Consent not only is not universally necessary for ethical clinical research, but it is also not sufficient. Norms such as social value of the research question, scientific validity of research methods, and appropriate balance of risks and benefits are all necessary for ethical clinical research. Nevertheless, a moral requirement to obtain informed consent remains vital for a wide range of clinical research, grounded in personal sovereignty.

Acknowledgment

Parts of this chapter have been based on the following articles: Miller, F.G. 2008. Research on medical records without informed consent. *Journal of Law, Medicine and Ethics* 36:560–66; and Miller, F.G., S. Joffe. 2006. Evaluating the therapeutic misconception. *Kennedy Institute of Ethics Journal* 16:353–66.

References

1. Annas, G.J., and M.A. Grodin. 1992. *The Nazi doctors and the Nuremberg Code.* New York: Oxford University Press.
2. Feinberg, J. 1986. *Harm to self,* 54–55. New York: Oxford University Press.
3. Weindling, P.J. 2008. The Nazi medical experiments. In *The Oxford textbook of clinical research ethics,* ed. E.J. Emanuel, R.A. Crouch, C. Grady, R. Lie, F.G. Miller, and D. Wendler, 18–30. New York: Oxford University Press.
4. Jones, J.H. 2008. The Tuskegee syphilis experiment. In *The Oxford textbook of clinical research ethics,* ed. E.J. Emanuel, R.A. Crouch, C. Grady, R. Lie, F.G. Miller, and D. Wendler, 86–96. New York: Oxford University Press.
5. Cobb, L.A., G.I. Thomas, D.H. Dillard, K.A. Merendino, R.A. Bruce et al. 1959. An evaluation of internal-mammary artery ligation by a double-blind technic. *New England Journal of Medicine* 260:1115–18.
6. Modell, W. 1962. Comment on 'Some fallacies and errors.' *Clinical Pharmacology and Therapeutics* 4:146.
7. Arras, J.D. 2008. The Jewish Chronic Disease Hospital case. In *The Oxford textbook of clinical research ethics,* ed. E.J. Emanuel, R.A. Crouch, C. Grady, R. Lie, F.G. Miller, and D. Wendler, 73–79. New York: Oxford University Press.

8. Faden, R.R., and T.L. Beauchamp. 1986. *A history and theory of informed consent,* 200–32. New York: Oxford University Press.

9. Beecher, H. 1966. Ethics and clinical research. *New England Journal of Medicine* 274:1354–60.

10. Katz, J., with A.M. Capron and E.S. Glass, eds. 1972. *Experimentation with human beings,* 10. New York: Russell Sage Foundation.

11 Ibid., 25.

12. Ibid., 38.

13. Ibid., 52.

14. Mill, J.S. 1972. *On liberty.* In *Utilitarianism, liberty and representative government,* 73. Everyman Library. London: J.M. Dent.

15. Kant, I. 1998. *Groundwork of the metaphysics of morals,* ed. M. Gregor, 37. Cambridge: Cambridge University Press.

16. Miller, F.G., and A. Wertheimer. 2007. Facing up to paternalism in research ethics. *Hastings Center Report* 37(3):24–34.

17. Ibid.

18. Appelbaum, P.S., L.H. Roth, and C. Lidz. 1982. The therapeutic misconception: Informed consent in psychiatric research. *International Journal of Law and Psychiatry* 5:319–29.

19. Dresser, R. 2002. The ubiquity and utility of the therapeutic misconception. *Social Philosophy and Policy* 19:271–94.

20. Fried, C. 1974. *Medical experimentation: Personal integrity and social policy.* New York: American Elsevier.

21. Appelbaum, P.S., L.H. Roth, C.W. Lidz, P. Benson, and W. Winslade. 1987. False hopes and best data: Consent to research and the therapeutic misconception. *Hastings Center Report* 17(2):20–24.

22. Appelbaum, P.S., C.W. Lidz, and T. Grisso. 2004. Therapeutic misconception in clinical research: Frequency and risk factors. *IRB* 26(2):1–8.

23. Appelbaum et al., "False hopes," 20.

24. Ibid., 20.

25. Ibid., 21.

26. Ibid., 21.

27. Ibid., 21.

28. Ibid. See also, Lidz, C.W., and P.S. Appelbaum. 2002. The therapeutic misconception: Problems and solutions. *Medical Care* 40(supplement): V-55–V-63; and Lidz, C.W., P.S. Appelbaum, T. Grisso, and M. Renaud. 2004. Therapeutic misconception and the appreciation of risks in clinical trials. *Social Science and Medicine* 58:1689–97.

29. Stiller, C.A. 1994. Centralised treatment, entry to trials and survival. *British Journal of Cancer* 70:352–62.

30. Braunholtz, D.A., S.J. Edwards, and R.J. Lilford. 2001. Are randomized clinical trials good for us (in the short term)? Evidence for a "trial effect." *Journal of Clinical Epidemiology* 54:217–24.

31. Peppercorn, J.M., J.C. Weeks, E.F. Cook, and S. Joffe. 2002. Comparison of outcomes in cancer patients treated within and outside clinical trials: Conceptual framework and structured review. *Lancet* 363:263–70.

32. Vist, G.E., K.B. Hagen, P.J. Devereaux, D. Bryant, D.T. Kristoffersen, and A.D. Oxman. 2005. Systematic review to determine whether participation in a trial influences outcome. *British Medical Journal* 330:1175.

33. Miller, F.G. 2008. The ethics of placebo-controlled trials. In *The Oxford textbook of clinical research ethics,* ed. E.J. Emanuel, R.A. Crouch, C. Grady, R. Lie, F.G. Miller, and D. Wendler, 261–72. New York: Oxford University Press.

34. Annas, G.J., and M.A. Grodin. 1992. *The Nazi doctors and the Nuremberg Code.* New York: Oxford University Press.

35. Sreenivasan, G. 2003. Does informed consent to research require comprehension? *Lancet* 362:2016–18.

36. Lidz, C.W., and P.S. Appelbaum. 2002. The therapeutic misconception: problems and solutions. *Medical Care* 40(supplement):V-55–V-63.

37. Appelbaum et al., "False hopes."

38. Flory, J., and E. Emanuel. 2004. Interventions to improve research participants' understanding in informed consent for research: A systematic review. *Journal of the American Medical Association* 292:1593–1601.

39. Miller, F.G. 2008. The ethics of placebo-controlled trials. In *The Oxford textbook of clinical research ethics,* ed. E.J. Emanuel, R.A. Crouch, C. Grady, R. Lie, F.G. Miller, and D. Wendler, 261–72. New York: Oxford University Press.

40. Wendler, D. 2004. Can we ensure that all research subjects give valid consent? *Archives of Internal Medicine* 164:2201–04.

41. Wald, N., M. Law, T. Meade, G. Miller, E. Alberman, J. Dickinson, G.E. Simon et al. 1994. Use of personal medical records for research purposes. *British Medical Journal* 309:1422–24; and Simon, G.E., et al. 2000. Large medical databases, population-based research, and patient confidentiality. *American Journal of Psychiatry* 157:1731–37.

42. Black, N. 2003. Secondary use of personal data for health and health services research: Why identifiable data are essential. *Journal of Health Services Research and Policy* 8(Suppl 1):36–40.

43. Woolf, S.H., S.F. Rothemich, R.E. Johnson, D.W. Marsland, J.V. Tu, D.J. Willison, F.L. Silver et al. 2000. Selection bias from requiring patients to give consent to examine data for health services research. *Archives of Family Medicine* 9:1111–18; Tu, J.V., et al. 2004. Impracticability of informed consent in the registry of the Canadian stroke network. *New England Journal of Medicine*

350:1414–21; and Buckley, B., et al. 2007. Selection bias resulting from the requirement for prior consent in observational research: A community cohort of people with ischaemic heart disease. *Heart* 93:1116–20.

44. Beauchamp, T.L., and J.F. Childress. 2001. *Principles of biomedical ethics*, 5th ed., 297. New York: Oxford University Press.

45. Gostin, L.O., and J.G. Hodge Jr. 2002. Personal privacy and common goods: A framework for balancing under the National Health Information Privacy Rule. *Minnesota Law Review* 86:1439, at 1454.

46. Ibid., 1455.

47. Ibid., 1441.

48. Feinberg, J. 1986. *Harm to self*, 54–55. New York: Oxford University Press.

49. Starr, P. 1999. Health and the right to privacy. *American Journal of Law and Medicine* 25:193–201, at 200.

50. Ibid., 201.

51. Rawls, J. 1999. *A theory of justice*, rev. ed., 96. Cambridge, MA: Harvard University Press.

52. Harris, J. 2005. Scientific research is a moral duty. *Journal of Medical Ethics* 31:242–48.

53. Mill, J.S. 1972. *On liberty*. In *Utilitarianism, liberty and representative government*, 74. Everyman Library. London: J.M. Dent.

Index